Topical Issues In Pain 5

Physiotherapy Pain Association

Topical Issues in Pain 5

Treatment
Communication
Return to Work
Cognitive Behavioural
Pathophysiology

Editor
Louis Gifford FCSP BSc MAppSc

Foreword
Lorraine Moores MSc MCSP

AuthorHouse™ UK Ltd.
1663 Liberty Drive
Bloomington, IN 47403 USA
www.authorhouse.co.uk
Phone: 0800.197.4150

This book was first published by CNS Press in 2006

Published by AuthorHouse 08/30/2013

ISBN: 978-1-4918-7669-5 (sc)
ISBN: 978-1-4918-7670-1 (hc)
ISBN: 978-1-4918-7680-0 (e)

Foreward

I am delighted to be writing the Foreword for this, the eagerly awaited fifth volume in the Physiotherapy Pain Association's Topical Issues in Pain Series. The PPA was established in 1994. In 1996 it was formally recognised as a Clinical Interest Group of the Chartered Society of Physiotherapy for Physiotherapists with a special interest in managing patients with both acute and chronic pain. The acknowledgement of a multidimensional understanding of pain and a biopsychosocial model supporting our treatment approach underlies the Association's philosophy.

So we are now twelve years on, and the PPA continues to move from strength to strength. The Association has, within a relatively short time, become a highly respected and active Clinical Interest Group with a Northern Branch (PPA North) set up in 2000. We now have a membership of some 600 physiotherapists, an active website (www.ppaonline.co.uk) and a high quality publication, PPA News, produced twice a year. Over the years a number of Study Days and Symposia have been run and the PPA has provided exceptional programmes at the CSP Annual Congress. To date, there have been seven Pat Wall Lectures at Congress with contributions from a number of leading experts in the pain field including Pat Wall himself in 1999 and Ronald Melzack in 2002. PPA members have also made significant contributions to workshops at the International Association for the Study of Pain's World Congress on Pain.

The Topical Issues in Pain series was launched in 1998 with the publication of TIP 1. This highly acclaimed series aims to provide health care professionals with up to date information about a wide range of issues in the management of pain. The PPA has now produced this its' fifth book - quite an accomplishment! I would like to thank Louis Gifford (Editor) on behalf of the PPA Executive Committee and the PPA membership for his hard work and unwavering enthusiasm and commitment in editing the Topical Issues in Pain series.

This volume is divided into five sections. Section one addresses treatment principles including manual therapy in the 21st century and the application of goal setting strategies. Section two outlines the importance of effective communication and describes the key communication skills that can optimise assessment and management of our patients. Return to work issues are the focus for section three. The role of physiotherapists working within vocational rehabilitation is outlined and illustrated with a case study. Occupational obstacles for patients returning to work and the benefits system are discussed. An overview of psychosocial approaches is provided within section four. The benefits of early intervention in reducing the risk of pain related problems such as fear of pain and work loss are highlighted. The successful integration of physiotherapy and clinical psychology practice within pain management rehabilitation is also discussed and outlined with case histories. Section five reviews the evidence for changes in the primary cortex in chronic pain and the implications for the treatment. Muscular activity in chronic pain is outlined in addition to molecular mechanisms within the spinal cord.

I would like to thank all the authors who have very kindly contributed to this volume. Your input is greatly appreciated. The TIP series as a whole brings together an extensive accumulation of research and a remarkable breadth of knowledge presented in a very understandable and practical way. If you don't already have the previous TIP books my advice is get them - you won't be disappointed!

Lorraine Moores
Physiotherapy Pain Association Chairperson
December 2005

Preface

If you were to go back ten years, would you have ever thought that in a very short time physiotherapists would be claiming to change motor and sensory mapping in the brain during and following treatment and management of pain and be taken very seriously? Would you have thought that physiotherapists would be actually researching these phenomena and starting to prove them? Would you have considered that the foundations of our understanding of how our treatment techniques might work or don't work could be so turned on their head? Would you have thought that a great many physiotherapists would be leading movements of change in working practices and treatments related to pain, pain management and return to work – that we would be starting to be listened to by main-stream medicine?

Physiotherapists are pulling ahead and some, are way ahead. These are those who base their day to day work practices around a multidimensional and biopsychosocial model of pain. Those who read, understand, feel at ease with and implement the kind of material found in the Topical Issues in Pain series! No arguments, no political manoeuvring, no in-fighting, but sound and well reasoned agreement around a very sound model secured by outstanding and continually growing scientific support – it's powerful, it fits, it works – but will it endure?

It is my firm and unashamedly passionate belief, that well informed physiotherapists, occupational therapists and clinical psychologists, are not just ahead of their own profession here, but also of many others involved in pain management and treatment too, i.e. General Practitioners, Orthopaedic Surgeons, Rheumatologists, Chiropractors, Osteopaths and the many alternative practitioners. The list should also include those who teach these practitioners their clinical skills too. On a day-to-day level these disciplines, for the most part, offer single 'things' to have, to take, or to experience, – tablets, injections, operations, manipulations, corrections, rebalancing, and more of the same, - with weak and unimpressive support from well constructed clinical trials. There is growing evidence that some can maim, that there are many side effects and that some cause unnecessary tissue damage and scarring. So why do they all endure?

Is it because they make intuitive sense, because they are uncomplicated, easy to explain, easy to teach and easy to learn? The knee is arthritic, worn-out, it needs replacing; the nerve is trapped it needs releasing.... Is it this simplicity that makes them all so appealing and so highly marketable? Is it also true that many are driven and maintained by market forces?

We now have a growing body of science to support the processes and practices used in Cognitive Behavioural treatment (CBT) based rehabilitation programmes. This growing support for CBT interventions bears a striking resemblance to the support that continues to accrue for the gate-control theory of pain put forward by Pat Wall and Ronald Melzack 40 years ago! Yes, – the support for CBT based programmes just keeps coming in, but why is CBT still so hard to find? Why hasn't it caught on? Why isn't it supported more? And above all, will it endure?

A big problem is that management approaches, like CBT, which are naturally embraced within the biopsychosocial model, are so difficult to market in the present climate. They may even be unmarketable because they require time, a great deal of highly trained practitioners time.
This time contains the complex skills of caring human interaction – 'People skills', very demanding human skills – empathy, listening, communication, teaching, planning, explaining, ingenuity, showing, reassuring, distracting, energising, engaging, motivating, rewarding, encouraging, goal setting, demonstrating and analysing... All the things that cannot easily be manufactured for a mass market, that take time to learn, that are difficult to teach and for which there is never likely to be a grateful sponsor to give support.

It seems astonishing that proven CBT based programmes for chronic pain or return to work programmes for pain sufferers should be so poorly funded, so thin on the ground and so poorly supported – when so many millions go into unproven or feeble treatments that frequently render the sufferer moribund, incapable and physically unproductive. What is it with this great call for evidenced based medicine? Where are the supporters and sponsors of these evidence based treatments? Where are the training programmes? Who's interested? Who really cares?

How can CBT, the biopsychosocial model and patient centred management approaches that embrace physical goal achievement and community rehabilitation endure without a sponsor, without a commercial product, without substance, without packaging and without speed of delivery?

It is my great hope, through books like this one and through individuals like those who have written here and set down their example, that this solid, well-constructed, model of practice that the Physiotherapy Pain Association members embrace, will endure. It has to, because it makes so much sense when time is taken to understand and learn. Simplistic models for pain related problems and the accompanying disability are unsatisfactory; they cannot endure if good science continues to influence.

I confidently predict that just as the gate control theory gradually gained support and recognition, so too will the biopsychosocial model and the relevant science. I also predict that a great deal of what is written in the pages of these small volumes contains many of the principles of management that will still be relevant in a great many years to come. It will take time, so let's be patient.

Louis Gifford
December 2005

Contributors

Jacqueline Adams DipCOT
Senior Occupational Therapist
Occupational Therapy Department
Elgar Unit
Newtown Hospital
Newtown Road
Worcester WR5 1JG

Anne Daykin PhD MApplSc MCSP
Research Physiotherapist
Section of Ageing and Health
Department of Medicine and Therapeutics
University of Dundee
Ninewells Hospital and Medical School
Dundee DD1 9SY

Ian Edwards BAppSc Physio, Grad Dip Physio(Ortho), PhD
Lecturer
School of Health Sciences
University of South Australia
Adelaide, South Australia

Louis Gifford FCSP BSc MappSc
Chartered Physiotherapist
Kestrel, Swanpool,
Falmouth, Cornwall TR11 5BD

Peter Gladwell MCSP, BSc
Clinical Specialist Physiotherapist
Biopsychosocial Medicine
Frenchay Hospital
Bristol BS16 1LE

Steve Goldingay MCSP BSc(Hons) Grad Dip Phys
Principal Therapist
Chronic Pain Rehabilitation Service
Kendrick Wing
Warrington Hospital
Lovely Lane
Warrington WA5 1QG

Angela Green MCSP MSc
Research & Development Therapist
Institute of Rehabilitation
University of Hull
215 Anlaby Road
Hull HU3 2PG

Nicola Hunter BSc MCSP CMIOSH
Chartered Physiotherapist
RehabWorks Ltd
St Andrews Street South
Bury St Edmunds
Suffolk IP33 3PH

David Jackson MCSP MSc
Research Facilitator
Institute of Rehabilitation
University of Hull
215 Anlaby Road
Hull HU3 2PG

Richard Johnson DClinPsychol
Clinical Psychologist
Manchester & Salford Pain Centre
Hope Hospital
Stott Lane
Salford M6 8HD

Mark Jones BS (Psych) P, Grad Dip Advan Manip Ther MAppSc
Program Director
Coursework Masters Programs in Physiotherapy
School of Health Sciences
University of South Australia
Adelaide, South Australia 5000

Francis Keefe PhD
Professor, Department of Psychiatry and Behavioral Sciences and
Psychology Social and Health Sciences
Associate Director for Research
Duke Pain and Palliative Care Program
Pain Prevention and Treatment Research Program
Box 3159 Duke Medical Center
Durham, USA NC 27710

Jennifer Klaber Moffett MCSP MSc PhD
Professor of Rehabilitation and Therapies
Institute of Rehabilitation
University of Hull
215 Anlaby Road
Hull HU3 2PG

George Koumantakis PhD MSc MCSP
Private Practitioner & Lecturer in Physiotherapy
Drosopoulou 6
Kypseli, 112 57
Athens, Greece

Lorraine Moores MSc MCSP
Clinical Specialist Physiotherapist
Manchester & Salford Pain Centre
Hope Hospital
Stott Lane
Salford M6 8HD

Penny Mortimer MCSP MSc
Clinical Physiotherapy Specialist
COPE (Centre of Pain Education)
Sutton Hospital
Cotswold Road
Sutton, Surrey SM2 5NF

Lorimer Moseley PhD BAppSc(Phty)(Hons)
Nuffield Medical Research Fellow
Department of Human Anatomy & Genetics & fMRIB Centre
University of Oxford
South Parks Road
Oxford OX1 3QX UK

Shilpa Patel BSc(Hons), MSc
Research Associate
Department of Health Sciences
Division of Pain Management & Anaesthesia
University of Leicester
Leicester General Hospital
Gwendolen Road
Leicester LE5 4PW

LisaCaitlin Perri BA
Clinical Psychology Graduate Student, Duke University
Pain Prevention and Treatment Research Program
Box 3159 Duke Medical Center
Durham, USA NC 27710

Steve Robson MCSP BSc(Hons)
Chartered Physiotherapist
Aspen Physiotherapy & Sports Injury Clinic
28 Front Street
Prudhoe, Nothumberland NE42 5DQ

Cindy Scipio BA
Clinical Psychology Graduate Student, Duke University
Pain Prevention and Treatment Research Program
Box 3159 Duke Medical Center
Durham, USA NC 27710

Gail Sowden BSc MSc
Consultant Physiotherapist
Primary Care Sciences Research Centre
Keele University
Staffordshire ST5 5BG

Stephen Thompson
Senior Lecturer
School of Biological Sciences
University of Plymouth
Plymouth, Devon PL4 8AA

Paul Watson PhD MSc BSc(Hons) MCSP
Senior Lecturer in Pain Management
Department of Health Sciences
University of Leicester
Gwendolen Road
Leicester LE5 4PW

Sharon Wilday MSc SROT DipCOT
Cognitive Behavioural Psychotherapist
Honorary Lecturer
University of Birmingham
17 Portland Road
Edgbaston
Birmingham B16 9NH

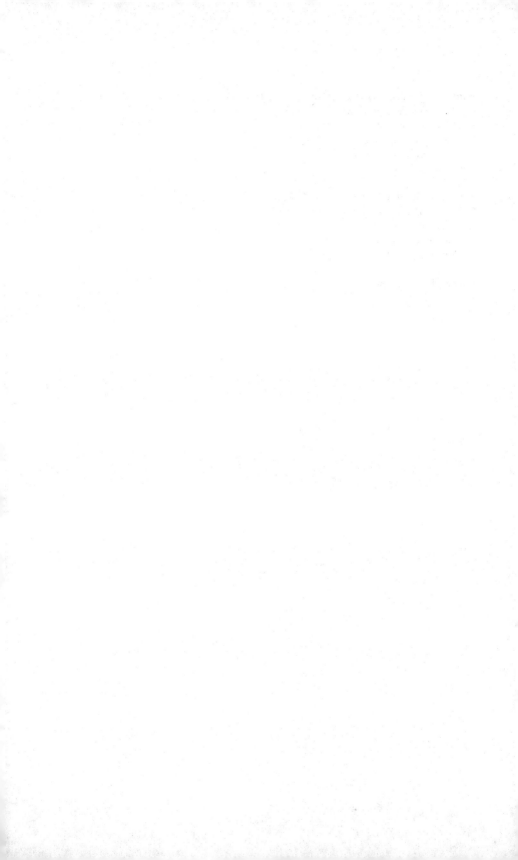

Contents

Part 3: Return to Work

Part 4: Cognitive-behavioural

Part 5: Pathophysiology

1

Treatment

1

Manual Therapy in the 21st Centuty

STEVE ROBSON AND LOUIS GIFFORD

Manual therapy in its various forms has been described throughout recorded medical history. The Greek physician Hippocrates described spinal manipulation as far back as the 5th century BC. More recently, the popularity of manual therapy both with clinicians and patients has continued to grow throughout the 19th and 20th centuries in line with the spread and growth of the chiropractic, osteopathy and physiotherapy professions. Today much of the theoretical basis used to prescribe and administer manual therapy is still drawn from the original teachings and philosophies of its early pioneers.

However, while many manual therapy treatment approaches have changed little since their inception, pain science and our understanding of pain has advanced rapidly. So rapidly in fact that the last decade has seen more progress in the pain sciences than throughout the preceding history of medicine. With these advances it is widely recognised that for the first time in medical history we have started to assimilate a 'pain knowledge base' founded on good scientific evidence as opposed to the theories and quasi-empirical approaches that came before.

Responding to the emergence of this recent scientific evidence, some authors have started to review the construct of manual therapy, and its actions and efficacy (e.g. Wright 1995, Souvlis et al 2004, Zusman 2002 & 2004). Undoubtedly understanding this better will help us to decide if, or when, manual therapy is an appropriate treatment for pain. Evidence on which to base clinical decisions is welcome news for many clinicians and patients alike, particularly among the current and often endless jungle of therapies vying to 'treat and cure' those suffering with pain, disability and illness.

Manual therapy defined

For the purpose of this discussion, manual therapy will be largely considered in two of its most commonly prescribed forms, namely, joint mobilisation and joint manipulation. Direct reference to the many other forms of manual therapy such as positional release, craniosacral techniques, muscle energy etc will not be made. However, these manual techniques can easily be considered in a similar context as they are highly likely to influence the same pathways of peripheral and central processing as mobilisation and manipulation. Thus, their overall relevance via a more palatable rationale should become clearer along the way.

Maitland (1986) defined mobilisation as "passive movements performed in such a way that at all times they are within the control of the patient so that the patient can prevent the movement if they so choose". In contrast manipulation techniques have been defined as those techniques used to force a joint beyond its presumed physiologic barrier and up to its anatomical barrier (Haldeman & Hooper 1999). Thus, they are beyond the conscious control of the patient and include such techniques as chiropractic adjustments, high velocity low amplitude (HVLA), grade 5, long-lever and thrust techniques. These techniques are often accompanied by an audible clicking or cracking sound.

Mobilisation and manipulation theories

The proposed mode of action and claimed effects of joint mobilisation and manipulation ranges, in some manual therapy disciplines, from being highly specific, to others which portray them in an all-encompassing 'cure all' approach. A review of the current evidence base is helpful when considering how these proposed theoretical approaches stand alongside current scientific evidence.

Mobilisation techniques are described in terms of utilising physiological and accessory joint movements either separately or together. For the unfamiliar, physiological movements are defined as those a person can carry out actively, for example flexion, extension and abduction. Examples of accessory joint movements include the small degrees of slide, glide, spin and roll inherent within joints during normal movement. Individual accessory movements cannot be self-initiated but can be performed passively by someone else.

Maitland (1986 &1991), Edwards (1992), Mulligan (1999) and Grieve (1988) describe mobilisation techniques in terms of treating mechanically derived joint problems. Particular techniques are described as restoring the 'position and function' of the joint's intra-articular structures therefore improving joint range of motion and relieving mechanically mediated pain.

Maitland (1986) and Mulligan (1999) describe mobilisation techniques specific to manoeuvring a 'painful' torn and displaced meniscus in such joints as the knee or temporomandibular joint thus altering the position of the meniscus allowing greater pain free range of motion. In the absence of normal meniscal healing there is no evidence offered to suggest that any change or reduction in the position of menisci is reliably sustainable in the long-term and subsequent recurrence or persistent displacement are commonplace with these injuries (Norris 1993, Apley & Solomon 1994, Dandy & Edwards 1998).

The basic tenet of mobilisation techniques describes them in terms of eliminating mechanical causes of pain by restoring normal joint range of motion, therefore removing the underlying mechanical irritant and thus achieving the cessation of pain. Despite the fact that many patients present with pain that fits the diagnostic criteria described for the prescription of such techniques, treatments using this approach do not always eliminate or alleviate pain (Frost et al 2004, UK BEAM trial 2004). Non-responders to these and other types of manual therapy do often display temporary or sustainable clinical improvements in joint range of motion but may also report little or no significant improvement in their overall pain presentation (Gifford 2004). If the cause of pain in these circumstances is purely mechanical as has been postulated, then logically pain should resolve commensurate with restoration of joint range of motion. Clearly the absence of pain relief despite clinical improvements in joint range of motion highlights the multi-dimensional nature of pain and the strong indication that pain is never likely to be a pure 'mechanical' entity.

The intervertebral disc

The clinical diagnosis of prolapsed intervertebral discs (PIVD) has often been cited as a reason to attempt the manipulative reduction of prolapsed disc material (Cyriax 1974). However, the related literature does not contain any definitive or reliable evidence to support the claim that discs can be reduced by manipulation or mobilisation procedures. The improvements in diagnostic imaging over recent years has in fact resulted in accumulating evidence to the contrary, thus confirming that intervertebral discs do not revert back to any semblance of their original structure following manipulation (Cassidy & Kirkaldy-Willis 1985, Bourdillon & Day 1987, Chrisman et al 1964).

5

Further, Gifford (2002), has reviewed the disc healing potential, or the 'potential' of the injured disc to change, and argues that its structure is virtually inert. He concludes that all the biological processes of change within the disc are extremely slow (measured in years, not days or weeks) and that even minor tears of the outer annulus lead to disruptive and degenerative changes throughout, – not healing/recovery (importantly he urges us to remember that even a degenerate disc is still a very strong structure though).

Despite these findings and arguments, some authors have continued to produce anecdotal reports of PIVD reduction based on observational single case studies (Cox et al 1993, Hession & Donald 1993). It is true that the profile of the intervertebral disc is altered during manipulation by the torsional forces involved, but there is no evidence to suggest that these transient forces are capable of reducing a bulging annulus or sequestrated nuclear material (Matthews & Yates 1969).

There is compelling evidence that the annulus fibrosis of intervertebral discs can be injured by manipulation procedures. Farfan (1977) demonstrated annular failure with relatively small forces when applying 'manipulative like torsion' to intervertebral joints. Anatomically the annulus is vulnerable in positions where significant torque is produced. Annular failure can occur with forces as small as 113Nm, this magnitude of torque is easily attainable by manipulators, particularly in positions of axial rotation, which 'slackens' 50% of the obliquely oriented annular fibres (Bogduk 1997). In this position half of the annulus offers little circumferential support and the annulus is markedly more susceptible to injury from manipulation techniques that produce annular torsion. With this in mind it will be no surprise to learn that the majority of manipulations resulting in annular failure contain a rotational component (Grieve 1994).

The possible role of the disc presents a fascinating paradox here: that even though manipulation can relieve pain, the thing that is being manipulated may actually be injured in the process! This argument can apply to any physically forceful exercise or manual treatment procedure.

Asymmetry, mal-alignment and movement dysfunction

The concepts of asymmetry, mal-alignment and movement dysfunction are criteria that have frequently been used to form the basis of structural diagnosis and subsequent treatment by manipulation and mobilisation techniques. Many of the theoretical approaches currently in use originated from osteopathy and chiropractic, often to be adopted with little enquiry by physiotherapy practitioners (Watson & Kendall 2000).

Osteopathic and chiropractic approaches were founded on the concept of somatic dysfunction, (DiGiovanna & Schiowitz 1991, Greenman 1996, Lee 1999, Nathan 1999) this is considered to be due to an impaired or altered function of the bodily framework (somatic system). Osteopathy considers this impaired function to be due to changes in skeletal, arthroidal and myofascial structures including their related vascular, lymphatic and neural elements.

In osteopathic literature the mnemonic ART is often used to describe the three classical diagnostic criteria deemed to be present with so called 'somatic dysfunction. "A" represents asymmetry, "R" range of motion and "T" tissue texture abnormality. Manipulation and mobilisation techniques are thus prescribed on the basis of observable or palpable asymmetry and considered alongside 'abnormal' range of motion (ROM) that is said to be detected by motion tests.

The clinical finding of 'structural asymmetry' is fundamental to this approach, which advocates an evaluation of the differences in position of anatomical landmarks. However, although many patients present with asymmetry this can be due to multivariate factors including, congenital and developmental anomalies as well as ageing and disease states (Bogduk 1997). Congenital and developmental anomalies can include the failure of one or more parts of a vertebra to develop (agenesis), failed vertebral union affecting the secondary ossification centres of vertebrae and also changes in the number or identity of vertebrae resulting in observations of lumbarisation, sacralisation or bony union elsewhere in the spine or pelvis. Other anatomical features such as cervical ribs and the adaptive process through which the clavicle on an individuals' dominant side develops naturally to be shorter and thicker than the opposite (non-dominant) clavicle, can all add to the 'appearance' of asymmetry (Lewis 2004). Many observable states of asymmetry such as torticollis, scoliosis and 'pelvic shift' occur temporarily during periods of healing and recovery.

It is arguable that asymmetry is commonplace, possibly even normal, and in the presence of some growth and disease states, a very adaptive process. This perspective thus applies in the presence of congenital or developmental anomalies as well as through disease states, ageing and also during healing and normal skeletal development. Asymmetry for many individuals must be considered to be 'normal for them' and therefore of questionable clinical relevance in many cases (Robson 2003). After all, asymmetry often persists after symptom resolution. These very important factors are fundamentally overlooked by this clinical approach (Freburger & Riddle 1999).

In addition to 'asymmetry' the 'ART' approach utilises motion tests said to detect 'movement dysfunction'. The motion tests described in much of the literature are predominantly for the spinal and pelvic regions (DiGiovanna & Schiowitz 1991, Greenman 1996, Lee & Walsh 1996, Lee 1999). It is claimed that the detection of abnormal spinal motion is possible by assessing 'perceived differences' in the coupled movements at spinal joints. Coupled movements are based on the principle of Newton's second law, which states that the motion of an object is directly proportional to the applied force and occurs in the direction of the straight line along which the force acts (Davis et al 1986). Clinically, segmental spinal motion testing is said to be possible by palpating over the transverse processes for perceived differences in motion at the underlying zygapophysial joints during spinal movements such as flexion and extension.

Primary movements of spinal joints do create small 'coupled' movements in other planes during bending and twisting, which minimises resistance to the primary movement. However, in-vitro measurements of coupled movements demonstrate that they are small, inconsistent and change with posture (Panjabi 1989, Cholewicki et al 1996). This is not consistent with claims made in much of the related literature or by proponents of this approach, who purport that coupled movements are a predictable and identifiable phenomenon that can be used to formulate diagnoses and plan treatment (DiGiovanna & Schiowitz 1991, Greenman 1996, Lee 1999).

Bogduk (1997) found that, 'there are average patterns of coupled movements, but not all individuals exhibit the same degree of coupling at any segment or necessarily in the same direction as average; nor do all normal individuals necessarily exhibit the average direction of coupling at every segment'.

In summary, motion tests based on spinal coupling have been shown to be both unreliable and invalid methods of assessing spinal function. Despite these findings some authors have continued to advocate this approach. For example, in her book 'The Pelvic Girdle,' Lee (1999) supports her decision to use this system by stating that 'even if the biomechanics of the lumbosacral junction were confirmed and conclusive, the potential for altered biomechanics to exist is high, rendering 'perceptive clinical observation of a patient as the most direct way to assess spine motion clinically, despite its lack of objectivity'.

Motion tests have also been described as part of the diagnostic procedure used to inculpate 'pelvic and sacro-iliac joint (SIJ) related pain and dysfunction. However, the very question of dysfunction and mechanically related pain at the SIJ's is in itself contentious. In the related literature the incidence of pelvic joint pain has been postulated to be as high as 96% down to less than 1% of those people presenting with lumbo-pelvic pain (Pulisetti

& Ebraheim 1999, Ressel & Rudy 2004). Anaesthetic joint blocks have often been described as the 'gold standard' method of implicating the SIJ as the primary pain source (Maigne et al 1995, Schwarzer et al 1995, Slipman et al 1998, Kokmeyer et al 2002). However, it is generally recognised that without image guidance, injection into the SIJ is not only technically very difficult but also unreliable (Pulisetti & Ebraheim 1999).

It is now evident that pain and tenderness/hypersensitivity to physical testing located in the region of the SIJ's may well be 'referred' rather than originating in the local structures. Referred pain and tenderness follow changes that occur in the spinal cord and higher centres of the central nervous system (CNS). Thus, second-order neurons in the dorsal horn of the spinal cord become sensitised by noxious afferent stimuli arriving from the periphery (for example from injured or pathological tissues and nerves in the lumbar spine) (see chapter 20). This afferent 'barrage' of sensory nerve activity may then lead to changes in the 'characteristics' of second-order nerve cells so that they become 'excited' by non-noxious stimuli arriving from neural networks that relate to other tissues. Hence, normal inputs from networks relating to the normal SIJ tissues may be processed as pain and in so doing not only make the area painful, but also, hypersensitive to touch and to physical tests. This normal tissue hypersensitivity phenomenon is termed secondary hyperalgesia in the pain science literature (Wall 1991, Fortin et al 1999, see also chapter 20). The clinical finding of SIJ area pain and tenderness has the potential to be a false positive as far as damage to the tissues of the SIJ are concerned. The finding may well be a simple manifestation of 'central sensitivity' rather than a true reflection of actual physical damage or pathology.

Some further consideration of central sensitisation and secondary hyperalgesia can be helpful when examining the mechanisms by which anaesthetic injection of the SIJ's might sometimes achieve pain relief. Anaesthetising first-order neurons in the region of the SIJ's can essentially 'shut off', or significantly reduce, sensory input to related second-order neurons in the dorsal horn. This reduced 'normal' input, in some cases, appears to be enough to bring about rapid change in central activity and as a result greatly reduce central sensitisation and thus the perception of pain (Melzack 1994). Interestingly and unsurprisingly, Pulisetti & Ebraheim (1999), found that the hypoalgesic effects of SIJ anaesthetic blocks wore off in 2-14 days in 90% of patients, which questions the long-term value of this technique in therapy.

The clinical reasoning process used here is no different to that used in other clinical scenarios such as calf tenderness secondary to primary lumbar L5/S1 nerve root derived pain (sciatica). Most clinicians would probably feel comfortable reasoning that the calf tenderness is 'referred' from the L5/S1 nerve root and dorsal horn sensitisation. Accordingly the calf would not be considered to be the primary source of pain. It seems that in the case of SIJ pain this clinical reasoning process is often ignored in favour of inculpating the SIJ as a primary source of mechanically related pain. Yet in the absence of inflammatory pathologies there is no sound evidence available to suggest that the SIJ's are a common site of mechanical dysfunction and/or pain.

The range of movement at the SIJ's is notably very small, even in those diagnosed with hypermobility. Studies of SIJ movement occurring around the transverse, longitudinal and antero-posterior axes found that the mean ROM was 1-2 degrees, with no individual ranges greater than 4 degrees (Sturesson et al 1998, Jacob & Kissling 1995). Studies of the commonly used pelvic and SIJ clinical motion tests have concluded that they are both an unreliable and invalid method of assessing and diagnosing dysfunction and / or pain related to these joints (Potter & Rothstein 1985, Dreyfuss et al 1996, Harrison et al 1997, Slipman et al 1998, Freburger & Riddle 1999, Levangie 1999, O'Haire & Gibbons 2000, van der Wurff et al 2000, 2000a, Riddle & Freburger 2002).

The poor reliability and validity of this approach is aptly demonstrated by the results of a study by Toussaint et al (1999) who carried out a series of standard manual SIJ dysfunction tests on 480 male construction workers and found that although 92.1% had tests deemed to be positive for dysfunction, yet these workers were completely asymptomatic. In summary, there is as yet no sound evidence to suggest that clinical approaches using asymmetry and joint motion testing to formulate diagnoses and treatment are either scientifically valid or reliable.

Joint cavitation phenomena

Joint manipulation is often accompanied by an audible 'popping' sound that has been said to result from cavitation within the joint. Greenman (1996) described the appearance of negative shadows on radiographs taken immediately after manipulative cavitation had occurred. These 'shadows' were said to be due to changes in the density of nitrogen gas resulting from manipulation, which it has been suggested, causes synovial fluid to change from a 'liquid to a gaseous state'. However, recent improvements in diagnostic imaging including computerised tomography (CT) have not identified any post-manipulative evidence of gas in the joint space or of any increase in the width of zygapophysial joint spaces (another claimed effect of manipulating these joints). These findings were the same whether or not traction was applied to the joint during manipulation (Cascioli et al 2003).

Meniscoid and capsular entrapment

Various theories surrounding entrapment of the articular capsule or meniscoid within zygapophysial joints have been proposed as a cause of spinal pain and dysfunction (Bogduk 1997). High resolution CT and MRI imaging has never identified meniscoid or capsular entrapment and both their presence and amenability to treatment via mobilisation or manipulation is entirely speculative.

'Subluxation' theory and evidence

Chiropractic philosophies of assessment and treatment were founded over 100 years ago based on the belief that joint subluxation or 'positional faults' occur, particularly at spinal joints, and that this 'abnormality' interferes with the body's health. Despite significant progress within orthodox medical sciences, chiropractic subluxation theory has changed little since Mr D.D. Palmer, a nineteenth century grocer and 'magnetic healer', claimed to have 'discovered' chiropractic. Chiropractic literature cites subluxation as a major contributory cause of many human conditions as diverse as pain, autism, epilepsy, hypertension, Bell's palsy and mental illness (Jamison 1987, Sandteur & Adams 1987,Goff 1988, Pistolese 2001, Alcantra et al 2003, Ressel & Rudy 2004). The list of diseases and ailments chiropractors consider to be related to subluxations is both extensive and extraordinary. The plethora of conditions claimed to be amenable to chiropractic treatment is almost endless. For example, Chiropractic literature includes such topics as a role for chiropractic therapy in influencing the body's immune system in people with acquired immunodeficiency syndrome (AIDS) (Lucido 1988) as well as in Parkinson's disease (Elster 2000 & 2004), multiple sclerosis (Elster 2004) and infertility (Rosen 2003, Shelley 2003).

One example of chiropractic education literature aimed at encouraging the general public to seek chiropractic treatment proclaims that, "subluxation is interference in your body that can lead to decay, dysfunction, and in some cases death" (www.discoversubluxation.com). This sinister and very worrying sounding statement is accompanied by the 'encouraging' message that regular chiropractic treatment to correct spinal subluxations can prevent this from happening! However, again, and perhaps reassuringly, there is no worthy evidence whatsoever to support chiropractic claims that visceral, immune or mental disease states emerge as a result of subluxation induced compression of autonomic nerves in the intervertebral foramen of spinal joints.

Rigorous literature searches of diagnostic scanning and radiological studies have failed to identify the heralded phenomenon of 'subluxation'. Interestingly and encouragingly, some chiropractic authors (Keating 1988, Keating et al 2005, Seaman 2004) have voiced their professional concern regarding the total absence of evidence surrounding the existence of subluxations, suggesting the need for more research and a move away from the existing chiropractic paradigm. Due to an absence of radiographic evidence Dalseth (1976) stated that 'the popularly used chiropractic x-ray diagnosis of positional faults or 'subluxations' is illusory'.

As this notably 'theosophical' chiropractic approach was founded on the proposed existence of subluxations, the subsequent lack of any reasonable evidence for 'subluxations' naturally nullifies all of the self-generated claims that have been made regarding the merits of chiropractic theory as it currently stands. It is not unreasonable to point out that a treatment cannot be prescribed to 'cure' something (subluxation) that does not exist.

A brief history of pain science

Since the 16th century specificity model of pain was proposed by Rene Descartes, the 'Cartesian' model has dominated the medical treatment of pain until recent times. Several 'pattern theories' followed Descartes model before publication of the now classic paper in 1965 by Melzack and Wall (1965) who described the 'gate control theory'. This was the first model to describe in any detail the involvement of descending pathways from the brain to spinal cord and their proposed role in modulating pain. To this day the gate control model has endured and expanded to include contemporary scientific knowledge. Our present understanding of pain offers a number of important factors in relation to physical medicine and manual therapy. As the preceding review of traditional manual therapy techniques indicates, many earlier theories have been expounded and nullified by a growing understanding of pain science. Much of the guesswork has been replaced by an expanding knowledge of the mechanisms specific to manual therapy that are capable of modulating pain.

It is known that the overall experience of pain involves the interplay of receptors, connecting neural pathways and processing within the central nervous system (CNS). There is no single un-modifiable, 'one-way only', 'Cartesian like' pathway in the nervous system responsible for pain. Pain is a highly complex amalgamation of 'in-parallel processing' of multiple sensory, cognitive and affective/emotional elements, all of which contribute to our pain experiences all the time, whether acute or chronic (Gifford 1998, 1998a). The fact that pain pathways are not 'hard wired', but modifiable, emphasises the importance and true holism of the biopsychosocial factors involved in everybody's experience of pain. Contrary to the way that many theoretical paradigms of pain-related musculoskeletal dysfunction shackled us firmly to the peripheral bodily tissues; current pain science directs us centrally to give our long overdue attention to the functioning of the brain, the nervous system and its inherent plasticity.

Despite limited and varying degrees of clinical success, manual therapy has become the preferred mode of treatment for many practitioners (UK BEAM trial team 2004). Evidence shows that some manual therapy techniques including mobilisation and manipulation can have effective pain relieving qualities. However, there is no evidence to suggest that pain relief resulting from manual therapy occurs via the traditional mechanically based theories discussed. As it has already been argued, if musculoskeletal pain problems were purely of a 'mechanical' nature, surely we would expect more consistent outcomes from every patient-manual therapy interaction? 'You-have-normal-range-of-movement-therefore-you-have-no-pain'just doesn't always follow. The very lack of consistency begs us to provide more credible explanations. At the same time, however, we need to have a reserved respect for the likelihood that when an individual has some movement impairment, homeostatic monitoring mechanisms may well be continually striving to promote 'mechanical' well-being and harmony. For example, by producing a pain response component whose only fulfilment is the restoration of normal movement, mechanical well-being and adequate intrinsic support. With perspectives like this though, there is a need for a wider appreciation of an individual's conscious and unconscious information monitoring and processing and the plethora of mechanisms that must gather to produce a response, – the very stuff that goes to make up the biopsychosocial approach argued for here.
It is recommended that if a more effective use of manual therapy is to be achieved and promoted there is an urgent need to incorporate much more of the current available pain science evidence into most manual therapists' clinical reasoning. This may well require an unpalatable and possibly radical shift of philosophy for a great many practitioners. The aim is to focus the inclusion of manual treatments more appropriately, and at the same time offer a sound and mature scientific framework that is acceptable and understood by the wider medical community and the general public alike, who, in the opinion here, have been mislead for far too long.

Pain related neurobiology

(for greater detail of pain neurobiology see chapters 18 and 20 this volume)

It is beyond the scope of this discussion to include an in-depth review of the neurobiology involved in the production of pain or the mechanisms involved in pain facilitation and inhibition; however a basic understanding of this is fundamental to maximising available therapeutic interventions. There is now compelling evidence to demonstrate how both transient and potentially permanent pain related changes take place within the CNS following tissue injury. This has provided considerable insight into the neurobiological basis of pain.

Central sensitisation

It is known that *first order* nociceptive specific (NS) neurones (nociceptors), not only undergo changes in their peripheral terminals following tissue injury, but also at their central terminals within the dorsal horn of the spinal cord. The process is called 'central sensitisation' by pain scientists (Wall 1991, Fields & Basbaum 1999, Woolf & Slater 2006). Further, synapsing *second order* 'NS' cells, that lie in the dorsal horn and project to the brain, also become increasingly more sensitised to incoming sensory impulse traffic (Woolf & Slater 2006). As already discussed in the sacro-iliac joint section earlier - once sensitised, modest or even normally sub-threshold stimuli from previously dormant collateral synapses that relate to input from quite normal structures, become capable of eliciting a response and hence producing pain. Thus sensory input from normal structures can be processed in terms of pain. These changes in the behaviour of NS first and second –order cells result from complex chemical and anatomical changes of the cell (see chapter 20). It is now well known that the second order NS cell's characteristics 'plastically' change to become more akin to those of so called 'wide dynamic range' (WDR) neurones (Wall 1991). WDR neurones, whose cell bodies are situated in the dorsal horn region of the spinal cord, normally respond to a 'wide' range of stimuli. Hence responses can occur from mechanical, chemical and thermal peripheral stimuli that range from non-noxious at one end of the spectrum to noxious at the other (Craig & Dostrovsky 1999). If any of these types of stimuli from the periphery reach the 'sensitised WDR like' central NS neurones the resulting output that surges upwards to the brain can be massively 'exaggerated' or amplified. Thus, minor input from the periphery via primary afferents subserving damaged tissue (primary hyperalgesia & mechanical allodynia), as well as input from surrounding and distant *undamaged* tissues (secondary hyperalgesia) can cause an explosive central reaction that may be processed in some situations as quite marked and severe pain. What is even more remarkable is the observation that sensitised dorsal horn cells are capable of producing spontaneous 'ectopic' output in the absence of any primary afferent input from the tissues at all (Barker et al 2003) – hence the potential for pain that is felt in tissues actually deriving from within the CNS (Gifford 1998a). The fascinatingly close parallel this has with the mechanisms thought to underlie phantom limb pain have been discussed at length by Gifford (1998a).

It is of great clinical significance that the sensitivity of the dorsal horn of the spinal cord is strongly influenced by descending pathways from the brain; and that these can act to both facilitate and inhibit dorsal horn activity (Wright 1995, Price & Bushnell 2004, see also chapter 20). Furthermore, the brainstem nuclei from which the descending pathways originate are extensively connected to, and influenced by many cortical and subcortical regions (Price & Bushnell 2004). As well as processing 'nociception', these higher brain regions are involved with processing psychological information such as thoughts, beliefs, emotions, attention, motivation and pain context. Collectively these psychological factors exert immense influence over descending pathways and the overall experience of pain (Zusman 2002, Price & Bushnell 2004). It is becoming evident that the way in which an individual psychologically responds to pain derived from nociceptive activity is likely to have a neurobiological impact throughout the whole of the nervous system involved. Powerfully, this is saying that psychological factors, like focus of attention, anxiety and fear, cause actual physical and neurophysiological changes in the nervous system that can lead to long term pain states (Gifford 2006). Hence, *chemical* changes, like the quality, amount and type of neurotransmitters, *physiological* changes for example in impulse processing and transmission; and actual *anatomical* changes in nerve cell architecture like axon growth and the formation of new synapses (Woolf & Salter 2006).

Increased focus on pain that links to pain anxiety and pain concern is likely to dampen the effectiveness of the descending inhibitory control system but at the same time facilitate the antagonistic descending excitatory control system. Thus concerned attention to pain may turn the 'pain-off' cells off and the 'pain-on' cells on (see discussion below and Fields et al 2006). The result of this is increased nociceptive activity and increased pain, - a very important ingredient that leads to long-term central hyperexcitability and the resulting chronic maladaptive pain. The mechanism by which this occurs is called 'Long-term-potentiation', a term that has been taken from the field of memory biology because of its remarkable similarity to the neurobiological processes observed in pain (e.g. Rose 1992, Pocket 1995, Ji et al 2003, Woolf & Salter 2006). It seems that pain gets established in the central nervous system in a way that is very similar to that occurring in memory acquisition (Gifford 1998a, 2006 and chapters 18, 20 of this volume).

Long-term potentiation

Long lasting nociceptive afferent stimulation of dorsal horn neurones can evoke long lasting 'central sensitisation' with the potential to lay down 'pain memories' (e.g. Gifford 1998a, Sandkhuler 2000). As discussed above, this involves actual chemical and anatomical changes of these cells, which are mediated by activation of inherent cellular protein kinases. Protein kinases are 'messenger molecules' found in neurones that stimulate gene transcription factors causing specific genes to 'switch-on' and express in favour of increased production of proteins that are used to form more receptor sites and new synapses on the post-synaptic cell membrane (see Chapter 20 this volume for detail). More receptor sites essentially act to 'strengthen' synaptic connectivity and hence, it's efficiency. This process is known as long-term potentiation or LTP (see LeDoux 2002, Zusman 2004). Thus, if LTP occurs at multiple sites it causes the formation of a new 'pain-memory pathway', it leaves an 'imprint' or 'memory-trace' in the CNS that has the potential to be easily reactivated or even maintained permanently in an active state. Thus, once pain 'gets into the system' it may be very hard to get rid of – consider how difficult it is to forget something and then you can appreciate how difficult it may be to get rid of a 'pain' imprint! It is very difficult to take your mind off an unpleasant memory, and if you do manage it, it doesn't take much to rekindle it again - just like those who suffer ongoing maladaptive chronic pain (see Gifford 1998a).

Cortical reorganisation

There is compelling evidence that the primary sensory and motor areas of the cortex are continuously changeable or 'plastic' throughout life (chapter 18 this volume). The more we use or do something – the greater the activity and the greater the density of neurones involved. Conversely, the less something occurs, the more its representational pathway tends to diminish (see chapter 189). Activity in cortical zones representing our various body regions is not only altered by injury but also by behaviourally relevant stimulation and training. Utilising this knowledge as part of a therapeutic approach when treating notoriously difficult conditions such as complex regional pain syndrome and phantom limb pain has produced some extremely impressive results (Flor et al 1997,McCabe et al 2003, Flor 2002, Moseley 2004). Some authors have described cortical changes related to pain in terms of the size and delineation of cortical somatic zones involving shrinkage and expansion as well as 'smudging' of these regions. However, the involvement and degree to which cortical reorganisation is responsible for causing pain is still uncertain. (discussed at length in chapter 18)

As discussed, the therapeutic application of this new knowledge requires a fundamental shift away from traditional clinical theories. Zusman (2004) referred to the importance of this when he discussed how achieving extinction (new synaptic learning) was about logically "teaching the nervous system (not muscles!) to instruct muscles on how to negotiate everyday movements without (undue) pain provocation" and thus enable the laying down of a 'new' adaptive motor 'memory' (extinction).

Flor (2004) has demonstrated how psychological processes, such as operant conditioning, classical conditioning and selective attention, influence cortical reorganisation and pain memory. These findings suggest a number of directions amenable to therapeutic interventions and these will be discussed later.

In summary, it is now known that neuroplastic changes take place at all levels within the central nervous system following injury. These changes occur in the regions of the spinal cord, brainstem, thalamus and cortex and they all play a vital role in the development and maintenance of pain (Price & Bushnell 2004). Psychological processes are capable of enhancing or diminishing the experience of pain and as we have seen, can strongly influence neuroplastic changes. It is becoming more and more apparent that despite the commonality of the neurobiological and psychological mechanisms involved in the development and maintenance of pain, each persons pain experience is likely to be made up of different quota's of each of these 'products'. In fact the content of these products will also be subject to change along with each individual's state of health and life experiences. It is hardly surprising that the formulaic 'recipe type' approaches of manual therapy and physical medicine have so far merely scratched the surface of a much deeper problem (Waddell 2003, Frost et al 2004, UK BEAM trial team 2004).

Pain relief following mobilisation and manipulation

Gate control

Good evidence exists to demonstrate how manual therapy can effectively stimulate central mechanisms resulting in *hypoalgesia*. One component of this involves activation of the spinal component of the gate control mechanism within the dorsal horn of the spinal cord. Rapid pain reduction via spinal gating can occur if large low-threshold A-beta fires are stimulated manually (or otherwise) in the periphery. A-beta fibres synapsing at dorsal horn cells have an inhibitory effect on the nociceptive output of these cells essentially reducing the flow of nociceptive output through the spinal gate

(Wall 1999a). One problem that has to be reconciled is that the process of central sensitisation described earlier results in A-beta fibre input being processed as pain, hence 'proprioceptively' and 'light-touch' exacerbated pain. Manual therapy therefore has the ability to aggravate pain when these underlying conditions occur.

There are two further important considerations with regards manual therapy and its relationship to pain-gate 'closing' potential.

Firstly: Loss of A-beta neurones may be an important consideration because they are notoriously susceptible to injury with subsequent dysfunction, degeneration and death. While it needs closer scrutiny, it is likely that anyone who has suffered a significant nerve root pain, e.g. sciatica or brachialgia, will have some kind of A-beta fibre impairment. Loss of A-beta fibres from the periphery means the loss of a normal, peripherally based, inhibitory mechanism at the pain gate. Hence, a clear tissue-based reason for the lack of effect/aggravating potential, of manual therapy input in many patients.

Secondly, the death of spinal cord inter-segmental neurones that are characteristically inhibitory (gate-closing) in nature has also been observed to occur in animal models of nerve-injury related pain (see Woolf & Salter 2006). Here, high levels of afferent nociceptive traffic following nerve injury leads to massive increases of excitatory amino acid release in the dorsal horn. Via 'excitotoxic' effects this massive over-load of chemicals can lead to the death of vulnerable intersegmental inhibitory interneurones – and hence to a loss of effectiveness of normal gate-control. Just from reasoning at this level it is hardly surprising that there are such a wide range of responses to pain treatments whose effects mostly derive from tissue based inputs.

Descending pathways

Further to the inhibition of nociceptive flow at the dorsal horn via input derived from the tissues, is the influence that the descending pathways from the brain are likely to have on the 'sensitivity' and 'plasticity' of the spinal cord processing mechanisms (Wright 1995, Fields & Basbaum 1999, Souvlis et al 2004, Zusman 2002, 2004,). A number of brain regions and descending pathways responsible for the hypoalgesia associated with manual therapy have been identified (Casey 1999, Fields et al 2006).

The periaqueductal gray (PAG) area is an important modulator of nociception. Activation of PAG nuclei and their related pathways via afferent stimulation is thought to be capable of activating descending inhibitory systems (Skyba et al 2003). 'Maitland grade 3 type' joint mobilisations are an example of 'afferent stimulation'. Other pain relevant inhibitory nuclei and pathways that are thought to be stimulated by the physical effects of manual therapy include those relating to the nucleus cuneiformis, locus coeruleus (LC), nucleus reticularis gigantocellularis (NGC), nucleus reticularis dorsalis (NRD) and rostral ventromedial medulla (RVM)(see chapter 20). The RVM is significant since it is a major source of brainstem axons projecting to the dorsal horn and is capable of both inhibiting and facilitating nociception via two classes of intrinsic neuron involved in 'switching' nociception on or off. Research indicates that the descending pathways identified utilise noradrenaline and serotonin (5HT) as their neurotransmitters, however the sensitivity of the RVM is also strongly influenced by both endogenous and exogenous opiates (endorphins & enkephalins) and is therefore also modulated by other non-mechanical stimuli (Wright 1995, Fields & Basbaum 1999, Souvlis et al 2004, Fields et al 2006).

Diffuse, or 'distant, noxious inhibitory control (DNIC)

Contemporary as well as ancient pain treatments use pain to relieve pain. Throughout history therapeutic counterirritation produced by such modalities as heat, cold, chemical irritants and intense mechanical stimuli have been used and documented. Contemporary physical therapy is not in short supply here either, Geoff Maitland has taught students for many years to: 'find what hurts and hurt it'. The technique usually involves the therapist driving their thumbs into the specific pain sensitive tissues with extreme vigour. A major aim of physical examination taught to most Physiotherapy students is to find the 'physical source' of the pain and focus treatment on the area. Many practitioners use manipulations and mobilisations that do hurt patients and of course can (but not always!) relieve symptoms for a while. Acupuncture, acupressure and transcutaneous electrical nerve stimulation has also been observed to produce varying levels of counterirritation and subsequent pain relief in human as well as animal experiments (see Melzack 1994 for an excellent review). Upon discovery of the PAG – RVM – dorsal horn modulatory pathway it was proposed that intense and noxious stimulation actually activated the descending inhibitory control systems and thus reduced nociceptive transmission to the brain from the level of the spinal cord. This effect appears to be mediated by the enkephalin group of endogenous opiates, which are known to be released at spinal and supraspinal levels (Fields et al 2006). In puzzling contrast to this it is also known, as one would expect, that cutaneous noxious stimulation can activate the pain 'on cells' and inhibit the pain 'off cells' at the RVM – hence pain now actually enhancing pain. Here, noxious stimulation in one part of the body *facilitates* nociception and pain in other parts of the body – think of the hypersensitivity of many chronic pain patients, – even minor discomfort produced by quite modest manual therapy away from the pain areas can produce marked exacerbations of their pain state. In other patients noxious stimulation using 'getting at the pain' techniques or vigorously and painfully manipulating well away from the area of pain can pleasingly activate quite significant analgesic effects. Most of us are familiar with the experience of stubbing a toe leading to the realisation that some pain elsewhere has been relieved.

DNIC is thought to occur via a 'surround' inhibition that heightens the contrast between the area being stimulated and the surrounding region. This would in effect increase the perceived intensity of pain at the area of stimulus but would also result in a net analgesic effect in the regions outside of the stimulated zone. It seems that the brain is well organised to focus all its attention on the item of most immediate concern, and put on-hold, or even completely re-evaluate, less important or less pressing issues for later consideration.

In summary, noxious stimulation from modalities including manual therapy activate multiple CNS networks. Some of these networks facilitate nociception and some inhibit it. Whether an individual's response to noxious stimuli is increased or reduced pain depends on factors like the location of stimulus, its duration, the circumstances in which it is delivered and the context and meaning of the noxious stimulus for that person. What they are thinking, feeling and focusing on during the treatment process may be a very important consideration (Thacker & Gifford 2002, Gifford 2006). We should also never forget to consider a vast spectrum of individual differences in sensitivity – one person's pleasure is another's pain. Unfortunately, just because one individual gets benefit from a painful intervention does not mean a similar problem for another individual will receive the same benefit from it! Further, a given individual's 'sensitivity-setting' may show a considerable *normal* fluctuation, day to day, hour to hour, minute by minute. Logically, all this means that for *any* physical treatment to have a positive effect there has to be a serious consideration of the patient's 'processing' or 'appraisal' of the situation – hence, 'top-down – before bottom-up' (Gifford 2006) – meaning work on tissues cannot begin (or is unlikely to succeed) until the brain is 'set-up' to accept it. It seems highly likely that whatever we do with patients must make sense to them if it is going to stand any reasonable chance of helping (Gifford 2006).

Habituation

There is compelling evidence that graded exposure to mechanical stimuli such as mobilisation techniques can reduce and sometimes abolish pain through the process of habituation. Habituation occurs as calcium ion channels on the presynaptic terminal of a nerve become less efficient following repeated stimulation and opening, this results in a marked reduction of the available calcium essential for the release of synaptic neurotransmitters. The subsequent decline in volume of neurotransmitter decreases the postsynaptic nerve potential and reduces the nerves ability to reach the threshold necessary for impulse generation. Essentially, habituation can be considered to be a decline of a conditioned response following repeated exposure to the conditioned stimulus (Jastreboff & Hazell 2004). Most therapists will have observed how pain can gradually subside or even change location during treatments using manual techniques or repeated exercise. This mechanism has been proposed by Gifford (2002b) to, at least partially, explain the changing pain response that can be achieved using the repeated movements advocated by the 'McKenzie approach'. Gifford (2004a, 2006) calls it the 'pain-boredom' effect or 'pain-boredom-acquisition processing', when explaining it to patients! For it to be successful one important 'top-down' ingredient is that the patient must feel comfortable and confident that repeatedly bringing on a pain is not harming.

Extinction

As already discussed, under certain conditions the CNS develops 'pain memories' through the process of LTP. New learning, involving the acquisition of 'painless memories', can bring about 'extinction' of an ongoing and maladaptive pain memory (Zusman 2004). Extinction involves the formation of a new memory via synaptic learning and LTP. In order for this new memory to be of any therapeutic value it needs to supersede the former pain memory in the ongoing 'competitive struggle' for perception dominance within the CNS. Therefore the stronger and more practiced the mode of learning the greater likelihood there is for extinction and clinical success. However, new memory acquisition / LTP does not eliminate an older memory and therefore old pain memories are still capable of 'breaking through' periodically or permanently into perception. This will be recognisable to clinicians as symptom 'flare ups' and the relapsing and remitting nature of many peoples pain.

Facilitation and inhibition of motor activity

A number of studies have reported manual therapy as having both inhibitory (Wright 1995, Zusman 1992) and facilitatory (Keller & Colloca 2000, Colloca & Keller 2001, Dishman et al 2002) effects on the motor system. However, some of these studies lack scientific validity, insofar as the experimental models used were based on hypothetical treatment approaches and clinical theories. As a comment and in contrast, descending, cortico-spinal 'motor' pathways, are known to send inhibitory and excitatory branches to the sensory and nociception processing regions of the outer layers of the dorsal horn (reviewed in Galea & Darian-Smith 1995). Hence an evolutionary elegant pathway whereby pain can be dramatically stopped in order to allow movement to proceed. Limping away in pain is of no survival value when a lion is chasing you! No wonder function-with-purpose has always been such a good painkiller.

Sympathetic nervous system (SNS) responses

Similarly, some studies performed on SNS responses to manual therapy have also lacked construct validity (Clinton & McCarthy 1993). However, Souvlis et al (2001) and Vicenzino et al (1999) have demonstrated an excitatory response of the SNS to grade 3 type mobilisation techniques, these include sudomotor (increased body temperature) and cutaneous vasomotor (blood vessel dilation) responses.

Placebo

As with many therapeutic interventions it is inevitable that varying degrees of placebo responses to manual therapy techniques will be observed. The Oxford dictionary (1996) defines the 'placebo effect' as a 'beneficial (or adverse) effect produced by a placebo and not due to any property of the placebo itself'. It is recognised that placebo is a complex interaction of biological, psychological and sociological processes (as already discussed), and there are a number of factors surrounding placebo that are pertinent to manual therapy.

- Foremost, it is a myth that 33% of patients receiving placebo treatment for painful conditions will respond to the treatment with at least 50% reduction of their pain. Placebo responses have been shown to vary between almost 0 – 100% depending on the circumstances of the study (Wall 1999, Roche 2002).
- Circumstances that can increase placebo response include the level of confidence and belief practitioners display and have in the treatment techniques they use and the perception of this by their patient's.
- The more 'powerful' a treatment appears to be, the greater the placebo response is to it.
- Placebo does not merely affect the psychological aspects of pain; it can initiate real physiological effects including analgesia and decreased tissue inflammation.

(The placebo response is discussed at length in Topical Issues in Pain Vol 4: Gifford 2002a)

Integrating evidence into practice

Current scientific evidence offers insight into a number of potentially appropriate treatment modalities for pain, including manual therapy. In order to incorporate this growing body of evidence into clinical practice a perpetually changing and adaptive approach to clinical reasoning is fundamental if maximum therapeutic benefit is the goal. Many of the current 'hands on' and 'hands off' techniques can be integrated with current evidence and utilised in treatment. However, as discussed, much of the past theoretical basis surrounding 'hands on' techniques is at best scientifically very shaky and most likely invalid, hence a somewhat urgent need for new paradigms and shifts in thinking. As each person's pain experience involves dynamic elements of biological, psychological and social factors, it is important that each of these elements will need to be entered into the clinical reasoning equation. It is not trite to suggest that paying mere 'lip service' to this process of reasoning is likely to result in poor outcomes.

As the basis of this discussion involves a review of manual therapy a detailed analysis of biopsychosocial assessment will not be made. However, current evidence indicates that a good working knowledge of red and yellow flags is essential and readers are referred to works by Roberts (2000), Watson (2000), Watson & Kendall (2000) and Gifford et al (2006).

Clinical guidelines (CSAG 1994, Waddell 2003) that are derived from much relevant research (e.g. Linton 1996, 1998, 2004) suggest that it is essential to carry out a comprehensive 'low-tech' physical examination of the involved neuromusculoskeletal system. This can be used to not only screen for red flags but also to provide information regarding the patient's neurological and musculoskeletal function, including the presence or absence of such factors as mechanical allodynia and/or hyperalgesia. These findings provide an overview of the patient's neuromusculoskeletal 'sensitivity' state. As psychosocial factors are likely to be critical in modulating levels of 'sensitivity' we advocate carrying out a full or modified psychosocial assessment during initial examination of all patients. This not only 'flags' those at risk of chronicity but also provides information to assist the clinical reasoning process and planning of treatment. Although the 1994 CSAG guidelines for back pain suggest adding a psychosocial assessment at 6-weeks for 'non-responders', recent evidence indicates that the neuroplastic changes associated with chronicity are in place within hours of tissue injury, it is therefore proposed that early detection of known associated psychosocial risk factors is vital when planning both initial and ongoing treatment.

Although 'yellow flags' were not specifically intended for planning manual therapy treatment, they can be of enormous benefit when assessing all patients with pain. An appreciation of each patient's attitudes, beliefs and behaviours offers insight towards their individual levels of distress and coping. To demonstrate this it is worth considering some typical psychosocial assessment findings of a patient with low back pain. These findings might include reports of high pain intensity, a belief that pain is beyond their control, fear that pain is harmful and must be abolished before returning to activity as well as fear avoidance behaviours including the cessation of exercise and withdrawal from some activities of daily living. If it is found, following assessment of a patient, that the sum of their yellow flag findings indicates high levels of 'sensitivity' and distress, it might be important to question the appropriateness and wisdom of administering a strong manipulative thrust technique to the patient. Clinical reasoning utilising the biopsychosocial model and approach would suggest that such a technique could well result in 'flaring up' this patients symptoms. The possible detrimental consequences of using manipulative treatment in these circumstances may appear blatantly obvious, but if no enquiry regarding yellow flags was made how else could this have been reasoned and predicted? If we now contrast this with the 'recipe like' reasoning implicit within the traditional manual therapy philosophies discussed earlier, this same patient and clinical circumstances could easily have resulted in a decision to prescribe and administer strong manipulation.

Clinically, it is important to view the physical findings for this 'sensitised' type of patient from a perspective that sees the observations of movement and testing as being a reflection of their overall 'bio-psycho-social status'. For example loss of range of forward bending could be interpreted in one or all of the following ways:

1. A clear physical impairment (for example ankylosed lumbar spine and tight hamstrings) = **'Bio'** (the range is the same whether awake and alert or under deep sedation of an anaesthetic.)

2. The amount of pain produced and the response to it = **bio-psycho**

3. A reflection of the patient's loss of confidence, fear of re-injury and fear of exacerbating the pain **(bio-psycho-social).**

Clinical reasoning using the biopsychosocial paradigm indicates that it might be more appropriate to begin patient management by enquiring and explaining about pain and thus initially attempting to reduce levels of fear and distress (Butler & Moseley 2003, Gifford 2006, Gifford et al 2006). It might also be reasoned that management could be commenced with a 'hands off' approach such as graded exposure, which aims to help patients challenge fears associated with factors like movement-related pain or injury by gradually encouraging the restoration of 'thoughtless fearless' functional movement (Gifford 2003, 2006). For the patient described, a 'hands on' technique like gentle soft tissue massage might be a more effective and appropriate treatment to start the 'desensitising' and confidence building process.

From the patient example, what seems to be imperative is the need for both an appreciation and acknowledgement of the patient's overall state combined with an understanding of the biopsychosocial factors that underpin it. This creates a much healthier multidimensional forum for sound clinical reasoning. Clinical reasoning that has its underpinnings firmly anchored in good science and sound clinical management is free from the constraints imposed by the mostly one-dimensional traditional treatment approaches that are widely taught and promoted.

Considering the evidence discussed earlier regarding the efficacy of manipulation and mobilisation, it hopefully becomes clearer how many current techniques can be utilised to assist with pain relief. The available evidence also strongly emphasises that manual therapy and other passive therapies are only one part of a much bigger biopsychosocial picture. Used judiciously manual techniques can sometimes offer a useful window of opportunity to assist patients with management and understanding of their pain but they are rarely likely to be the sole answer in the long-term.

A new paradigm for manual therapy

Available evidence now outlines a number of pain relevant neurophysiological mechanisms that are amenable to manual therapy. For example, mobilisation and manipulation techniques like those described by Maitland (1986 & 1991) involving passive types of physiological and accessory joint movements can be used to stimulate inhibition of pain processing in the dorsal horn, as well as 'triggering' descending inhibitory pathways acting at the level of the spinal cord.

However, it is hard to see how the rather transient nature of a manipulation technique could produce significant levels of habituation. The oscillatory or sustained nature of many mobilisation techniques may well lend themselves towards achieving clinically effective states of habituation if the context in which they are performed is subtly altered. For example, as LTP has qualities of both specificity and associativity, any new synaptic learning (LTP) would need to result in some useful functional improvement for the patient if it is going to have any clinically meaningful value. New synaptic learning would be of little use to a patient if it were associated with lying face down on a therapists couch while mobilisations were performed on their lumbar spine. However, if the patient can see and feel that it is possible to bend forward with no pain and hence start to 'learn' pain-free movement, then this could have enormous functional significance. Experimenting with various mobilisation techniques while asking the patient to move can produce better and less painful movement. Some familiar examples of the sorts of techniques that can be used include 'so called' sustained natural apophyseal glides (SNAGS) and mobilisation with movement (MWM) (Mulligan 1999). Used in the right context, for example with lots of explanation combined with therapist assistance and reassurance, these types of techniques can sometimes help patients challenge feared or restricted movements.

Additionally it has been demonstrated that 'psychological products' such as classical and operant conditioning and selective attention and verbal cueing (Flor 2002a) are all capable of modulating neuroplasticity, including that of the cortical regions. This suggests the need for incorporation of a number of adjunct techniques while performing manual treatments. Thus, various forms of verbal encouragement, positive reinforcement and positive use of selective attention can be incorporated. Selective attention is fascinating, since simply asking the patient to focus their attention on a neutral or non-threatening stimulus such as pain free joint mobilisations can reduce or stop the supply of some of the 'psychological fuel' necessary for pain perception. However, in order to ensure that the patient is not being encouraged to concentrate on a painful or threatening stimulus (thus reinforcing their pain) it can be helpful to make basic enquiries during the administration of mobilisation techniques. This might include questions such as, 'does that feel okay'? 'Would you like me to use more or less pressure'? Or statements like; 'It's important that you feel comfortable with what I'm doing'. 'If it is causing pain I want it to be a type of pain that you feel is doing it good if at all possible'. 'This is much better if it's nice pain rather than nasty pain'.

As LTP requires regular periods of 'training' to achieve and maintain new synaptic learning, the prescription of exercises specific to restoring part or all of 'missing' functional movements is fundamental to achieving successful rehabilitation. It has been demonstrated that cortical reorganisation requires behaviourally relevant training and does not occur with passive stimulation (Jenkins et al 1990). Therefore isolated passive treatment in the form of mobilisation or manipulation is unlikely to be helpful in cases of chronic pain, regardless of the dosage of passive treatment administered. This emphasises the vital importance of an all-encompassing biopsychosocial approach, including exercises and training that achieve functional rehabilitation specific to each patients requirements and in particular their desired activities of daily living. Recent evidence has helped to outline both the indications and limitations of manual therapy.

The safety of mobilisation and manipulation techniques

As far as we are aware there is no evidence to suggest that serious tissue based injuries occur with 'reasonable' grades of mobilisation techniques. On the other hand, there is little doubt that even modest mobilisation techniques administered to patients with significant peripheral neurogenic or maladaptive central sensitivity are easily capable of 'stirring up' pain and associated symptoms. Knowledge of maladaptive pain mechanisms and the potential they have to cause significant flare-ups *without* tissue damage must surely help therapists and patients to have a better and more confident understanding of the situation. As we all know, it is never pleasant to stir up a patient's pain, especially with the belief that some ghastly damage has occurred.

The literature does contain numerous studies detailing incidents and accidents resulting from spinal and pelvic joint manipulation. Stevinson et al (2001), Grieve (1994), Dupeyron et al (2003) and Assendelft et al (1996) identified vertebrobasilar artery (VBA) injuries, intervertebral disc prolapse / sequestration and cauda equina syndrome as the most common accidents following manipulation. Other documented manipulation related accidents include death, stroke, nerve root compression, paraplegia, vertebral fractures and embolisms. It is pertinent to note that there are as yet no designated pre-manipulative screening protocols capable of eradicating these manipulative accidents (Haldeman et al 2002).

The average age of those patient's suffering VBA related strokes following cervical spine manipulation is 38-years old, this is far lower than that of national 'stroke averages'. This is particularly worrying in light of the otherwise 'rare' occurrence of this type of stroke in young people. There are conflicting reports in the related literature surrounding the incidence of manipulative accidents. Risk factors have been quoted to be between 1 in 20,000 to 1 in 4,000,000 manipulations performed. Until recently it has been difficult to ascertain a realistic incidence of manipulative accidents. This has largely been due to the significant under reporting of these events. However, Dupeyron et al (2003) studied the incidence of manipulative accidents occurring to patients who went on to present to 133 physicians including neurologists, neurosurgeons, and rheumatologists over a 2-year period. They found that the incidence of VBA accidents alone was 30 times higher than that in published series. Potentially, this indicates that the risk of serious manipulative accidents could be as high as 1 in every 666 manipulations performed.

In view of the incidence of 'side effects' associated with spinal and pelvic joint manipulation, it is probably fair to assume that if these techniques were subject to the same clinical trials and scrutiny as new drugs, their

27

licensing would be rejected on the basis of their inherent risk of injury. Furthermore, there is no evidence whatsoever to suggest that manipulation techniques have any superior clinical effect above and beyond alternative non-injurious mobilisation techniques. In view of the available evidence regarding benefit and risks, it is our belief that there are no circumstances in which it would appear appropriate to recommend the use of manipulation in clinical practice.

A willingness to change?

Jones (1995) stated that 'the principal fault behind many of the colossal misdirection's throughout scientific history has been the blind acceptance of what is written or professed as the truth at the time'. Historically, Cartesian reasoning and a preoccupation with various 'guru' driven theories have exerted a considerable and prevailing directional influence over the 'physical therapies'. However, even when elements of the 'truth' begin to emerge good clinical reasoning can still prove difficult if we don't know what clinical approach to adopt or which professionals to believe.

Currently the dissemination of 'best evidence' appears to be somewhat haphazard and while being met with enthusiasm in some quarters is feared and even reviled in others. The sheer volume of intra and inter-professional debate surrounding the emerging evidence base over recent years has highlighted this situation. Much of the criticism directed at evidence-based practice by some clinicians has contained the accusation that it removes a therapist's 'flair' and individual freedom to practice those techniques they feel are instinctively right for their patients. Most realistic clinicians probably agree that while clinical practice does need to directly reflect pain science it should not be so pedantic as to confine practitioners to only what is known. However, professionalism can never be equated to a 'green light' enabling unquestioned administration of any technique that is currently 'in Vogue'. Neither should it provide an open door for proponents of manual therapy (or other) techniques to attach 'evidence based' labels to their clinical approaches regardless of reliability and validity. Clinical management based on the growing biopsychosocial evidence allows practitioners to adapt and change their clinical reasoning and treatments to suit each patient's individual circumstances and thus provides a platform for the clinical practice of true 'therapist flair'.

Successful integration of scientific evidence into clinical practice not only requires a paradigm capable of incorporating perpetual change; it also requires honesty on the part of each clinician involved and genuine professional altruism. As this involves some very human qualities, the process is always open to unconscious and conscious misdirection during pursuit of personal, financial, professional or political gains.

References:

Alcantra J, Plaugher G, Van Wyngarden DL 2003 Chiropractic care of a patient with vertebral subluxation and Bell's palsy. Journal of Manipulative and Physiological Therapeutics 26(4):253

Apley AG, Solomon L 1994 Concise system of orthopaedics and fractures (2nd Edn). Butterworth Heinmann, Oxford

Assendelft WJ, Bouter LM, Knipschild PG 1996 Complications of spinal manipulation: a comprehensive review of the literature. Jour Fam Pract 42(5): 475-480

Barker RA, Barasi S, Neal MJ 2003 Neuroscience at a glance (2nd Edn). Blackwell, Oxford

Bogduk N 1997 Clinical anatomy of the lumbar spine and sacrum. (3rd Edn). Churchill Livingstone, Edinburgh

Bourdillon JF, Day EA 1987 Spinal Manipulation. (4th Edn). Heinemann, London

Butler DS, Moseley GL 2003 Explain pain. Noigroup publications, Adelaide

Cascioli V, Corr P, Till AG 2003 An investigation into the production of intra-articular gas bubbles and increase in joint space in the zygapophysial joints of the cervical spine in asymptomatic subjects after spinal manipulation. Journal of Manipulative and Physiological Therapeutics 26(6):356-364

Casey KL 1999 Forebrain mechanisms of nociceptors and pain: analysis through imaging. Proceedings of the National Academy of Science USA 96:7668-7674

Cassidy JD, KirKaldy-Willis WH 1985 Spinal manipulation for the treatment of chronic low back and leg pain: an observational study. In Buerger AA, Greenman PE (Eds), Empirical approaches to the validation of spinal manipulation. CC Thomas, Illinois 119-148

Cholewicki J, Crisco JJ, Oxland TR et al 1996 Effects of posture and structure on three-dimensional coupled rotations in the lumbar spine. A biomechanical analysis. Spine 21:2421-2428

Chrisman OD, Mittnacht A, Snook GA 1964 A study of the results following rotary manipulation in the lumbar intervertebral disc syndrome. Journal Of Bone And Joint Surgery 46A: 517-524

Clinton EMF, McCarthy PW 1993 The effect of chiropractic adjustment of the first rib on the electric skin response in ipsilateral and contralateral human forelimbs. Complimentary Therapies in Medicine 1:61-67

Colloca CJ, Keller TS 2001 Electromyographic reflex responses to mechanical force, manually assisted spinal manipulative therapy. Spine 26:447-457

Cox JM, Hazen LJ, Mungovan M 1993 Distraction manipulation reduction of an L5-S1 disc herniation. Journal Of Manipulative & Physiological Therapeutics 16(5):342

Craig AD, Dostrovsky JO 1999 Medulla to thalamus. In: Wall PD, Melzack R (Eds) Textbook of pain (4th Edn). Churchill Livingstone, Edinburgh 183-214

CSAG 1994 Clinical standards advisory group: Back pain. HMSO publications, London

Cyriax J 1974 Textbook of Orthopaedic Medicine, (8th Edn). Balliere Tindall, London

Dalseth I 1976 Chiropractic and radiological diagnosis. Tidsskrift for Den norske laegeforening 11:642-644

Dandy DJ, Edwards DJ 1998 Essential orthopaedics and trauma (3rd Edn). Churchill Livingstone, Edinburgh

Davis D, Kimmet T, Auty M 1986 Physical education: theory and practice. Macmillan education Australia, South Melbourne: 206-207

DiGiovanna EL, Schiowitz S 1991 An osteopathic approach to diagnosis and treatment. JB Lippincott, Philadelphia

Dishman JD, Ball KA, Burke J 2002 Central motor excitability changes after spinal manipulation: a transcranial magnetic stimulation study. Journal of Manipulative and Physiological Therapeutics 25:318-325

Dreyfuss P, Micaelson M, Pauza K et al 1996 The value of medical history and physical examination in diagnosing sacro-iliac pain. Spine 21:2594-2602

Dupeyron A, Vautravers P, Lecocq J et al 2003 Complications following vertebral manipulation – a survey of French region physicians. Ann Readapt Med Phys 46(1): 33-40

Edwards BC 1992 Manual of combined movements – Their use in the examination and treatment of mechanical vertebral column disorders. Churchill Livingstone, Edinburgh

Elster EL 2000 Upper cervical chiropractic management of a patient with Parkinson's disease: A case report. Journal Of Manipulative & Physiological Therapeutics 23(8): 573-577

Elster EL 2004 Eighty-one patients with multiple sclerosis and Parkinson's disease undergoing upper cervical chiropractic care to correct vertebral subluxation: A retrospective analysis. Journal of Vertebral Subluxation Research, Aug:1-9

Farfan HF 1977 Pathological basis for manipulative therapy. In : Proceedings of the 3rd Conference International Federation of Orthopaedic Manipulative Therapists, Vail, Colorado:135

Fields HL, Basbaum AI 1999 Central nervous system mechanisms of pain modulation. In: Wall PD, Melzack R (Eds), Textbook of pain (4th Edn). Churchill Livingstone, Edinburgh 309-329

Fields HL, Basbaum A, Heinricher M 2006 Central nervous system mechanisms of pain modulation. In: McMahon S, Koltzenburg M (eds) Wall and Melzack's Textbook of Pain (5th Edn). Elsevier,Churchill Livingstone, Edinburgh 125-142

Flor H 2002 Painful memories: can we train chronic pain patients to 'forget' their pain? European molecular biology organization reports 3(4):1-4

Flor H 2002a The modification of cortical reorganization and chronic pain by sensory feedback. Applied Psychophysiology and Biofeedback 27(3):215-227

Flor H, Braun C, Elbert T et al 1997 Extensive reorganisation of primary somatosensory cortex in chronic back pain patients. Neuroscience letters 224:5-8

Fortin JD, Washington WJ, Falco FJE 1999 Three pathways between the sacroiliac joint and neural structures. AJNR Am J Neuroradiol 20:1429-1434

Freburger JK, Riddle DL 1999 Measurement of sacroiliac joint dysfunction: a multicenter intertester reliability study. Physical Therapy 79(12):1134-1141

Frost H, Lamb SE, Doll H et al 2004 Randomised controlled trial of physiotherapy compared with advice for low back pain. BMJ 329:708-711

Galea MP, Darian-Smith I 1995 Voluntary movement and pain: Focusing on action rather than perception. In: Shacklock MO (Ed). Moving in on Pain. Butterworth-Heinemann, Chatswood 40-52

Gifford LS 1998 The mature organism model. In: Gifford LS (Ed). Topical Issues in Pain 1. Whiplash - science and management. Fear-avoidance beliefs and behaviour. CNS Press, Falmouth 45-56

Gifford LS 1998a Central mechanisms. In: Gifford LS (Ed). Topical Issues in Pain 1. Whiplash - science and management. Fear-avoidance beliefs and behaviour CNS Press, Falmouth 67-80

Gifford LS 2002 An Introduction to evolutionary reasoning: - Diet, discs, fevers and the placebo. In: Gifford LS (Ed) Topical Issues in Pain 4. Placebo and nocebo. Pain management. Muscles and pain. CNS Press, Falmouth 119-144

Gifford LS (Ed) 2002a Topical Issues in Pain 4. Placebo and nocebo. Pain Management. Muscles and Pain. CNS Press, Falmouth

Gifford LS 2002b Editorial: Therapist and patient fear of bending: Does the McKenzie approach - need a shift? Physiotherapy Pain Association News, December (14):3-8

Gifford LS 2003 Perspectives on the biopsychosocial model – part 3: Patient example – using the shopping basket approach and graded exposure. In Touch, Journal of the Organisation of Chartered Physiotherapists in Private Practice 102:3-15

Gifford LS 2004 Unnecessary fear avoidance and physical incapacity in a 55-year-old housewife. In: Jones MA, Rivett DA (Eds). Clinical Reasoning FOR Manual Therapists. Butterworth Heinemann, Edinburgh 61-86

Gifford LS 2004a Editorial: Re-writing 'Colonel Bogey' - can chronic pain be forgotten? Physiotherapy Pain Association News May (17):3-6

Gifford LS 2006 'Gifford's Aches and Pains': Patients, pain explanations, management foundations and concepts. CNS Press, Falmouth, In Press

Gifford LS, Thacker M, Jones M 2006 Physiotherapy and Pain. In: McMahon S, Koltzenburg M (Eds). Wall and Melzack's Textbook of Pain, (5th Edn). Elsevier, Churchill Livingstone, Edinburgh 603-617

Goff PJ 1988 Chiropractic treatment of mental illness; a review of theory and practice. Research Forum 4:4-10

Greenman PE 1996 Principles of manual medicine (2nd Edn). Williams & Wilkins, Baltimore

Grieve GP 1988 Common vertebral joint problems (2nd Edn). Churchill Livingstone, Edinburgh 303-307

Grieve GP 1994 Incidents and accidents of manipulation and allied techniques. In Boyling JD, Palastanga N (Eds). Grieve's Modern Manual Therapy (2nd Edn). Churchill Livingstone, Edinburgh 673-692

Haldeman S, Hooper PD 1999 Mobilization, manipulation, massage and exercise for the relief of musculoskeletal pain. In: Wall PD, Melzack R (Eds). The Textbook of Pain, (4th Edn) Churchill Livingstone, Edinburgh 1399-1418

Haldeman S, Kohlbeck FJ, McGregor M 2002 Stroke, cerebral artery dissection and cervical spine manipulative therapy. Journ Neurol 249(8):1098-1104

Harrison DE, Harrison DD, Troyanovich SJ 1997 The sacroiliac joint: a review of the anatomy and biomechanics with clinical implications. Manipulative Physiol Ther 20(9):607-617

Hession EF, Donald GD 1993 Treatment of multiple lumbar disc herniations in an adolescent athlete utilising flexion distraction and rotational manipulation. Journal Of Manipulative & Physiological Therapeutics 16(3):185-192

Jacobs HAC, Kissling RO 1995 The mobility of the Sacro-Iliac joints in healthy volunteers between 20 and 50 years of age. Clin Biomech 10:352-361

Jamison J 1987 Hypertension case finding and management in chiropractic clinics. European Journal Of Chiropractic 35:151-155

Jastreboff PW, Hazell JWP 2004 Tinnitus Retraining Therapy. Cambridge university press, Cambridge

Jenkins WM, Merzenich MM, Ochs MT et al 1990 Functional reorganisation of primary somatosensory cortex in adult owl monkeys after behaviourally controlled tactile stimulation. Journal of Neurophysiology 63:82-104

Ji R-R, Kohno T, Moore K A et al 2003 Central sensitization and LTP: do pain and memory share similar mechanisms? Trends in Neurosciences 26(12):696-705

Jones M 1995 Clinical reasoning and pain. Manual therapy 1:17-24

Keating JC 1988 Science and politics and the subluxation. American Journal of Chiropractic Medicine 1:107-110

Keating JC, Charlton KH, Grod JP et al 2005 Subluxation: dogma or science? Chiropractic & Osteopathy 13(17):1-27 (www.chiroandosteo.com/content/13/11/17)

Keller TS, Colloca CJ 2000 Mechanical force spinal manipulation increases trunk muscle strength assessed by electromyography: a comparative clinical trial. Journal of Manipulative and Physiological Therapeutics 23:585-595

Kokmeyer DJ, van der Wurff P, Aufdemkampe G et al 2002 The reliability of multitest regimens with sacroiliac pain provocation tests. Journal Of Manipulative and Physiological Thertapeutics 25(1):42-48

Le Doux J 2002 Synaptic Self: How our brains become who we are. Penguin Books, New York

Lee DG, Walsh MC 1996 Workbook of manual therapy techniques for the vertebral column and pelvic girdle. (2nd Edn). Friesen printers, Altona, Manitoba

Lee DG 1999 The pelvic girdle, Churchill Livingstone, Edinburgh

Levangie PK 1999 Four clinical tests of sacroiliac dysfunction: the association of test results with innominate torsion among patients with and without low back pain. Physical therapy 79(11):1043-1057

Lewis J 2004 Posture and subacromial impingement syndrome: does a relationship exist? In Touch, Journal of the Association of Chartered Physiotherapists in Private Practice108:8-17

Linton SJ 1996 Early interventions for the secondary prevention of chronic musculoskeletal pain. In: Campbell JN (Ed). Pain 1996 - An updated review Refresher course syllabus IASP Press, Seattle 305-311

Linton SJ 1998 The socioeconomic impact of chronic back pain: is anyone benefiting? Pain 75:163-168

Linton SJ 2004 Environmental and learning factors in the development of chronic pain and disability. In: Price DD, Bushnell MC (Eds). Psychological methods of pain control: Basic science and clinical perspectives. Progress in Pain Research and Management Vol 29. IASP Press, Seattle 143-167

Lucido VP 1988 AIDS: why it should concern us. Journal of the American Chiropractic Association 25:5,8-9

Maigne JY, Aivaliklis A, Pfefer F 1995 Results of sacroiliac joint double block and value of sacroiliac pain provocation tests in 54 patients with low back pain. Spine 21(16):1889-1892

Maitland GD 1986 Vertebral manipulation (5th Edn). Butterworth Heineman, Oxford

Maitland GD 1991 Peripheral manipulation (3rd Edn). Butterworth Heineman, Oxford

Matthews JA, Yates DA 1969 Reduction of the lumbar disc prolapse by manipulation. British Medical Journal 3:696-697

McCabe CS, Haigh RC, Ring EFJ et al 2003 A controlled pilot study of the utility of mirror visual feedback in the treatment of complex regional pain syndrome (type 1). Rheumatology 42:97-101

Melzack R, 1994 Folk medicine and the sensory modulation of pain. In: Wall PD & Melzack R (Eds). Textbook Of Pain, (3rd Edn). Churchill Livingstone, Edinburgh: 1209-1217

Melzack R, Wall PD 1965 Pain mechanisms: a new theory. Science 150:971-999

Moseley G L 2004 Graded motor imagery is effective for long-standing complex regional pain syndrome: a randomised controlled trial. Pain 108(1-2):192-198

Mulligan BR 1999 Manual therapy ; "nags", "snags", "mwms" etc, (4th Edn). Plane view services Ltd, Wellington

Nathan B 1999 Touch and emotion in manual therapy, Churchill Livingstone. Edinburgh

Norris CM 1993 Sports injuries diagnosis and management for physiotherapists. Butterworth-Heinmann Ltd, Oxford

O'Haire C, Gibbons P 2000 Inter-examiner and Intra-examiner agreement for assessing sacroiliac anatomical landmarks using palpation and observation: pilot study. Manual therapy 5(1):13-20

Oxford compact English dictionary 1996 Oxford university press, Oxford

Panjabi M, Yamamoto I, Oxland T et al 1989 How does posture affect coupling in the lumbar spine? Spine 14:1002-1011

Pistolese RA 2001 Epilepsy and seizure disorders: A review of literature relative to chiropractic care of children. Journal Of Manipulative & Physiological Therapeutics 24(3):199-205

Pockett S 1995 Spinal cord synaptic plasticity and chronic pain. Anesthesia and Analgesia 80:173-179

Potter NA, Rothstein JM 1985 Intertester reliability for selected clinical tests of the sacroiliac joint. Physical therapy 65(11):1671-1675

Price DD, Bushnell MC 2004 Overview of pain dimensions and their psychological modulation. In: Price DD, Bushnell MC (Eds) Psychological methods of pain control: Basic science and clinical perspectives. Progress in pain research and management Vol 29 IASP Press, Seattle 3-17

Pulisetti D, Ebraheim NA 1999 CT-guided sacroiliac joint injections. Journal of Spinal Disorders 12(4):310-312

Ressel O, Rudy R 2004 Vertebral subluxation correlated with somatic, visceral and immune complaints: an analysis of 650 children under chiropractic care. Journal Of Vertebral Subluxation Research, October:1-23

Riddle DL, Freburger JK 2002 Evaluation of the presence of sacroiliac joint region dysfunction using a combination of tests: a multicenter intertester reliability study. Physical therapy 82(8):772-781

Roberts L 2000 Flagging the danger signs of low back pain. In: Gifford L (ed) Topical Issues In Pain 2, CNS Press, Falmouth: 69-83

Robson SM 2003 Manipulation – an evidence based perspective. Physiotherapy Pain Association News, Dec(16):12-17

Roche PA 2002 Placebo and patient care. In: Gifford LS (Ed) Topical Issues In Pain 4. Placebo and Nocebo. Pain management. Muscles and pain. CNS Press, Falmouth 19-39

Rose S 1992 The making of memory: From molecules to mind. Bantam Press, London

Rosen MG 2003 Sacro occipital technique management of a thirty four year old woman with infertility. Journal of Subluxation Research, Dec (17):1-4

Sandetur R, Adams E, 1987 The effect of chiropractic adjustments in the behaviour of autistic children. American Chiropractic Association Journal of Chiropractic 24:21-25

Sandkuhler J 2000 Learning and Memory in pain pathways. Pain 88(2):113-118

Schwarzer AC, Aprill CN, Bogduk N 1995 The sacroiliac joint in low back pain. Spine 20(1):31-37

Seaman DC 2004 A contemporary view of subluxation that is consistent with the founder's views: a commentary. Journal of vertebral subluxation research Aug:1-4

Shelley J 2003 Healthy pregnancy in a previously infertile patient following D.N.F.T. chiropractic care: A case report. Journal of Subluxation Research, Dec(8):1-7

Skyba DA, Radhakrishnan R, Rohlwing JJ et al 2003 Joint manipulation reduces hyperalgesia by activation of monoamine receptors but not opioid or GABA receptors in the spinal cord. Pain 106:159-168

Slipman CW, Sterenfeld EB Chou LH et al 1998 The predictive value of provocative sacroiliac joint stress manoeuvres in the diagnosis of sacroiliac joint syndrome. Arch Phys Med Rehabil 79(3):288-292

Souvlis T, Vicenzino B, Wright A 2001 Dose of spinal manual therapy influences in SNS function. Musculoskeletal Physiotherapy Australia (MPA) Biennial conference, Adelaide

Souvlis T, Vicenzino B, Wright A 2004 Neurophysiological effects of spinal manual therapy. In: Boyling JD, Jull GA (Eds). Grieve's Modern Manual Therapy (3rd Edn), Elsevier, Churchill Livingstone, Edinburgh 367-379

Stevinson C, Honan W, Cooke B et al 2001 Neurological complications of cervical spine manipulation. Jour Rehab Soc Med 94(3):107-110

Sturesson B, Selvik G, Uden A 1989 Movements of the sacro-iliac joints; a roentgen stereophogrammetric analysis. Spine 14:162-165

Thacker M, Gifford L S 2002 A review of the physiotherapy management of complex regional pain syndrome. In: Gifford LS (Ed). Topical Issues in Pain 3. Sympathetic nervous system and pain. Pain management. Clinical effectiveness. CNS Press, Falmouth 119-142

Toussaint R, Gawlik CS, Rehder U et al 1999 Sacroiliac dysfunction in construction workers. Jour Manip and Physiol Therap 22(3):134-138

UK BEAM Trial Team 2004 United Kingdom back pain exercise and manipulation (UK BEAM) randomised trial: effectiveness of physical treatments for back pain in primary care. BMJ, doi: 10.1136/bmj.38282.669225.AE

Van der Wurff P, Meyne W, Hagmeijer RHM 2000 Clinical tests of the sacroiliac joint, a systematic methodological review. Part 1: Reliability. Manual therapy 5(1):30-36

Van der Wurff P, Meyne W, Hagmeijer RHM 2000a Clinical tests of the sacroiliac joint, a systematic methodological review. Part 2: Validity. Manual therapy 5(2):89-96

Vicenzino B, Cartwright T, Collins D, Wright A 1999 An investigation of stress and pain perception during manual therapy in asymptomatic subjects. European Journal of pain 3:13-18

Waddell G 2003 The back pain revolution (2nd Edn). Churchill Livingstone, Edinburgh

Wall PD 1991 Neuropathic pain and injured nerve: central mechanisms. In: Wells J, Woolf C (eds) Pain mechanisms and management, British Medical Bulletin, Churchill Livingstone, Edinburgh: 631-643

Wall PD 1999 The placebo and the placebo response. In: Wall PD, Melzack R (Eds) The Textbook of Pain, (4th Edn). Churchill Livingstone, Edinburgh 1419-1430

Wall PD 1999a Pain: The Science of Suffering (2nd Edn). Weidenfield & Nicholson, London

Watson P 2000 Psychosocial predictors of outcome from low back pain. In: Gifford LS (Ed). Topical Issues In Pain 2, CNS Press, Falmouth: 85-109

Watson P, Kendall N 2000 Assessing psychosocial yellow flags. In: Gifford LS (Ed). Topical Issues In Pain 2, CNS Press, Falmouth: 111-29

Woolf C J, Salter M 2006 Plasticity and pain: role of the dorsal horn. In: McMahon S, Koltzenberg M (Eds) Wall and Melzack's Textbook of Pain. Elsevier Churchill Livingstone, Edinburgh 91-105

Wright A 1995 Hypoalgesia post-manipulative therapy: a review of a potential neurophysiological mechanism. Manual Therapy 1:11-16

Zusman M 1992 Central nervous contribution to mechanically produced motor and sensory responses. Australian Journal of Physiotherapy 38:245-255

Zusman M 2002 Forebrain-mediated sensitisation of central pain pathways: 'non-specific' pain and a new image for MT. Manual Therapy 7(2) 80-88

Zusman M 2004 Mechanisms of musculoskeletal physiotherapy. Physical Therapy Reviews 9:39-49

Web pages referred to in this chapter:

www.discoversubluxation.com
www.chiroandosteo.com/content/13/11/17

2

A Practical Guide to Goalsetting

PETER GLADWELL

The aim of this chapter is to introduce the principles and practice of goalsetting within physical rehabilitation. The process of setting a goal with a patient integrates a wide range of theoretical and practical issues. For example, goalsetting has a central role within the Cognitive-Behavioural approach, and this will be discussed. There are also clear links between goalsetting and the development of self-efficacy, and the mastery of fear using a graded exposure approach. Other important aspects of goalsetting within rehabilitation include links with acceptance issues, with pacing and the avoidance of Activity-Cycling, and with the role of goals as outcome measures. The chapter is written in such a way as to be readable for a physical therapist with little knowledge of the Cognitive Behavioural approach. It is not intended to be an in-depth analysis of the theoretical issues. The chapter can be thought of as a clinically oriented "guided-tour" around goalsetting which acts as an introduction to the key issues. This chapter intersects and overlaps with many other chapters in previous volumes of Topical Issues in Pain.

Goalsetting: The Evidence Base

Much of the material presented is based upon discussions with countless patients and clinicians over the past ten years, and as such, no one "owns" goalsetting or can be specifically credited for its creation. Indeed, goalsetting is part of a complex healthcare intervention, and as such is not simply investigated using Randomised Controlled Trial (Dieppe 2004). An interesting case study presented by Linton et al (1999) hints at its effectiveness.

These researchers used six patients, randomly allocated to develop an exercise programme either by negotiating their exercise goal with the therapist, or having the goal set by the therapist. The condition was then reversed, using a different exercise. All six made larger percentage increases in exercise repetitions during the negotiated phase. Further exploration of the role of goalsetting using qualitative methods would be valuable. Goalsetting has been studied more extensively in stroke rehabilitation, and a recent qualitative study in this area by Parry (2004) offers insights into the difficulties which physiotherapists have in adapting their practice to incorporate goalsetting.

A Definition

A useful starting point is a definition from Chambers dictionary: a goal is a noun, meaning "an end or aim to effort or ambition". It is obvious from this definition that a goal can describe both the destination and the journey. One can set a goal that offers "an aim to ambition", but the experience of having and pursuing a goal is very different process from the final achievement of the goal. Clinically, many patients who set goals will later find themselves on a different path than the one they anticipated travelling along when the goal was first set. It is our role as physiotherapists to facilitate the process of goalsetting whilst being sensitive to the fact that the people we are working with are involved in a dynamic process. In exploring their potential for the future, the goalsetting process should allow them to be able to continuously review their priorities and to move onto more appropriate goals as rehabilitation unfolds.

Goalsetting within Rehabilitation and within a Self-Management Approach

Rehabilitation is a term usually applied to the process of returning to fitness and function following injury or illness. The term can imply a return to a previous lifestyle and level of activity. In this situation, goalsetting is usually focussed upon the activities that the patient used to do but is not currently managing.

However, many physiotherapists work with patients who are not expecting to return to their previous lifestyle because of their ongoing health problems. In this situation, rehabilitation goals may not be so easily defined. The patient may be considering new activities, having given up old ones because of the health problem. This is where goalsetting needs to be dynamic and flexible. This may involve exploration of a new role for the patient, when their previous role has been altered or abandoned. One patient involved in a goalsetting and rehabilitation programme described herself as "being in the process of recreating herself". Here then is an illustration of an interaction between goalsetting and a possible redefinition of the individual's identity that sometimes occurs. Goalsetting can expose and may help reflect the person's values and priorities.

Functional goalsetting can be a powerful reinforcement for exercise behaviour, if the links between exercise and function are explored with the patient (Figure 1). We can select exercises that might facilitate improvements in physical function, and work with the patient to integrate improvements gained through exercise into improved function. Within this interplay between increased exercise performance and increased function we can also develop setback plans (e.g. how to avoid a setback, and how to cope with one if it happens). Often, a plateau in improvement will occur. How might we help our patients to manage this phase?

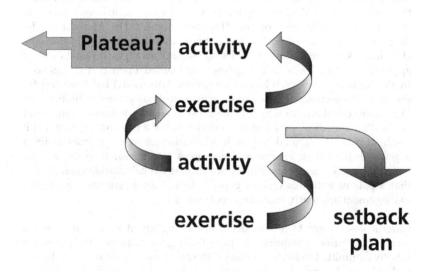

Figure 1. A Rehabilitation Flowchart, indicating the positive interaction between exercise and goalsetting for activity, incorporating a plan for setbacks and a plan for a plateau.

Goalsetting: Setting the Scene

Goalsetting can begin once there is an agreement between the patient and the clinician that it is an appropriate area to explore. In some circumstances, this agreement is easily reached. In the example below, the patient has attended for assessment, and as part of the clinical interview the therapist asks the patient what they were hoping to gain from coming to see the therapist.

Therapist: "When you came here today, was there something specific that you were hoping that I might be able to help you with?"
Patient: "I have been thinking about starting to ride my bicycle again, but I wasn't sure if it would be sensible to try, given the problems I have been having with my knee. I was hoping that you might advise me, and perhaps help me to work out how I could go about starting".

In this scenario, goalsetting is clearly on the agenda from the start. Note that asking the patient what *they* wanted from the contact was a vital initial step: if we assume what our patients want, we may never meet their needs.

Goalsetting may not be appropriate if the patient only wishes to have the therapist "make them better again", to take on a healing role, to "wave the magic wand". We, and our patients, grow up in a culture that understands the curative role of Medicine, operating within a paradigm often referred to as the "Medical Model" or the "Disease Model". The Medical Model describes a process whereby the patient attends with symptoms, the clinician takes a history and elicits signs, and arranges investigations if appropriate. This leads to a diagnosis, and based upon that diagnosis a treatment is chosen which leads to recovery. This model has been helpful for treating infectious diseases and fractures, but has serious limitations for long-term conditions for which a cure is not available. Patients often do not realise that a medical, or 'curative', solution is not a realistic hope, or that it might at best offer limited benefit. It is common for many patients to direct a great deal of their energy and resources into a searching for a cure. Unsurprisingly, the clinical experience of many rehabilitation therapists is that a patient with this type of belief is less likely to engage with a self-management approach, including goalsetting.

Careful assessment facilitates decision-making about how best to move forwards. Pertinent enquiries include finding out whether the patient is wholly committed to finding a cure. If the assessment indicates that there is unlikely to be an effective treatment to relieve their symptoms a rehabilitation or self-management approach may be of interest. On the other hand this may not be acceptable if they are stubbornly focussed upon a curative treatment. Self-management could still be explained and outlined, with an offer to return for help with self-management if they are unsuccessful in their aim of finding a cure. A variety of interactions have been proposed that can help these types of patients move on from their passive, 'looking for a cure' approach to a more active, self-managing approach. These include the 'Motivational Interviewing' approach (Miller & Rollnick 2002), an approach that incorporates evidence relating to the 'Readiness for Change' model (Kerns & Rosenberg 2000).

The most frequent situation is where the patient would like a cure, but also is realistic about the odds of finding one. Here the patient may be willing to try a self-management approach alongside a symptom-relieving treatment trial. For example, when a treatment such as TENS is offered, it takes only a moment to suggest that if the TENS is effective in controlling their pain it could be used to help in getting going again with some activities. A potential list could then be generated and discussed. This allows a quick insight into the kind of goals the patient might have. At the next appointment, if the treatment has been helpful, enquiries can be made as to whether or not the goals were achieved. It is important to appreciate that the provision of symptom relief does not automatically lead to an increase in function. For example, the patient might be concerned that any increase in function will cause an unacceptable exacerbation in symptoms, or lead to further/lasting damage?
Even if treatment is unhelpful, it can still be fruitful to follow up the brief discussion that established the potential goals. Discussing the obstacles to progress with the goal can be of value (see below).

The assessment process for a self-management programme usually involves reaching an agreement with the patient that they have a chronic health problem that is not amenable to currently available treatments. Once this occurs agreeing to goal setting and self management becomes a good deal easier. Often, patients have tried numerous treatments and already reached the conclusion that spending more time, energy and money in the search for a cure is pointless. In contrast, some never quite give up hope of a cure, and may rely upon their hope as a way of coping with their ongoing distress. Despite this, these patients may still agree that they want to develop their self-management skills, and even agree to suspend their search for a cure whilst attending the programme.

Some patients are unable to think of a goal. They may be in significant distress, disabled by their symptoms, and unable to consider how they might move forwards in their life whilst their symptoms persist. These 'fragile' patients require a great deal of skill to assess and manage. Their inability to set a goal may reflect their low confidence in their ability to achieve (i.e. low self-efficacy: see below, in the section headed "A Goal Should Be Achievable"). In this situation, it can help to ask,
"If someone could wave a magic wand and get rid of your symptoms, what would you do differently?"

Some therapists ask:
"If you woke up tomorrow with no symptoms, what would you do differently?"

Be warned however that the idea of suggesting that they might wake up with no symptoms can unproductively kindle false hopes!
Clearly, if they answer that they would not do anything differently, then the role for help with self-management is immediately restricted since they are very unlikely to productively engage in a goal-orientated programme.

It might be the first time anyone has asked, in a healthcare setting, what they want and they may require time to consider what their goals might be. Allowing time for reflection and review is therefore important.
Another helpful line of questioning can be to ask them what they have lost since the onset of the condition. This allows a focus on upon any deterioration in their quality of life, which then might lead to a consideration of some of these losses as potential goals. It can be helpful to broaden the patients thinking by exploring a range of possible goal situations, such as work, leisure and recreation, social activity, self-care and domestic activity.

The introduction of goalsetting at the assessment stage helps to establish a clear agenda for the time that the therapist will spend with the patient. In contrast if the assessment only focuses upon the symptoms that the patient has, the patient can be forgiven for thinking that the therapists' sole interest is the resolution of those symptoms.
Using the Problem Oriented Medical Record, with its' emphasis on the patients' "problems", can feel like a negative experience at times. Goalsetting helps shift the assessment towards a more positive focus and can be refreshing for therapists used to the POMR system (see the section below about goals as outcome measures).

Setting a SMART Goal

Once the therapist has reached an agreement with the patient that goalsetting is an appropriate area to explore, the goalsetting process can begin. The acronym "SMART" is widely used and is a useful focus for the goalsetting process.

SMART stands for:

Specific
Measurable
Achievable
Rewarding
Time-limited

I am not aware of the history of the acronym, but there are several variations on this theme. For example, the "R" is sometimes used to stand for "realistic", but this would seem to duplicate the word "achievable". I prefer the word "rewarding" because it ties in with the behavioural aspect of the Cognitive Behavioural approach (more on this later).

A Goal Should Be Specific

From the outset, a goal should be described in terms of what the patient might **do**. In other words, what **behaviour** are they aiming to develop? It is not specific to say that they want to "be" happy... the question is, what do they plan to **do** that will bring them happiness? It is not specific to say that they want to be relaxed: their goal could be to "practice a relaxation technique", which is a behaviour. It is interesting that Fordyce (1976) in his influential text "Behavioural Methods for Chronic Pain and Illness" did not describe the goalsetting process in depth, nor did he use the word "goal" as something that the patient was to focus upon. He saw the treatment goal of the therapist as helping the patient to increase, or decrease, the frequency of a clearly identified "target behaviour". So, for Fordyce, if our input leads to an increase or decrease in the frequency of the "target behaviour" then we are on the right track. But, if the "target behaviour" (goal) has not been described specifically enough, both patient and therapist run the risk of losing track of progress (or lack of it). Fordyce clearly recognised that human behaviour involves movement, and he therefore recognised the important role of physical therapists in supporting patients to move more, and/or to move (behave) differently.

Later advances in the Behavioural Model included theories such as the Self Regulation Theory, as described by Keefe & Lefebvre (1999). Self-regulation theory highlighted the role of the patient in monitoring, evaluating and reinforcing their own behaviour. This inevitably frames the therapist-patient interaction as a collaborative one, with the patient taking responsibility for setting and taking care of his or her own goals. Therapists can facilitate this firstly by helping patients seek realistic goals and then by problem solving the practical set-up of the process of achieving them. For example, if a goal is to do more ironing, we might need to be specific about whether the ironing is done standing or sitting, and even which items of clothing are ironed. This might seem pedantic, but details like this can mean the difference between a successful and an unsuccessful attempt (see below, "Goals as Indicators of Obstacles to Change").

A Goal Should Be Measurable

How many, how far, how long...?

This point echoes Fordyce's concern above. How many shirts are currently being ironed, and how often? How much further does the person want to walk, and does the walk involve rest periods? Does speed of walking matter? Fordyce argued that it is better to measure the behaviour in terms of a "movement cycle" rather than a time period. In other words, what is the best unit of measurement for the activity? For ironing, a "movement cycle" might be a complete shirt for some people, or for others, perhaps just half a shirt. To choose as the "movement cycle" a completely full ironing basket is unlikely to be successful (although I have met patients who have become used to setting this as their goal in the past, and are reluctant to change). In Fordyce's approach, each successful movement cycle should at first be rewarded, in order to increase the frequency in that behaviour. In the example above, a short rest, and a sense of achievement could reward each half shirt ironed.

Although it can be better to choose some divisible part of the movement in defining a goal, sometimes a time period is more appropriate. For example, visiting a pub with a friend for half an hour, or sitting at a computer for five minutes is likely to be effective. The use of timers can be quite valuable for this kind of goal, and the use of mobile phones with integral timers and alarms can be an advantage.

A Goal Should Be Achievable

This aspect of goalsetting would seem to be straightforward, but in reality it is more complex. Are the horizons of the patient limited by their current beliefs about their abilities? Or are they remembering a previous level of ability (the full basket of ironing in the example above), and setting their sights accordingly?
Earlier, the term self-efficacy was mentioned. Self-efficacy is a measure of a person's confidence in their ability to perform a given behaviour. For example, how confident are you that you can run a mile? Or two miles? Or three miles? Obviously, your level of confidence (self-efficacy) is likely to reduce as the mileage increases. There is a correlation between self-efficacy and function. Someone who has high self-efficacy about a specific behaviour is more likely to do it, and someone who has low self-efficacy is less likely to do it.

Successful achievement of a goal is likely to increase self-efficacy in that behaviour. In the case of a long-term goal (e.g. running a marathon, or writing a book), self-efficacy may need to be increased by setting smaller targets, or "proximal goals". Albert Bandura (1997) was highly influential in developing theories and evidence about self-efficacy, and he states that "proximal goals mobilize self-influences and direct what one does in the here and now". A distal goal is his term for a long-term goal: "distal goals alone are too far removed in time to provide effective incentives..." These concepts can be clinically useful for us: if a patient wants to get back to work, but this might take six months, what are the "proximal goals" that can be worked on which might increase his or her self-efficacy about the "distal" goal of returning to work? If the patient cannot identify these proximal goals but remains fixated upon the distal goal, we might need to spend some time in exploring the options with them.

A Goal Should Be Rewarding

This is a consideration that underpins the Behavioural aspect of the Cognitive-behavioural Model. If a behaviour leads to a consequence that increases the frequency of the behaviour, then that behaviour is likely to increase in its frequency. In this situation, the person behaving is being rewarded by the consequence of the behaviour. Rewards are not always obvious: we do not only increase our behaviour frequency because we are rewarded at every "movement cycle" by a chocolate biscuit! Our rewards might be more complex: a sense of independence, a feeling of getting somewhere, a financial gain, a relief of boredom or guilt (an example of negative reinforcement) are some examples.

Human beings are not straightforward, and are more complex than any psychological model. Our cognitions make the "rewarding" of goals more intricate. How many people will continue with an activity in spite of a significant increase in symptoms because stopping might feel "weak", like "giving in"? In this case, the "reward" of feeling like we have "beaten" the condition might give a powerful short-term reward. As therapists, however, we know from clinical experience that this kind of motivation can at times lead to a flare up of symptoms followed by a prolonged recovery involving a period of decreased activity that may be of longer duration than the period of activity. This is known as "Activity Cycling", or the "Boom and Bust" pattern of activity: see Figure 2. We might help our patients to identify this pattern of behaviour, and their "reward" might then be to realise that they have managed an activity successfully and "outwitted" the condition, avoiding the prolonged exacerbation of symptoms.

We may also do well to help our patients to reflect on their achievements. For example, we often pause too briefly to consider our achievements, and quickly move on to consider the next challenge: our patients are no different. They may also minimise their achievements: "it's nothing compared to what I used to manage" is a frequent response. This approach can undermine progress, and a strategy to deal with this comparison with the past is required if progress is to be made. The role of the patient in reinforcing his or her own behaviour is emphasised by self-regulation theory (see Keefe & Lefebvre 1999). Rewards do not always have to be complex: there is nothing wrong with the occasional chocolate biscuit as a reward!

Sometimes it can be difficult to identify rewarding goals, or to identify additional rewards if a goal which is less immediately rewarding is achieved. In response to the question, "what might you do to treat yourself?" some people might easily come out with a long list: a hot bath, a glass of something nice, a good book, a favourite video, time out to relax, shopping for something special... the list can be extensive. However, others can find this question very challenging, for a range of reasons. When the patient has limited financial and physical resources, it is all too easy to prioritise more practical concerns and overlook the things that bring more direct pleasure. It is important to help patients understand the importance of planning a "treat" when a goal is achieved.

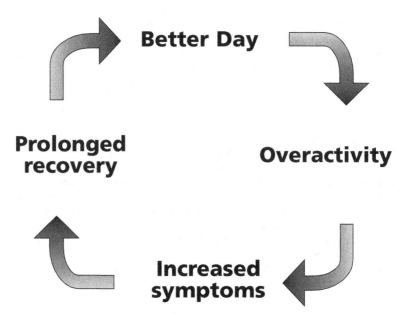

Figure 2. Activity Cycling, or the Boom and Bust cycle. This can lead to deconditioning, and a loss of confidence in activity. The period of recovery is typically more prolonged than the period of overactivity.

A Goal Should Be Time-Limited

When should the goal be achieved by? Is the time limit next week, next month, or Christmas? Without a clear timeframe, a goal can be delayed indefinitely. Often, we are working with people who find the goals that they have set to be challenging. If starting work on the goal is delayed for some reason, then this delay itself can be a reward for inaction. We are all likely to have experienced anxiety about a particular situation, only to have our anxiety relieved when the situation is avoided. For those who occasionally teach, an example might be a presentation that is cancelled: our stress levels drop when we hear we do not need to do it, and the feeling of relative relaxation is like a reward in itself. This type of reward is a form of negative reinforcement: an aversive situation is avoided by non-confrontation of the anxiety-provoking situation, but, there is a risk of avoidance-learning. The sooner we get on and do the presentation, the better, and if we can use relaxation skills to minimise our anxiety about the presentation, then that is better still.

The time-limited aspects of an agreed goal echo the comments earlier about proximal and distal goals. When we trained to be physiotherapists, the distal goal was to be a physiotherapist, but there were many interim goals, including reading, essays and placements that were the "proximal goals" with a shorter time frame. If we overlook "proximal goals" then the distal goal slips from our grasp.

Goals and Targets, and Odds of Success

One way of increasing the likely success of a goal is to break down the goal into smaller targets. Bandura's "proximal goal" has an overlap with the concept of a "target".

An example would be a goal to return to work. This requires a range of abilities, for example: to manage the journey, to negotiate successfully with one's manager and work colleagues regarding one's abilities and limitations, to tolerate the postures and movements required at work and to manage the work-related stresses. To start to work on this larger goal, smaller targets might be:

- driving half way to work and back, out of rush hour
- practising the walking that will be required at work
- setting aside some time every day to use the home computer, to prepare for longer periods later.

Whilst it is vital that a goal is generated by the patient, not the therapist, we can use our knowledge of posture and fitness to help them to set targets.

Following a discussion about this, it can be helpful to ask how confident the patient feels about the agreed next target. A simple visual analogue scale is useful:

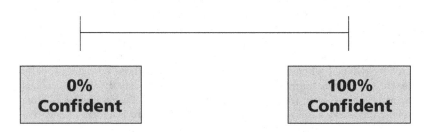

0%
Confident

100%
Confident

What is an acceptable level of confidence? As a guide, I would be concerned about setting targets that have less than a 50% confidence rating, and in the initial stages of rehabilitation, the greater the odds of success, the better. Remember that self-efficacy predicts functional ability, and is a measure of someone's confidence about managing an activity. If a patient's prediction is that they are likely to achieve their target, then they are likely to set more difficult targets in the future if they are successful. If they predict failure, and they do fail, a conclusion that they might draw is that they were right to doubt their ability in the first place. Too hard a target can lead to decreased self-efficacy, especially if it is associated with repeated failure to achieve.

Goals, Targets and Fear-avoidance

The role of fear of harm, and of fear of increased pain, is now well established in the development of chronic incapacity related to pain (Vlaeyen & Linton 2000). Early research suggests that this might be relevant for people with other health conditions, for example Chronic Fatigue Syndrome (CFS) and ME (Silver et al 2000, Nijs 2004). People who have a higher level of concern that an activity or exercise might cause damage, or might cause an exacerbation of their symptoms, are more likely to become more disabled. This fear can reach phobic proportions for some people, but is more often seen at a lower level.

What has this got to do with goalsetting, however? There are several ways in which goalsetting is relevant for someone who has become fearful of movement (kinesiophobic). Firstly, the thorough assessment described above (that allowed the therapist and the patient to consider the role of goalsetting) will have identified whether there might be significant element of kinesiophobia, which might limit the patient's function. During the clinical interview, a comparison should be made between the patients' premorbid level of activity and exercise and their current level. This quickly indicates the degree of disability caused. Also, asking the patient about their experiences of activity and exercise since the onset of their symptoms will let the therapist know how they have approached physical activity. Was the attempt successful or not, and what was the result of the success or failure?

Example:
A person recovering from mild CFS/ME had done well to build up to a walking distance of three miles. Impatience to make progress then led them to turn this walk into an alternating jog/walk, each managed alternately for about 200 metres. Unfortunately, this rate of increase was too rapid, and a relapse occurred, which thankfully was brief. As a result, the patient became fearful to do any jogging at all. Following discussion, they realised that the error was not the jogging, but too much jogging, and set a more realistic target to jog for one hundred metres within the three-mile walk.

A brief review of a person's past physiotherapy experience is also helpful during the assessment. It is important to allow the patient to speak freely by wording the question in such a way that they feel comfortable to let you know how they actually responded.

Example:
Therapist: "Have you ever met up with a physiotherapist before?"
Patient: "Yes, before I had surgery".
Therapist: "I know that not everyone who sees a physiotherapist has a positive experience. How did you get on?"
Patient: " Well, I'm sure that they meant well, but every time I did the exercises I could hardly sleep afterwards. I just thought that it couldn't be doing any good, so I stopped going".
Therapist: "Do you remember what you were doing in the way of exercise?"
Patient: " I had to do side bends as far as I could go, and bend forwards, ten times each. The thing is, it was bending that first started my back problem off".

In this example, we have learnt that the patient has a concern about the safety of bending, and that prescriptive exercise has been unhelpful for them. We also have an indication that their pain can continue to be worse for some time, once aggravated by activity. To gain their trust, we may need to work carefully to establish a level of trust in our approach. To continue the dialogue, the therapist might say:

Therapist: " It sounds as if you have lost confidence in bending".
Patient: "I have, because it causes so much pain afterwards".
Therapist: "Some people I have seen find that the loss of confidence becomes a problem in itself".
Patient: "I know what you mean. It does put me off doing some things."

Therapist: " I wonder what it might be like for you to feel more confident about movement?"

Patient: "I think it might help, but I would still have to contend with the pain".

Therapist: "So it would be helpful to feel more confident, but you would still have to be sensible about how much you did."

Patient: "I suppose so".

Therapist: "If there was a safe way for you to build up your confidence again, what might you do differently as a result?"

Patient: "Well, it would be nice to be able to care for my dog again. My children have taken over that job, and my dog is not getting groomed as well as I would like".

Here, we have an opportunity to start a contract between the therapist and the patient which addresses the patient's fear using functional goalsetting. If this patient came to see you, how might you go about negotiating the smaller targets that would allow them to make progress with the larger goal of grooming the dog? How might you help the patient to understand that an increase in symptoms does not equate to harm?

Again, it is important to remember that the patient needs to be setting the goals, and deciding on the targets, and our role is to guide them based on our knowledge of ergonomics, and what might be a successful progression. If a patient's determination to make progress gets the better of them, they may be tempted to jump over some of the "stepping stones" that would otherwise lead them more gradually towards success, and increased confidence. Physiotherapists working in this way can often find themselves negotiating with the patient to make slower progress than might have been tried in the past. This can be very challenging for physiotherapists who are used to prescriptive exercise setting and pushing the patient on to do more. Adjustment in this role can take time to achieve successfully.

During the goalsetting process with someone who has become fearful of harm or injury, progress is measured by a gradual increase in confidence (or decrease in fear), and by an increase in function. Symptom levels are not a useful guide to the rate of progress, provided the patient is satisfied that they are not slipping into a pattern of "Activity Cycling", overdoing it one day and having a prolonged decrease in activity afterwards.

Goals and Baselines

In order to avoid unhelpful Activity Cycling, a useful link can be made with the skills used in setting baselines for exercise and activity (Muncey 2002). The patient needs to know how much of an activity can be managed at a time, without increasing the odds of a persistent increase in symptoms that leads to reduced activity the next day. If they can walk for two minutes on one day, four on the next, and three the day after, an average of three minutes per day has been achieved. Based upon clinical experience with fear-avoidant chronic pain patients, a baseline that is set below this average is likely to be more successful. There are several reasons for this, all of which need to take into account the normal variation of symptoms from day to day. A patient might not feel able to keep up the average on a daily basis, but are more likely, more willing and more confident to manage a lower level, say 50% of average. This is particularly helpful if there is a significant level of fear of increased symptoms after the activity: hence, confidence can be gained at the lower level before an attempt is made to increase a little every day. Patients may learn by Respondent Learning (Keefe & Lefebvre 1999) to associate an activity with an increase in symptoms. Working at a low baseline should allow them to experience an activity without a significant increase in symptoms, so that the learned association can be broken. Data needs to be gathered before the baseline goal level can be ascertained and started on.

Example:
Patient: "I'd like to walk further, but if I try to do more, I always end up suffering for it. It's difficult to know from day to day how much to do… it's only the next day that I find out if I have overdone it or not."
Therapist: "You are describing a common problem for a lot of the people we see here. Their pain doesn't really help them know when to stop, because of the delay before the pain gets worse".
Patient: "That's right. My doctor said 'stop if it hurts', but that doesn't help me that much."
Therapist: "What if we worked out what you could manage on an average day, and use that as a guide? Perhaps if you started out aiming to keep to something below that average, it would help to control the ups and downs you have been having. They sound a bit like a roller-coaster ride".

There are many reasons why people choose to do more than they perhaps should at times, including the opportunity to feel normal for a while, to keep up with others, to catch up on jobs, guilt about others doing more to help them… the list is long, and addressing these issues is beyond the scope of this chapter. However, I hope that I have indicated that goalsetting inevitably links to pacing, setting baselines, avoiding risks of exacerbations of symptoms, and a whole host of personal motivators that lead to Activity Cycling.

Goals as Indicators of Obstacles to Change

Time spent at each appointment reviewing progress with goals can reap rewards, especially if it helps us to understand why our patients might not be making progress. We cannot expect the process of change to be easy: if it were easy, they probably would have achieved their goals without our help. A clear examination of any obstacles to progress allows us to focus attention upon relevant problem-solving strategies. Problem-solving itself is a large subject, but there are some key points to consider. For example, is the obstacle to progress related to any of the following factors, known informally as the "Four P's":

Planning: was the plan of action insufficient, and does it need to be modified? For example, a goal to go swimming might not be progressing because the patient is unsure about how they will manage to prepare a meal later that day. They may need to refine the plan, perhaps by preparing food the day before, or inviting themselves round to a friend's to eat... whatever the solution is, it has to be the right solution for the patient, and it is helpful if they can generate the solution themselves.

Pacing: was the goal attempt consistent with the principles of good pacing? For example, a goal to go swimming might not be progressing because the patient is concerned about whether the journey to the pool itself will exhaust them. A possible solution might be to allow time to rest before changing to swim. .

Prioritising: is the goal actually high enough on their list of priorities to be tackled? It might be that the goal is otherwise sound, but that at the present time there are other life events that prohibit progress. It might be that these other life events also mean that the contact with the physiotherapist is poorly timed, and might be best delayed until a later date. Having said that, we all know from our personal experience that there is rarely a "best time" to start to change our behaviour, and that a delay in making a difficult change can lead to further procrastination (see earlier discussion about negative reinforcement). A discussion regarding priorities might be relevant: If the patient did not achieve the change, how would that be for them? Would that be acceptable for the time being?

Positioning: does the obstacle relate to positioning issues? For example, does the patient only swim breaststroke, and find the position uncomfortable? If so, problem solving around the use of goggles to allow them to immerse their face might help. Would side-stroke more manageable? Does the positioning problem relate to pacing as well: could they manage a width, with a rest afterwards? Could progress be achieved by incorporating stretches to allow the swimming position to be achieved more easily? Multiple approaches to problem solving may need to be applied to overcome the obstacle.

Record Keeping and Goals

There are several advantages to keeping a written record of progress with goalsetting.

- The process of writing the goal down allows the "SMART" process to be used and checked to see if it is Specific, Measurable, Achievable, Rewarding and Time-limited? If it isn't, does it need revising?
- A written record is also a form of commitment, especially if a goal chart (Appendix 1) is to be displayed in a public place in the patient's home.
- Commitment to oneself and to others that a goal will be attempted can be a powerful motivator.
- A goal chart can also help attempts and outcomes to be evaluated. Was the outcome successful, or were there obstacles to change that need to be considered?
- Record keeping emphasises the responsibility of the patient in self-monitoring of behaviour, which is one of the three cornerstones of Self-regulation theory.

Goals As Outcome Measures And Indicators of Treatment Cessation

The goals that are negotiated early on in rehabilitation can act as outcome measures. Simply reviewing the list of goals with the patient and discussing the progress can be enough. Goals might have been fully or partially achieved, and some might still be available for the future. Still others might have been explored during treatment and decisions taken to lessen their priority or even abandon. A goal that has not been achieved is not necessarily a failure, especially if a revised goal that is more achievable or more rewarding has been substituted. Sometimes, this can be a sign that acceptance of the current situation has taken place.

For example:
Therapist: "When we first met, one of the goals you set was to return to playing tennis."
Patient: "Looking back, I can see that was unrealistic. I'd love to be able to play again, but to be honest I need to be looking forward to other forms of exercise. I am managing well with my walking goal, and if I continue, I think I can substitute short country walks with friends and still get the social contact I used to get from tennis."

Just because the tennis has not been achieved, this cannot be seen as a treatment failure, because this patient has moved on to more appropriate goals. This 'failure' is one of the shortcomings of a formalised goal-oriented outcome measure like the Goal Attainment Scale (GAS) (Heavlin et al 1982), which has been validated in a Pain Management Programme (Fisher & Hardie 2002). The scale was developed within a mental health setting, and requires an initial decision to be taken as to how much progress might be made with each goal. Final progress is scored according to whether progress is above or below the expected mark. Another linked shortcoming of the GAS for physical rehabilitation is that the process of setting a baseline is often a vital part of goalsetting. How can a patient be expected to predict how much progress they might make if they have not yet collected any data on what they can currently manage?

A more sophisticated measure of goal attainment is the Canadian Occupational Performance Measure (COPM) (Law et al 1998). This is often used by Occupational Therapists, and allows for two aspects of measurement: the patient's rating of their performance, and their satisfaction with that performance. The patient is asked to score their current performance on a 10cm VAS from 1 to 10, and then to score their satisfaction in the same way. Whist many patients tend to have a correlation between poor performance and poor satisfaction, the measure allows for assessment of any differences between the two. In the example above, the patient might have rated their tennis performance and satisfaction as low at the start of treatment. At the end of treatment, their performance will still be low, but their satisfaction with that performance may have increased. In other words, they are less distressed by their limitations, and more focussed upon other goals.

The scoring element of COPM can be a quick method to assess progress with a goal and the complete assessment form allows for a thorough review of a wide range of areas of goalsetting. It is worthwhile for physiotherapists to become familiar with this type of assessment measure, even if it is not routinely used. It is one of many examples of Occupational Therapy practice that we can learn from to help our patients maximise the benefits gained from their exercise programmes. If we can help someone with a long-term condition make the connection between the exercise programme that they have been developing and their increasing functional ability achieved through goalsetting, then we will have maximised the benefits of the exercise, and improved our physiotherapy outcome.

Acknowledgements:

I would like to thank the staff of the Frenchay Pain Management Programme for their role in the development of these ideas over the past six years. I would also like to thank Vicki Harding for her helpful comments on the first draft of this chapter. I would also like to recognise the many patients who have helped me to understand how to help others to Goalset more effectively.

References

Bandura A 1997 Self-efficacy: the exercise of control. Freeman, New York
Dieppe P. 2004 Complex interventions. Musculoskeletal care 2 (3): 180-186
Fisher K, Hardie RJ 2002 Goal attainment scaling in evaluating a multidisciplinary pain management programme. Clinical Rehabilitation 16: 871-877
Fordyce, WE 1976 Behavioural methods for chronic pain and illness. Mosby, St. Louis
Heavlin WD, Lee-Merrow SW, Lewis VM 1982 The Psychometric Foundations of Goal Attainment Scaling. Community Mental Health Journal Vol 18, 3, 230-241
Keefe FJ, Lefebvre JC 1999 Behaviour therapy. Textbook of pain 4th Edn. Eds: Wall PD & Melzack R
Kerns RD, Rosenberg R 2000 Predicting responses to self-management treatments for chronic pain: application of the pain stages of change model. Pain 81 (1): 49-55
Law M, Baptiste S, Carswell-Opzoomer A, McColl M, Polatajko, H & Pollock N 1998 Canadian Occupational Performance Measure manual (3rd. Edn.) Ottawa, ON: CAOT Publications ACE
Linton SJ, Jannert M, Overmeer T. 1999 Whose goals should guide? A comparison of two forms of goal formulation on operant activity training. Journal of Occupational Rehabilitation 9 (2): 97-105
Miller WR, Rollnick S. 2002 Motivational interviewing: preparing people for change (2nd Edn.) Guildford Press, New York
Muncey H 2002 Explaining pain to patients. Topical Issues in Pain Vol 4: 157-66
Nijs J, De Meirleir, K, Duquet, W 2004 Kinesiophobia in chronic fatigue syndrome: assessment and associations with disability. Archives of physical medicine and rehabilitation 85: 1586-92
Parry R 2004 Communication during goal-setting in physiotherapy treatment sessions Clinical Rehabilitation 18: 668-682
Silver A, Haeney M, Vijayadurai P, Wilks D, Pattrick M, Main CJ 2000 The role of fear of physical movement and activity in chronic fatigue syndrome. Journal of Psychosomatic Research 52: 485-493
Vlaeyen JWS, Linton SJ 2000 Fear-avoidance and its consequences in chronic musculoskeletal pain: a state of the art review. Pain 85: 317-332

Appendix 1

GOAL CHART

Name: Date:

Clearly state your long-term goals:

Goal 1:

Goal 2:

Goal 3:

Goal 4:

Goal 5:

Now break your goals down into small, achievable targets:

Week	Goal 1 targets set:	Results achieved:
1		
2		
3		
4		
5		
	Goal 2 targets set:	Results achieved:
1		
2		
3		
4		
5		

Remember: goals should be "SMART":
- Specific: is your goal too vague? If so, try to be clearer about it.
- Measurable: how will you know if you have achieved your goal?
- Achievable: how likely are you to be successful?
- Rewarding: will you enjoy the results?
- Time limited: when do you want to have achieved your goal?

3

Communication and Assessment: What are the issues for physiotherapists?

STEVE GOLDINGAY

Introduction

Communication skills are an essential feature of effective clinical practice in many fields of health care and are especially important in the assessment and management of people in pain. As it has been stated: "It is hard to overemphasise the importance of focused, sensitive and skilled communication in the assessment of chronic pain patients" (Main & Parker 2000). For physiotherapists striving to develop a biopsychosocial perspective to their work, the need for skilful communication in assessment has been underlined (Main & Watson 2002) and there have been calls for improving communication skills as an essential first step in developing cognitive-behavioural techniques within physiotherapy practice (Klaber Moffett 2003). The perceived need for education and training in communication skills within mainstream musculoskeletal physiotherapy may be more controversial, however. Whereas few physiotherapists would disagree with the importance of good communication, many might question the need for addressing communication as a distinct area for continued professional development, arguing instead that communication will evolve naturally as physiotherapists develop their knowledge base, "hands on" skills and clinical reasoning. After all, training in communication skills features in physiotherapy undergraduate curricula, but there appears to be little provision for its development at postgraduate level.

The key question, therefore, is not so much whether communication skills are important, but whether further education and training in communication is necessary, or even desirable.

This chapter aims to explore the communication issues associated with the process of musculoskeletal assessment and in so doing will seek to challenge the view that good communication skills develop automatically during a physiotherapist's career. It will illustrate how traditional approaches to assessment in musculoskeletal therapy, along with certain common communication habits, can lead to inhibition of patient disclosure and so undermine the accuracy of assessment. Some of the common obstacles to effective communication will be outlined. In the following chapter, the key skills of information gathering, including those of promoting disclosure and structuring the interview, will be described, as will some strategies for improving communication skills.

Why do communication skills matter?

There is now a sizeable body of research into communication between health practitioners and patients. Much of this has investigated the doctor – patient relationship, particularly in the fields of primary and oncology / palliative care. Considerable work has been done to define the key determinates of effective communication and also to describe where communication can go wrong. It is generally accepted that there are many problems associated with poor communication with patients, especially for the medical profession. For example, 80% of patient complaints arise from ineffective communication and problems with doctor communication are regularly raised in patient focus groups (Towle 1998). Many of the specific problems identified in the communication literature have been collated and described (Kurtz et al 1998). There appears, for example, to be difficulties for doctors with screening patients' problems, such that important complaints and concerns remain undisclosed at the end of the consultation. Other problems relate to the use of jargon and to the quantity and quality of information provided, with subsequent detrimental effect on patients' understanding and recall of what was discussed.

On the other hand, potential benefits from improved communication for both patients and clinicians have been described (BMA 2003, Maguire & Pitceathly 2002). These include:

- Greater accuracy in the identification of patient's problems
- Improved patient understanding of the condition and of their options for investigation and treatment
- Increased adherence to treatment, including recommendations for behavioural change
- Improved health outcomes, including reduced vulnerability to anxiety and depression
- Greater patient satisfaction with the consultation

Many professional bodies within the medical profession have endorsed the importance of communication skills by provide training and assessment as part of their evaluation for membership. These include the various Royal Colleges of General Practitioners, Physicians and Surgeons (BMA 2003, Galasko 1999).

For physiotherapists, the need to give attention to communication has been accelerated by the emergence of patient-centred perspectives on care and by initiatives such as the Expert Patient Programme. In effect, these developments promote patients as active partners in the care process, so that they become informed and involved in decision-making about their care. In addition, these approaches encourage health professionals to recognise the value of the knowledge and skills that patients bring to the encounter. The significance of this for communication will become apparent later.

Biopsychosocial assessment: the integration of two perspectives

Nobody visits a doctor – or a physiotherapist - with just a symptom. They also have ideas, concerns and expectations related to the symptom (Tate 2003). In the context of musculoskeletal pain, individuals' reactions to their pain play the most important part in the development of disability (Watson, 2000). The biopsychosocial perspective therefore demands that information of a psychosocial nature acquired during assessment is given at least **equal clinical significance** to that of pain itself. Essentially, it mitigates any tendency to regard "psychosocial questions" as peripheral to the "proper" physiotherapy task of attending to, treating and abolishing the patient's pain.

By using a biopsychosocial framework, the physiotherapist is challenged with assessing the patient's problems from two perspectives (fig. 1). The "bio" (or medical) perspective is concerned with the gathering of facts from which inference about possible causes of pain and subsequent treatments can be made. This will include screening for clinical red flags and may also include the gathering of information related to a particular approach or paradigm (e.g. 'Maitland'). The psychosocial or patient's perspective is concerned with the patient's responses to pain - areas such as beliefs about the cause of pain, concerns about the future, expectations about what might help - and so on. Physiotherapists therefore need to integrate these two perspectives into one approach.

Medical perspective – disease	Patient's perspective – illness
Sequence of events	Ideas and beliefs
Symptom analysis	Concerns
Relevant systems review	Expectations
	Effects on life
	Feelings

Fig. 1 Exploring the patients' problems from 2 perspectives (Kurtz et al 2003)

Factors that discourage assessment of the patient perspective

The traditional structured interview format

Students of all disciplines are encouraged to develop their history-taking skills by following a structured interview format (e.g. fig 2). This has many advantages for training, particularly in the earlier phases. However, its contents and the way in which it has been taught may also have unwittingly contributed to the development of unhelpful communication styles and created difficulties for assessing the patient perspective (Kurtz et al 2003).

- Chief complaint
- History of the present complaint
- Past medical history
- Family history
- Personal and social history
- Drug and allergy history
- Functional enquiry / systems review

Fig. 2 Content guide for the Traditional Medical History (Kurtz et al 2003)

Firstly, the structured interview has often excluded explicit assessment of the patient perspective and in so doing has failed to deliver the thoroughness that it has sought to provide. In these circumstances, crucial psychosocial information may be perceived to be of secondary clinical significance. Secondly, the way in which history taking has been taught has exclusively focused on the data itself, rather than the means by which it is collected.

That is, the content of the interview has taken priority over the process of conducting the interview. Clinical supervisors and teaching faculty will have supported this process by emphasising the need to swiftly acquire and then to present the key biomedical data. Furthermore, the process of documentation, using the key headings, reinforces the sequence by which a history is taken and defines the domains of enquiry pursued. In the "traditional medical interview", doctors ask a series of quick, closed questions and encourage patients to provide brief, precise and objective replies (Dillon 1997).

Are there problems for physiotherapists in communication associated with the current use of structured interview formats in the musculoskeletal field? Although therapists rarely follow precisely the sequence of topics in such a format, it does nevertheless indicate the subject areas to be explored and the direction in which the interview should go. Consider, for example, a typical content summary for the subjective assessment (fig.3).

Area of examination	Information gained
Body chart	Type and area of current symptoms, depth, quality, intensity, abnormal sensation, relationship of symptoms
Behaviour of symptoms	Aggravating factors, easing factors, severity and irritability of the condition, 24 hour behaviour, daily activities, stage of the condition
Special questions	General health, drugs, steroids, anticoagulants, recent unexplained weight loss, rheumatoid arthritis, spinal cord or cauda equina symptoms, dizziness, recent X-rays
History of present condition	History of each symptomatic area, how and when it started, how it has changed
Past medical history	Relevant medical history, previous attacks, effects of previous treatment
Social and family history	Age and gender, home and work situation, dependents and leisure activities

Fig 3 Summary of subjective examination (Petty & Moore 1998)

There are a number of specific points that can be made about this example:

1. There is little emphasis on the patient perspective
2. The nature of the 'need to know' information encourages the use of closed and directive questioning from the outset
3. In terms of sequence, primacy is given to exploring matters related to the identification of pathology. Information about social and work life, for example, comes last, so that the learner may perceive these matters to be of secondary importance.

There is also the expectation that musculoskeletal physiotherapists should be able, by the end of the subjective interview, to decide on "the source of the symptoms or dysfunction (i.e. the structure at fault)" and to decide on strategies for the physical examination (Petty & Moore 1998). Given the pressures of time and many physiotherapists' anxieties about omitting physical examination from the initial consultation (and indeed some patients' expectations), the psychosocial elements of the interview may be sacrificed to focus on the "core elements" related to pain.

Communication characteristics that inhibit disclosure

The implication of the above is that the physiotherapists may focus on their musculoskeletal therapy agenda to the detriment of exploration of the patient perspective. In addition to this, therapists may find themselves using a variety of strategies or styles that have been found to prevent or discourage patients from expressing their concerns (CRC 1999). Some of these strategies are highlighted in list 1.

One other important consequence of focusing narrowly on causes of pain and tissue dysfunction during assessment is a tendency to miss the underlying significance of the line of enquiry and so lack empathy with the patient at key moments. For example, a therapist may fail to notice that questions seeking information about the mechanism of injury may be upsetting for the patient, particularly if the incident is disturbing to recall (e.g. "Which way was your head turned at the point where the car hit you from behind?").

1. Over reliance on the use of **closed questions**, which only allow the respondent to provide brief answers about a very specific line of enquiry, such as "yes", "no", or "better", "worse".
2. The inability to pick up and respond to **patient cues**. Patients will often drop hints or cues as to their thoughts and feelings, even when the therapist uses a high control style. Hence, useful lines of enquiry, usually of a psychosocial nature, are missed.
3. The provision of **premature advice or reassurance**, before the full background information is ascertained, particularly in relation to the patient's past experiences and current beliefs.
4. The use of **blocking**, where the therapist will switch the subject when the patient raises a particularly difficult area.
5. The tendency to **minimise** or **make light** of difficult topics, particularly in relation to the patient's feelings, by confirming the inevitability of feeling a certain way, or by 'jollying along'.

List 1. Strategies that inhibit patient disclosure

Physiotherapist communication styles

The few studies that have investigated this area suggest that musculoskeletal physiotherapists may indeed take a therapist-centred style, analogous to that deployed in the traditional medical interview described above. Thornquist (1990), for example, undertook a qualitative study looking at the first encounters between physiotherapists and patients. Using video recordings and semi-structured interviews, she was able to compare the communication methods and styles of 3 different kinds of physiotherapist, including manual (musculoskeletal) physiotherapists. She described how manual therapists tend to dictate the content and form of the dialogue and regularly adapt the information provided by the patient to their own frame of reference. Of significance was the failure of manual physiotherapists to respond to leads provided by the patient, responding instead by introducing further topics to the dialogue. Thornquist represented this schematically (fig. 4) whereby a different letter indicates each topic and the number designates who opens the topic and subsequently who responds.

Therapist:	A1	B1	C1			F1			G1	
Patient:		A2	B2	C2	D1 E1		D2 E2 F2			G2

Fig.4. Schematic representation of typical dialogue between manual physiotherapist and patient (Thornquist 1990)

In another study conducted in New Zealand, Haswell et al (1997) audio taped the first encounter between 14 different manipulative physiotherapists (average 16 years as a physiotherapist and all holders of the Diploma in Manipulative Therapy) and their patients. The tapes were transcribed and each utterance was categorised into one of eight kinds of communication. The results demonstrated the predominance of closed over open enquiry (in a ratio of 4:1) and minimal emphasis on the kind of communication skills that allow patients to express their thoughts and feelings.

The ways in which physiotherapists block patient disclosure can be further illustrated by reviewing transcriptions of audio recordings of initial assessments made in a typical physiotherapy outpatient department. For example, the following extract shows how the quest for definitive answers regarding the patient's aggravating and easing factors and diurnal patterns of pain intensity has lead the therapist to repeatedly use a series of closed and directive questions. Subsequently, a number of patient cues, or topics of potentially fruitful enquiry (highlighted in bold), are ignored:

Therapist:	…and what about walking, walking make you feel better did you say, walking round or…?
Patient:	It didn't on the last one *(last episode of pain)*, but sometimes it does. If **I've been sitting and I get up and I turn, I can click my back. Whoever's sat in the office with me can hear it.**
Therapist:	Does that make you feel better, or not particularly, make you feel worse?
Patient:	No, nothing
Therapist:	OK. What about lying down? Lying down makes it feel better or worse, or not make any difference?
Patient:	I can lie on my sides. **Whereas on my back I couldn't do or on my front I couldn't do.**
Therapist:	So you don't like lying on you back or on your front?
Patient:	My front's probably my worst.
Therapist:	But lying on your side, would it actually make you feel better if you lay down on your side or…?
Patient:	Yes.
Therapist:	OK. Any particular side?
Patient:	No.
Therapist:	No. What's it like first thing in the morning? Is it at its worst, at its best or have you not noticed any pattern?
Patient:	Last time I had it, **my doctor told me to get out of bed on my side rather than getting straight up…** so I tend to do that.
Therapist:	Do you feel worse in the mornings, or better, or not make any difference?

Patient:	Varies
Therapist:	Pottering around, do you feel stiffer in the mornings then you get a bit easier, or do you not notice any difference?
Patient:	No, no
Therapist:	OK it doesn't get sorer or anything like that towards the end of the day?
Patient:	*(long pause)*......No
Therapist:	What else do you do that makes it feel worse? Anything you do that makes it feel worse? Or anything you avoid doing because you know it's going to hurt?
Patient:	I don't lift particularly heavy things if I can help it. **It can be something as silly as pulling on my leather riding boots** and the strain of...probably the position I'm in, but the strain of, you know, getting the riding boots quite tight, pulling them on, that can just......it **just feels like something**.......*(both patient and therapist speak at once)*
Therapist:	OK. Fine. Anything you know that makes it feel better, anything you do?
Patient:	Heat.
Therapist:	Heat. OK. Nothing else? Are you better staying still or moving around generally?

In the following extracts from the same interview, the patient provides leads regarding the cause of pain (in bold) which are not followed up:

Therapist:	You say you've had a problem with your back before. When did your first episode happen?
Patient:	I had a car crash roughly 1990, something like that, and it wasn't until I went for my medical for my claim that the X-ray of my back....**he said I'd got problems with my discs that would come to light later on.** I had physio at BUPA then.
Therapist:	...and you had pain then did you when you went to the physio at BUPA?
Patient:	Yes. He just said it was **severe whiplash.**
Therapist:	....and that's just the one episode of physio that you've had
Patient:	Yes
Therapist:	...and did it settle down completely?

And later in the interview:

Therapist:	You've had an X-ray done recently?
Patient:	Last November, I came off one of my horses jumping and the hospital X-rayed me because they thought there was something broken somewhere. **All they said they found was that one of my discs looks a little bit...I think she said closer than the others. She thought that might just be me and not the injury.**

Therapist:	Right OK. So you fell off your horse and landed on your bottom or something?

The following transcripts from another interview illustrate how reassurance (in bold) is attempted without the nature of the patient's concerns being fully elicited. Therefore, the reassurance provided may not have had the intended effect.

Therapist:	So how long have you had this problem for?
Patient:	I've had problems with my back for about 2 or 3 years now - I first started having pain at the bottom of my back, like a deadened pain, and then it's only within the last 12 months I get pain round my hip and down the side of my leg...
Therapist:	So some in your back.....and probably in the last year do you think....
Patient:	Yes, I've had trouble with my hip and my leg. Now I've had an X-ray on my hip but it didn't show anything, but she said it doesn't always come up on an X-ray...
Therapist:	**...doesn't necessarily mean your pain is from your hip either, where your pain isn't necessarily a reflection of where it's coming from, so you can't always take an X-ray as being black and white....**
Patient:	Yes...Yes
Therapist:	So is there anything you think has caused your pain, is there any incident or anything...?

Later, the therapist misses an opportunity to explore the patient's response to the X-ray findings (in bold) and subsequently provides further advice and reassurance (again, in bold). If the full nature of the concern has not been addressed, it is likely that the provision of this kind of information at this stage will only serve to discourage disclosure of other concerns later on.

Therapist:	What's the doctor said to you about your back problem? Has he sort of explained or told you what....
Patient:	He said it was general wear and tear that's basically all he said and when I went to see the specialist she sent me for the X-ray on my hip and she said **nothing came back on that**
Therapist:	Is that just you hip you've had X-rayed? You've not had your back X-rayed?
Patient:	No, I've only had my back done once....
Therapist:	...in 2002?
Patient:	Yes.
Therapist:	That's fine...OK...So if I can just put on this body chart where your pain is. So where does it start?
Patient:	The lower, the lower part of my back, the bottom...

Therapist:	..and then you said it goes into your left side
Patient:	Yes I have, it's this hip and I have a pain down the side of my leg
Therapist:	**A lot of pain in your leg can come from your back. Don't think you've always got to have a hip problem. It can all radiate from your nerves.**
Patient:	Yes, she did explain that to me....
Therapist:	So don't worry too much that other joints are involved
Patient:	But I find as well that if I've been on my feet all day then it's worse at the night time and that's when I get a pain in my leg......

Obstacles to effective communication

It is worth reflecting on the various obstacles to effective communication that exist for physiotherapists working in the musculoskeletal field. Broadly speaking, they can be categorised into **personal** obstacles, relating to the therapist, **environmental** obstacles, including the organisational culture in which the therapist works, and obstacles arising from **patients'** perceptions and beliefs.

Personal

Attitudinal
- The therapist may not agree with the extent to which psychosocial variables should be assessed and managed. Hence, physiotherapists' beliefs about their role will influence their approach to assessment and consequently the communication styles and techniques used.
- Individuals may also not value the importance of communication as a legitimate and worthwhile pursuit for professional development.

Lack of knowledge and skills
- The therapist may be relatively unpractised at exercising the kind of communication skills that promote disclosure.
- In addition, the therapist may have difficulties in structuring the interview and finding the right balance between their own and the patient's agenda.
- There are issues around the boundaries of professional practice and therapists may be uncertain about addressing certain topics, expressing fears that they may be inappropriately undertaking counselling or psychology roles.

Lack of self-confidence
- Many therapists believe that they have neither the training nor experience in pain management to undertake psychosocial assessment and confidently handle the issues that arise as a result.

Beliefs about the perceived negative consequences of "probing"
- Therapists may fear precipitating strong emotions in the patient, such as distress or anger, and that this might cause some form of "psychological damage" to the patients and potentially to themselves. In the face of strong emotion, the therapist may feel uncomfortable or helpless and sense that the credibility of their helping role is undermined. They may also believe that it is irresponsible to provoke such reactions in relation to difficult issues that they cannot deal with
- There may be considerable worries about getting emotionally 'burned out' or even depressed as a consequence of routinely accessing the 'inner world' of people in difficulties
- Therapists may also fear getting too close to the patient

Environmental

- Therapists express concern that they do not have sufficient time to deal with psychosocial issues, viewing these as extra pressures to be contained within limited time resources for each patient. It is also hard to bring a discussion to a close if the patient is upset or in particular difficulty, causing problems with keeping to schedule. Waiting lists and targets may also lead to some departmental resistance to regularly extending appointment times
- There are considerable problems in achieving privacy in many physiotherapy departments. Disclosure may be inhibited by the proximity of others, with only a curtain in between cubicles.
- Physiotherapists extending their skills into psychosocial assessment and management usually require support through supervision, mentoring and through sharing their experiences with peers. This kind of support may not be adequate.
- The culture of learning, as propagated by senior staff and clinical supervisors, may continue to overlook the importance of psychosocial data and subsequently communication skills. Hence, students and less experienced physiotherapists enter the "real world" of practice by being encouraged to approach assessment according to a particular school of thought or paradigm within musculoskeletal therapy. As described previously, the pre-eminence of bio-medical or pain-related data encourages styles of enquiry that tend to prohibit exploration of the patient perspective.

Patient beliefs and perceptions

- Preconceived ideas about the nature of the role of physiotherapists may limit the extent to which patients are prepared to discuss matters that they believe are not directly related to pain.
- Some patients may believe that problems related to pain are inevitable and are therefore not worth addressing.
- They may not wish to be perceived as inadequate.
- There may be the perception that physiotherapists are very busy and would not wish to be burdened.

Summary

It appears that the communication styles associated with pursuing the source of symptoms and tissue dysfunction during musculoskeletal assessment are not suited to the task of promoting disclosure of the patient's perspective. Approaches that use pain as the primary variable of clinical significance will tend to encourage a high control style, where the content of the encounter is determined exclusively by the physiotherapist and information provided by the patient is gauged according to its relevance to the physiotherapist's precise agenda. The development of a biopsychosocial approach to assessment requires not only that the content of the assessment changes to accommodate the patient's perspective, but that attention is paid to the process of assessment, using techniques that promote patient disclosure and being able to share the agenda with the patient without losing control of the interview.

Acknowledgements:

With grateful thanks to the physiotherapists and patients who agreed to be audio recorded

References

British Medical Association 2003 Communication skills education for doctors: a discussion paper. BMA publications unit, London

Cancer Research Campaign 1999 Assessing Patients With Cancer. The Content, Skills and Process of Assessment. Training Manual. Psychological Medicine Group, Christie Hospital, Manchester

Dillon J 1997 Questioning. In: Hargie O (ed) The Handbook of Communication Skills. 2nd edn Routledge, London and New York 103-133

Galasko CSB 1999 Communication with patients, letter to BMJ 12 February

Haswell et al 1997 Basic Interviewing Skills: how they are used by manipulative physiotherapists. New Zealand Journal of Physiotherapy August 11-14

Klaber Moffett J 2003 Introducing cognitive-behavioural techniques in physiotherapy, letter to PPA News Issue16

Kurtz S et al 1998 Teaching and Learning Communication Skills in Medicine. Radcliffe Medical Press, Oxford

Kurtz S et al 2003 Marrying Content and Process in Clinical Method Teaching: Enhancing the Calgary-Cambridge Guides. Academic Medicine 78 (8):802-809

Maguire P, Pitceathly C 2002 Key communication skills and how to acquire them. British Medical Journal 325 (28 September):697-700

Main C, Parker H 2000 Social and cultural influences on pain and disability. In: Main C and Spanswick C (eds) Pain Management An Interdisciplinary Approach, Churchill Livingstone, Edinburgh 43 – 61

Main C, Watson P 2002 The distressed and angry low back pain patient. In: Gifford L (ed) Topical Issues in Pain 3. Sympathetic nervous system and pain. Pain Management. Clinical Effectiveness. CNS Press, Falmouth 175–200

Petty N, Moore A 1998 Neuromusculoskeletal Examination and Assessment: A handbook for therapists. Churchill Livingstone, Edinburgh

Tate P 2003 The Doctor's Communication Handbook 4th edn Radcliffe, Oxford

Thornquist E 1990 Communication: What happens during the First Encounter between Patient and Physiotherapist? Scandanavian Journal of Primary Health Care 8:133-138

Towle A 1998 Continuing medical education: Changes in health care and continuing medical education for the 21st century. British Medical Journal 316 (24 January) 301-304

Watson P 2000 Psychosocial predictors of outcome from low back pain. In: Gifford LS (ed) Topical Issues in Pain 2. CNS Press, Falmouth 85-109

4

Communication and Assessment: The skills of information gathering

STEVE GOLDINGAY

Introduction

The previous chapter described how the adoption of an approach focused on pain and tissue dysfunction can lead to communication styles that inhibit patients from talking about their ideas, concerns and expectations about their problems. It was suggested that by adopting a biopsychosocial perspective to their work, physiotherapists would need to extend their communication skills in order to accurately and efficiently assess psychological and social issues. This chapter aims to describe those key communication skills that can directly or indirectly aid the process of assessment. These skills are commonly described in a wide variety of texts and training manuals, but much of the material here is based upon the work of the Cancer Research UK's Psychological Medicine Group (see Contacts) and the Calgary-Cambridge method (Silverman et al 1998). Their relevance to the musculoskeletal field has been illustrated here by the use of related examples. Additionally, there is brief discussion of factors that may positively influence communication, such as confidently handling professional boundaries and techniques for evaluating communication performance.

Human communication is a highly complex process and it is acknowledged that there is no 'ideal' way of communicating. As such, the skills described are not intended to provide a formula for effective communication. Instead, it is hoped that physiotherapists will learn to appreciate and experiment with the 'tactics' that tend to promote patient disclosure and subsequently their understanding of the patient perspective.

The structured interview format

Communication may be enhanced by the use of an interview format that specifically addresses the patient's perspective. A typical content summary for such a format is provided in Fig. 1. Due to the potential scope of assessment, it is acknowledged that initial enquiry may need to be directed according to the findings of an appropriate screening questionnaire, or else that the assessment process is staggered over several sessions.

Area of examination	Information gained
Orientation	Nature and location of symptoms, patient's story from onset to present, expectations of physiotherapy, questions & concerns about problem
Previous intervention	Investigations and understanding, treatments and effects, advice received, causal beliefs
Medical history	Co-morbidity and effect on function, special questions (red flag screening), medication
Effects on function and participation	Current social and employment situation, typical day, effects on work, restrictions on activity, assistance required, aids and adaptations, downtime, sleep
Coping strategies	Current coping strategies: active and passive, perceived consequences of change (e.g. increasing activity, exercise, pacing)
Socio-economic	Effect on finances, benefits, medico-legal
Effect on family	Beliefs, responses, nature of support provided
Emotion	Nature and extent, effect on motivation
Pre-examination	Body chart, behaviour of symptoms

Fig. 1 Content summary of structured interview for biopsychosocial assessment

This format differs from the content summary of the subjective examination illustrated in the previous chapter by its significant emphasis on psychosocial enquiry and also by positioning this enquiry before detailed questioning about the pain itself. This is useful for encouraging investigation of the patient perspective. However, a flexible approach is required, as this sequence is not meant to suggest a hierarchy of importance of topics. Nevertheless, the biopsychosocial approach requires a shift of emphasis away from a therapist-centred agenda to one that accommodates the ideas, concerns and expectations of the patient. Therefore, questions and answers related to tissue pathology / dysfunction need to be incorporated into the wider picture. It is helpful to regard "traditional physiotherapy" as being integrated into the biopsychosocial perspective, rather than the other way round.

Styles of Questioning

The way in which questions are asked strongly influences the quality of information that is obtained. When the facts about a particular topic are required, closed or directive questions are most useful. **Closed questions** allow a "yes" or "no" answer e.g. "does walking make your pain worse?" whereas **directive questions** focus patients onto a specific topic, but allow only limited expression e.g. "When did your pain get as bad as it is now?" However, when the patient perspective is needed, **open questioning** is the best means of encouraging expression of thoughts and feelings. **Open directive questions** guide patients to a specific topic but in a way that allows free expression. In relation to initiating lines of enquiry within biopsychosocial assessment, for example, open directive questions are most useful – they have also been referred to as "stem questions" e.g. "what are you currently doing to relieve your pain?" (Main & Watson 2002).

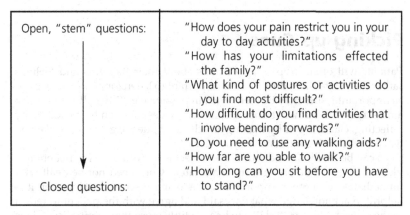

Open, "stem" questions:	"How does your pain restrict you in your day to day activities?"
	"How has your limitations effected the family?"
	"What kind of postures or activities do you find most difficult?"
	"How difficult do you find activities that involve bending forwards?"
	"Do you need to use any walking aids?"
	"How far are you able to walk?"
Closed questions:	"How long can you sit before you have to stand?"

Fig. 2 Example of open to closed questioning technique:

Developing a style that moves from open to closed questioning ensures that patients are given opportunities to convey their feelings or viewpoints about a topic even before all the factual information is acquired (fig. 2). The physiotherapist therefore establishes the patient perspective earlier and then gradually moves to establish details.

Listening

Active listening is one of the hardest skills to acquire, as it involves not just attending to the words that are being spoken but also the underlying messages that the speaker is trying to convey. Listening requires effort – it is not a passive activity – and an essential component of active listening is the process of making sense of the message. One of the problems is that although it is possible to understand speech at rates of up to 600 words per minute, the average person speaks between 100 and 140 words per minute (Adler & Rodman 2003). This provides a great deal of mental spare time for preparing the next question (or perhaps daydreaming!) rather than paying attention to the patient. This spare time needs to be dedicated to understanding the message. Effective listening is associated with picking up on patient cues, facilitating patient responses, using appropriate non-verbal behaviour and ensuring that the patient is not interrupted. In addition, the use of paraphrasing and summarising focuses the physiotherapist to understand and remember the patient's messages, as well as demonstrating the physiotherapist's interest and respect for what is being said.

In addition to listening, good observation skills will help the physiotherapist attend to the non-verbal communication and the ways in which this adds meaning to the messages conveyed e.g. through facial expression, tone of voice, body posture, eye contact and so on.

Picking up Cues

Patients will often drop 'cues' or hints about their thoughts and feelings rather than state them directly. It is important to listen for and pick up cues, as important issues may be mentioned in passing e.g. "My G.P. says it's just a muscle strain, but what does she know?" Cues can then be picked up by reflecting, clarifying or by making an educated guess e.g. "Sounds like you don't have much confidence in your G.P.?"

Cues can be easily missed, but if the subject is important to the patient it is likely that it will be brought up again later. Cues need not be dealt with immediately if another important area is being discussed. However, it is helpful to acknowledge what was said and agree with the patient to return to the subject later e.g. "I'd like to know a little more about your discussions with your G.P. so could we come back to that later? You were talking about what you believe to be causing your pain....."

Building rapport

There are several aspects to the process of engaging the patient that are necessary conditions for effective communication:

Using appropriate non-verbal behaviour
It is important to develop habits of non-verbal behaviour that communicate attention and interest in the patient's story. These include:
- Making regular eye contact and ensuring that consulting or writing notes does not interfere with the patient's willingness to continue talking
- Using nods, gestures and body movement (such as leaning forwards) to signal interest in what the patient is saying
- Ensuring a relatively close physical distance between physiotherapist and patient without an obstacle such as a plinth in-between

Accepting the patient perspective
The physiotherapist needs to suspend judgement and accept the legitimacy of the patient's viewpoint, even if they do not agree with what is being said. With many patients, it is helpful for the physiotherapist to state that they believe that the patient's pain is real.

Demonstrating empathy
There are 3 elements to this:
1. Actively listening to what the patient is communicating
2. Making sense of it and what it means
3. Communicating that back to the patient

In addition, it is useful for the physiotherapist to use brief phrases that demonstrate that they are trying to understand the patient's predicament and appreciating how difficult things are for them. It is not necessary to fully understand or agree with what the patient is saying.

Providing support
Aspects of a supportive approach include showing concern and a willingness to help where possible, acknowledging and appreciating any positive coping strategies that the patient is already using and emphasising the importance of partnership in tackling problems.

Facilitating patient responses and developing accurate understanding

Facilitating

It is important that words or gestures are used that encourage the patient to continue talking. This shows that the physiotherapist is listening and that what the patient is saying is important.
E.g. "yes", "right", "go on".

Paraphrasing

This is where the physiotherapist uses their own words to restate their understanding of the patient's message, without adding further detail. The use of paraphrasing aids effective listening and also demonstrates the physiotherapist's interest and concern to the patient.

Paraphrasing might reflect the ideas the physiotherapist believes the patient has expressed:

Patient: "I don't understand it. The consultant held up the scan and said there was nothing wrong"
Interviewer: "You're thinking something's been overlooked?"

Or it may reflect their understanding of the patient's feelings:

Patient: "I really thought he was going to get my back right"
Interviewer: "You were disappointed...."

In order to make paraphrasing sound more natural, one of three approaches may be used:

(a) changing the patient's wording:

Patient: "My GP says listen to my body, and then the last physio tells me to exercise through the pain barrier"
Interviewer: "It's confusing to know what to do for the best."

(b) offering an example of what the patient is talking about:

Patient: "Nobody appreciates what it's like to be in the pain I'm in"
Interviewer: "Like when your wife complains all the time about the decorating..."

(c) reflecting the underlying theme of the patient's remarks:

Patient:	"...I've not been so low recently. My doctor told me to try to get fitter so I walk to get the paper everyday. I'm also pottering around in the garden a bit more."
Interviewer:	"You've felt a lot better since you've started building up your activities...?"

Summarising

At key points in the interview, such as at the end of a particular line of enquiry, the physiotherapist can summarise or recap the information or messages gained in that section of the discussion. This gives the physiotherapist the chance to consolidate their understanding and shows the patient that they are being listened to. It aids accuracy by allowing the patient to add to, refute or confirm the information provided in the summary. Summarising is especially useful in conjunction with screening (see below).

Clarifying

It is often important to find more information about what the patient has just said. This is especially true when there may be ambiguity with regard to a word or phrase. The physiotherapist must not assume that the patient's understanding of a word or phrase is the same as their own.

Patient:	"I don't bother going to see my doctor anymore, I just keep getting fobbed off"
Interviewer:	"Can you tell me what you mean by fobbed off?"

Patient:	"Obviously I have to take it easy at the moment"
Interviewer:	"Take it easy.......?"

This is particularly true for phrases with medical connotations.

Patient:	"I've got a slipped disc in my back"
Interviewer:	"Can you tell me what you understand by your slipped disc?"

Reflecting

The patient's own words may be used as a means of clarifying something, or simply to facilitate discussion.

Patient: "My doctor said he couldn't understand why I am in so much pain"

Interviewer: "He couldn't understand........?"

Screening

At points in the interview where specific topics have been addressed and lines of enquiry are closing, it is useful to check whether there is anything else that is bothering the patient before moving on, or checking that all the important information has been acquired.

Interviewer: "You've told me how your pain restricts you.....*(list problems)*....is there anything else which is particularly concerning you?"

Making an educated guess

Leading from what the patient has already described, it may be possible for the physiotherapist to guess as to what the patient is thinking or feeling. The physiotherapist may simply describe their perception of what's going on for the patient. Once again, understanding is enhanced, as the patient's can either confirm or refute the suggestion, or add more detail to it.

Patient: "....and it was only after I complained about having to do the lifting work three times that I was moved onto stocktaking duties."

Interviewer: " It seems to me that you're pretty angry about the way you've been treated at work...?"

Patient: "Well, actually no, they've been pretty good overall since then. It was just the one guy who didn't believe me to start with and he's moved on now anyway."

Interviewer: "Ok. You say your employers have been 'pretty good' – tell me more about that."

Use of silence

Patients may need time to find the right words, so it is important to resist the temptation to jump in to help them out.

Indicating the reason for asking the question

It may help the physiotherapist to give a brief indication as to why the topic is important for them, particularly when broaching more difficult topics or if there is suspicion that the patient is unclear as to why certain topics are being addressed. This often means explaining how the issue links with functional activities.

Interviewer: "People sometimes tell me that when they have had to cut right back on their usual activities (give examples) that they can get fed up and low in mood, or frustrated or angry about things. Does any of this apply to you?"

Interviewer: "In order to get a better picture, I sometimes need to understand your understanding of things. I know you're not a doctor but do you have any clues or theories as to why your pain has persisted all this time?"

Behaviours to avoid

Question style

As stated above, closed or directive questions, although useful for establishing facts, are not useful for eliciting disclosure of thoughts or feelings. In addition, the physiotherapist should also try to avoid **leading questions** which tend to stifle disclosure of the patient's own thoughts and feelings and in the worst case leads to false information.

Interviewer: "The X Ray on your back was normal so there's nothing of great significance to worry about, is there?"

In addition, **multiple questions** are easily used with the enthusiasm for information, but the various parts are rarely answered.

Interviewer: "What does your husband think about your problem..........and what does he do when your pain is very bad?"

There can also be times when the physiotherapist asks a number of questions along a particular theme, but where there are important distinctions between the questions and the specific point of the enquiry is lost.

77

Interviewer   "Is there anything you can't do, anything that you're really struggling with at home or anything you want to get back to doing that you were doing before?"

Blocking

The physiotherapist may switch the subject when they cannot face a difficult problem or area of concern.

Patient: "I really don't know how I'm going to cope if I lose my job"
Interviewer: "So what else makes your pain worse?"

Jargon

Using medical jargon runs the risk of the patient not understanding, being frightened or investing a different meaning to what was intended

Interviewer: "So the scan shows that you've got three degenerative discs in your low back..."

Premature advice or reassurance

It is quite common for physiotherapists to offer "expert opinions" early in the interview, before all the information has been acquired. It usually better to postpone advice or reassurance until the precise nature of the concern or problem has been ascertained and then to provide it in the context of a broader understanding gained by the end of the assessment. For example, a physiotherapist may give lengthy exercise advice before the problems associated with the patient's previous attempts to do so have been elicited.

Minimise or normalise fears

This can discourage patients from expressing their thoughts or feelings, because it reinforces the inevitability of having those fears and so possibly the sense that discussing them would be a fruitless activity.

Patient: "If it continues to get worse I know I'll be out of my job before too long."
Interviewer: "It's normal to think like that after what's happened to you."

Jollying along

Deliberately trying to maintain a light-hearted atmosphere ensures that the physiotherapist distances themselves from potentially difficult issues and so discourages the patient from expressing their concerns

Patient: "I really don't know how I'm going to cope if I lose my job"

Interviewer: "Whoa – just think though, no getting up at 6 a.m.! What other shifts do you do?"

Structuring and controlling the interview

There are significant challenges for musculoskeletal physiotherapists in controlling the content and direction of discussion during the course of an assessment interview. Exploring patients' thoughts, feelings and beliefs and responding to their concerns implies the need to achieve a balance between the physiotherapist's and the patient's own agenda. Often, of course, there will be a significant overlap between the two. However, as the patient is encouraged to talk, there is the danger that they begin to dictate the agenda, as the therapist 'allows' them free rein to talk about whatever's on their mind. It is vitally important for the therapist to remain mindful of their own agenda whilst responding to the concerns of the patient. Balancing the professional and patient agenda, therefore, is a significant challenge and takes considerable skill.

1. The physiotherapists can mention the **time available** at the beginning of the interview (and if necessary during it). This has the effect of focusing the minds of both therapist and patient.

2. During the interview the physiotherapist can establish the habit of asking them self **"have I achieved my purpose in relation to this particular issue?"** Being mindful of this question will help to ensure that a topic has been satisfactorily covered before moving on. It will also help prevent being unnecessarily sidetracked by the patient into irrelevant territory.

3. When stopping the patient, the physiotherapist should explain why they are doing so to help the patient understand. Use of the hands may be helpful. A **negotiating** style can assist the interviewer to redirect the interview.

- "If I could just stop you there. You've told me a lot of important things, but there are a number of other topics I'd like to ask you about before we finish today – is that OK? Could I ask you what kind of activities you find especially difficult?"

4. The combined use of **summarizing** and **screening** can help the physiotherapist to decide whether to move the patient on.

- "If I could stop you there for a moment, you've told me that.....*(summary)*....is there anything else which is important for me to know?"

5. The use of **'signposting'** and **negotiation** to move from one topic to the next is helpful for keeping the interviewer's mind focused whilst taking the patient from one subject to another (rather than moving abruptly from one to the next).

- "Ok. You've told me about how your pain affects your work – could I ask you how your problem has affected your family life?

Changing subjects smoothly can also be achieved by **summarising** the key points from the last issue and building a 'bridge' to the next area of discussion.

- "So you've told me how you are concerned that you may have slipped a disc in your back and that a friend of yours had the same thing and needed an operation. I just wonder what you think might happen to you if you tried to increase your activities now?"

6. The **reason for asking specific questions** may also be outlined helping the patient to understand the importance of the line of enquiry.

- "In order to make a plan for your recovery, I think it would be useful to see what activities you can still manage so that we can build from these."

Scope of physiotherapy practice

Accessing the 'inner world' of the patient runs the chance of the patient disclosing information which is difficult to deal with and can not be directly addressed by a physiotherapist e.g. workplace bullying, marital problems, alcohol abuse. The physiotherapist may have concerns about the extent to which they should pursue specific topics or what to do with information that they are given.

Two important points may help here:
- The physiotherapist should keep in mind the question – "to what extent does the problem they are telling me about impact upon physical function?"
- The physiotherapist can inform the patient at the earliest opportunity, or at the appropriate moment, those areas that they can directly assist with and those areas that they can't. It is realistic to appreciate that some problems elicited will not have immediate solutions.

It is therefore legitimate to pursue a line of enquiry where the problem appears to directly influence the patient's ability to function e.g. overprotective spouse, low motivation. Helping the patient to articulate their concerns will assist them in understanding the nature of their problem more precisely and will inform the goal setting process. It also helps in building trust and a stronger empathic therapeutic relationship. However, as stated, the therapist needs to acknowledge and inform the patient of the limits of their ability to assist - and so set boundaries to the intervention.
The nature of the precise boundary of clinical practice for physiotherapists is likely to be a source of some considerable discussion and possible contention. However, one working demarcation can be illustrated by the following example. A patient may present with an apparent obsession with keeping their house clean and tidy sufficient to prevent any change in pacing of daily activities. Helping the patient to recognise the link between their apparent high standards and inability to pace activities falls within the scope of physiotherapy practice. However, attempting to change the patient's view on the importance of this level of housework does not.

Handling more difficult situations

There may be times when patients become highly emotional. They may be angry at the way they have been 'let down' by the health care system. Or else they may be tearful when describing the contrast between their current and previous lifestyles. It is important to remember that it is highly unlikely that the patient will be somehow damaged by such displays of emotion. On the contrary, patients may benefit by being able to express their feelings and articulate whatever is on their mind.

The following points may be helpful:

- Give the patient time. Do not be tempted to jump in and finish their sentences or "jolly them along".
- Awkward silences are OK. In these situations choose your moment to simply reflect back what you are seeing or hearing e.g. "it's hard to talk about it", "it makes you angry".
- Tell the patient that it is OK to be upset or angry
- Demonstrate empathy – reflect back the messages you think the patient is trying to convey
- Distinguish between your own emotional responses to the patient and what is best for the patient
- Identify any "yellow flags" at the root of their feelings e.g. misconceptions, mistaken fears or beliefs
- Negotiate the timing of any information, opinions or advice that you would like to give

Developing effective communication

Departmental factors

There are many external factors that will influence physiotherapists' capacity to develop their communication skills. Some of these factors relate to the ethos of the department in which they work and the perceived legitimacy of routinely exploring the patient perspective. Communication skills are more likely to flourish in a department that promotes a culture of biopsychosocial assessment and management. For example, the use of psychosocial screening questionnaires creates the expectation that the patient perspective is a core component of assessment and authenticates patient disclosure of psychosocial information. In addition, the department may enable suitable conditions for enhancing communication, such as extended appointment times for appropriate patients so that important discussion can be completed, or even the allocation of areas where privacy is enhanced, such as quiet rooms or corner cubicles, where interruptions are kept to a minimum. In addition, physiotherapists may be able to experiment with their structured interview format – since assessment forms incorporating headings and prompts to explore the patient's perspective will underpin efforts to improve communication. An environment where psychosocial issues are routinely discussed, both formally (e.g. through case studies) and informally, will promote an atmosphere of peer support, and will reinforce the need to develop the necessary communication skills for patient management. This may be enhanced by links with pain management services so that important advice and guidance can be provided to enable physiotherapists to develop their confidence in handling more difficult issues using the appropriate communication strategies.

Education and Training

Teaching of communication skills should aim to dissociate didactic and experiential methods, and match the level of challenge to the experience and/or aptitude of the physiotherapist. Creating an adequate knowledge base is the first step and can be achieved through didactic teaching and discussion. However, developing the key communication skills requires the opportunity to learn and rehearse skills, such as provided by **role-play**, which can be best achieved by workshops with limited numbers of participants.

Role-play

This provides the most useful method by which the key skills can be practiced and rehearsed in a safe environment. In addition, by playing the role of a patient, the therapist can gain valuable insight into how someone with pain might think and feel. However, there are many challenges inherent in setting up effective role-play, not least because of the concerns and fears of the participants. Broadly speaking, the greater the level of complexity the role-play provides, the greater the potential rewards for the participants, but also the harder it is for the facilitator to ensure that what happens is both effective and safe.

Paired role-play

The simplest form is paired role-play where participants take turns in playing interviewer and interviewee using prepared scenarios. Participants are usually least reluctant to engage in this form of activity since their performance is not placed under direct scrutiny. The introduction of an observer, however, can initially make participants uneasy. Feedback by peers can be a very useful means of gaining insight on performance and so enhance the skills being practiced, but there is often the fear is that the experience may be effectively a humiliating critique of what went wrong. To ensure that the experience of feedback is a positive one, the following rules should be applied:

- Discussion should be "paused" at key moments in the interview for feedback to take place. This is to make sure that a manageable amount of material is discussed at any one time.
- The observer should firstly describe what went well – this is so that good practice is acknowledged and reinforced.
- The observer should then describe what could have been done differently. That is, they should be able to offer an alternative approach to any of the strategies used and not merely criticise what happened.

- The interviewee or 'patient' can remain 'in role' and offer insights by describing how they felt at key moments in the interview, for example, their reaction to a particular line of questioning.

Group role-play

Bringing an entire group together for role-play provides more opportunities and presents significant challenges. One advantage is that the group will offer a greater variety of perspectives to the same interview, so that valuable discussion can be facilitated. Two issues where several viewpoints are useful are:

- Feedback as to precisely what went well
- The impact of various communication strategies used upon the 'patient'

In order for the group role-play to be successful, however, several 'safety' features need to be deployed. Considerable confidence and skill is required to effectively facilitate group scenarios. It is recommended, therefore, that the facilitator takes time to prepare thoroughly and undertakes the task with like-minded and supportive physiotherapists!

The facilitator should:

1. Ensure that participants are aware before they enter the training the nature of the role-play that will be used. Participation needs to be voluntary!
2. Use a demonstration role-play initially, where the facilitator plays the interviewer and periodically steps out of role to facilitate discussion.
3. Allow 'patient' volunteers plenty of time to prepare, and discuss the role-play with volunteers beforehand (some days before, if appropriate). They can be encouraged to weave together autobiographical details as well as their own clinical experience to inform their presentation, but warned not to include personal 'inflammatory' material, which may undermine their capacity to effectively remain in role.
4. Encourage the group to take equal responsibility for what happens, including assigning tasks to individuals.
5. Halt the role-play at key points and ask the group to describe what went well before alternative approaches are offered. Feedback should also be elicited from the interviewer as to their perception of their performance, including their thinking behind certain communication strategies.
6. Ask the group to provide suggestions for the next steps in how the interview is to proceed. Encouraging precision can enhance group responsibility, for example, if a participant suggests that the interviewer should "ask about the family", the precise wording of the question should be elicited.

7. Signal to the role-players that it is OK to get stuck or lose track of the line of enquiry. The role-play can be halted by the participants themselves, or by the facilitator if it obvious that they are in difficulty. Once again, the group can provide support to the interviewer by commenting positively on their performance and suggest ways to recommence the role-play.

Use of audio or video recording

Recordings of actual initial assessments provide valuable information and material for reflection. By listening to the recording, the key communication skills and strategies used can be identified and the impact that they appeared to have upon the patient discerned. It will usually be possible to establish that particular lines of enquiry had been omitted or overlooked and the recording can be used to establish whether important patient cues had been missed. As with any process that places clinical practice under scrutiny, it is helpful to identify what went well and why it went well. This balances any tendency to dwell on the least successful aspects of the interview.

In order to obtain this material, the patient needs to give their fully informed consent. The Appendix provides an example of a patient information form and accompanying consent form that conforms to current requirements governing confidentiality and consent.

Attendance on Communication Skills Workshops

The Cancer Research UK lead 4-6 workshops per year (see Contacts). These workshops provide excellent opportunities to develop the skills of effective communication with patients.

Summary

This chapter has attempted to highlight the various skills and strategies that physiotherapists may use in order to improve the accuracy of their assessments, particularly in relation to the understanding of the patients' perspective. It has been suggested that the need to acquire effective communication skills goes hand-in-hand with the development of the biopsychosocial perspective. Because of the extensive nature of the communication field, the focus of this chapter has been on the practical approaches to skills development, rather than a more theoretical discourse of the topic.

Strategies related to the process of assessment have been described, but equally there are useful approaches to enhance other aspects of the encounter, such as promoting patient recall and adherence to recommendations made by the physiotherapist.

Developing communication skills are a core component of clinical practice, but their acquisition does not appear to happen automatically with 'patient mileage'. Communication skills training, therefore, perhaps linked to pain management approaches, would provide a fruitful means of clinical and professional development.

References

Adler R, Rodman G 2003 Understanding Human Communication. 8th Edition. Oxford University Press, New York

Main C, Watson P 2002 The distressed and angry low back pain patient. Appendix. In: Gifford L (ed) Topical Issues in Pain 3. Sympathetic nervous system and pain. Pain Management. Clinical Effectiveness. CNS Press, Falmouth 193–200

Silverman J, Kurtz S, Draper J 1998 Skills for Communicating with Patients. Radcliffe Medical Press, Oxford

Contacts

Denise Pyke
Comunication Skills Workshop Administrator
Tel: 0161 446 3683
e-mail: denise.pyke@man.ac.uk

Cancer Research UK Psychological Medicine Group
Stanley House
Christie Hospital NHS Trust
Withington
Manchester M20 4BX

Useful Websites

www.listen.org
　　Website of the International Listening Association - a professional organization whose members are dedicated to learning more about the impact that listening has on all human activity.
www.skillscascade.com
　　A collection of resources to promote and support the teaching of communication skills in health care.
www.motivationalinterview.org
　　Resources for those seeking information on Motivational Interviewing

Appendix

North Cheshire Hospitals Chronic Pain Management Service

Information for patients on the recording of interviews

I would like to take the opportunity of making an audio recording of discussions with your physiotherapist today. The following information will help you to decide whether or not you wish to give your consent to this recording being made. I do stress, however, **that you do not have to agree to being recorded and that this would not affect the quality of care that you receive.** Please read the following information carefully.

The purpose of making the recording is to help physiotherapists assess their communication skills more accurately. **The recording will be used for this purpose and not for making decisions about your care.** If suitable, recorded extracts may be used for training physiotherapists. No part of the recording would contain references to your name or any other information which would identify you personally. In this situation your further specific consent would be sought.

The recording would not form part of your medical record and would be erased once it has fulfilled the purpose for which it was made. However, it would be treated with the same level of confidentiality as your medical record. All recordings are securely stored and are only available for my use.

Even if you agree to being recorded you may withdraw your consent at any time during the interview, at which point the recorder will be turned off and the recording erased at the earliest opportunity. Your consent will also be confirmed at the end of the interview.

Thank you for reading this information. If you have any further questions please do not hesitate to ask me.

Steve Goldingay
Specialist physiotherapist (chronic pain)

CONSENT FORM for audio recording of interview
North Cheshire Hospitals NHS Trust

Patients surname .... Other Names ....

Date of Birth   /   /   Unit Number .... Sex (please tick) M ☐ F ☐

Contact details (for further consent, if required) ....

....

MEMBER OF CLINICAL STAFF (this part to be completed by the member of clinical staff who is to make the recording)

• Type of interview to be recorded for which written evidence of consent is appropriate:

....

• I confirm that I have explained the recording and the purpose for which it will be used to the patient in terms that in my judgement are suited to the understanding of the patient.

Signed .... Date ....

Name of member of clinical staff ....

PATIENT (this part to be completed by patient)

1. Please read this form and the information sheet Information for patients on the recording of interviews very carefully.
2. If there is anything you don't understand about the explanation, or if you want more information, please ask the member of clinical staff named above
3. Please check that all the information on the form is correct. If it is, and you understand the explanation, then sign the form.

I am the named patient:

I agree
• to what is proposed which has been explained to me by the member of staff named above.

I understand
• that the audio recording to which I have agreed will only be used for assisting physiotherapists to assess their communication skills more accurately
• that the recording will not form part of my medical record and can be erased when no longer required.
• that it will be given the same protection of confidentiality as my medical record.
• that it may be useful for teaching physiotherapists and that my consent will be specifically sought if any recording is used for this purpose

Signed .... Date ....

Consent confirmed at end of recording   **YES / NO**

Recording No.: .... Date erased: ....

5

Communication within therapeutic encounters: Message received and understood?

ANNE DAYKIN

Introduction

Communication is a fundamental tool for the effective management of pain. It is the key to access our patients' sensations, functional limitations, expectations, beliefs and concerns. Communication lies at the heart of shared decision-making, health behaviour change and patient enablement leading to their active participation with the management of pain. The CSP have again recognised communication as a core standard of physiotherapy practice (CSP 2005).

Within a therapeutic encounter there is always a two-way flow of communication between patients and health care professionals (HCPs) in order to achieve a shared therapeutic goal. Tuckett et al (1985) draw our attention to the important point that a consultation between a patient and a HCP is a meeting between the beliefs and expectations of both parties. Thus, to allow an exchange or sharing of these beliefs and expectations is a priority. Without such an exchange, there can be no certainty that the therapeutic encounter will be 'successful' in the opinion of the patients. In addition, HCPs and patients are at risk of talking and acting at cross-purposes. Establishing the patients' beliefs and expectations is a central recommendation within a biopsychosocial assessment and is a feature of evidence-based patient-centred consultations.

However, not all physiotherapists establish their patients' beliefs and expectations. Musculoskeletal outpatient physiotherapists and their patients with chronic low back pain (LBP) were observed and interviewed at designated stages throughout their therapeutic encounters (Daykin & Richardson 2004).

The physiotherapists claimed an implicit awareness of their patients' beliefs and expectations through noting their patients' behaviour and through their own "gut feelings". As they had not explicitly asked their patients, this awareness was only partial and sometimes misguided according to the narratives of their patients. Table 1 provides excerpts from transcripts of pre and post assessment interviews with Mary a Senior I and her patient Mr G.

	Mr G's Pain Beliefs	Mary's Interpretation of Mr G's Pain Beliefs	Mary's Pain Beliefs Regarding Mr G
Causal Attributions	I think that I did some damage to my back when I was actually lifting something (6) Mr G mentioned work, putting on weight, nerves, arthritis on his x-ray It would be nice to know which the actual, or where the actual problem is (969-970)	Well he relates it originally to an injury (7) He's been told by the consultant before he came to see me that he had wear and tear within his back so from that he must have a pretty good idea you know (21-22)	The x-ray identifies L3-4 as being visibly osteoarthritic. I feel that he does have some degenerative change within his back (102-103)
Treatment Expectations	Mainly exercises to actually em, build up the muscle in the back I suppose to support the spine (293-294) And maybe I don't know whether they do like infrasound or anything like that on the back…just a load of sound waves isn't it? Something similar to like whales do or something like that (502-503, 507-508)	Em, I haven't actually discussed that much with him (173)	Indication would be to treat to try and resolve the particular problems that present at the moment which are the stiffness that I felt below the active level that's painful, and then by loosening that up hopefully reduce the discomfort at the over active level the L3-4 level and then get him on a home exercise programme to maintain flexibility of the lower lumbar vertebrae (110-114)

	Mr G's Pain Beliefs	Mary's Interpretation of Mr G's Pain Beliefs	Mary's Pain Beliefs Regarding Mr G
Expectations of a Cure	Obviously where arthritis is concerned nothing I suppose I don't know (453-455) If you found the right thing then hopefully you know if your back is how it should be then there would be no more pain (861-863)	I don't think he's looking for a cure. Or at least I hope he's not looking for a cure (laugh) because if it is a degenerative change osteoarthritic change we're not going to give that. Em, I think most people do attend for physiotherapy hoping that we will actually be able to sort out all their problems (174-178)	So it's not going to be a condition that will cure. It's going to be something that he will have to live with (103-106) So he'll be self-managing. He may not be 100% pain free but he will definitely be self-managing (104-105)

Table 1: An outline of the beliefs of Mary (Senior I) and her patient Mr G regarding causal attributions, treatment expectations and expectations of a cure (line numbers of transcripts within parentheses)

It can be seen that Mary assumes that Mr G has received a satisfying explanation because he saw a consultant prior to attending physiotherapy. However, Mr G seems to have multiple theories regarding his pain and is still seeking a meaningful explanation. Mary has not discussed Mr G's treatment expectations and is uncertain regarding his expectations of a cure. If Mr G's expectations are not met then his satisfaction with the management of his pain problem is likely to be poor.

Mary's beliefs regarding the cause of Mr G's pain are based on a structural-pathology model and as can be seen later these beliefs are reflected in the explanations she gives Mr G. Facet or posterior intervertebral joint osteoarthritis is not a helpful clinical diagnosis as the correlation between radiological findings and patients' sensations are weak. Mary's beliefs are guiding her clinical reasoning towards treatment decisions that are not evidence-based. Note that there is no mention of psychosocial risk factors in this encounter. This example suggests that Mary and Mr G's communication has not allowed an exchange of beliefs and expectations and this may have a detrimental effect on the management of Mr G's LBP.

Components of Interpersonal Communication

The components of interpersonal communication fall broadly into three categories. These are verbal (words only), paralinguistic (tone of voice, silence etc) and non-verbal (gestures, behaviours etc). Subconsciously we all pay as much attention to *how* someone tells us something as to *what* they say (Waddell 2004).

A) Verbal Communication

Verbal forms of communication are dependent on language and the words we use. Whilst interacting with our patients we draw on techniques that encourage them to talk in some detail about their expectations, beliefs and condition. These techniques, amongst others, are questioning style, reflection and summarising.

i) Questioning style

Everybody will have heard of a closed question that asks for specific information and so fosters short answers: 'So you think the wear and tear is causing your back problems?' An open question allows the patient to answer in whatever way they like and so encourages them to talk and expand on the subject. Examples of open questions which can be used to explore the psychosocial elements of a patients' problem are (Main & Watson 2002):

'Do you have any clues or theories as to why the pain is persisting?'

'I know you're not a doctor, but what do you think is the cause?'

What explanations have you been given about your pain?'

Very simple open questions can provide illuminating information regarding the patients' beliefs.

ii) Reflection

Reflecting on what the patient has said acts as a cue for them to elaborate on a particular theme, belief or feeling. Reflection techniques such as using keywords or paraphrasing can be used instead of questions that can divert the conversation according to the beliefs of HCPs and not to those of their patients.

An example of reflection through using keywords:

I'm always reading things, I read that someone did a bungee jump once with a bad back and cured it.

A bungee jump?

Yes, so I did one! But it didn't cure me (laugh) in fact it hurt a bit more afterwards

An example of reflection using paraphrasing:
I'm always reading things, I read that someone did a bungee jump once with a bad back and cured it.
You read that bungee jumps cure bad backs
Yes, so I did one! But it didn't cure me (laugh) in fact it hurt a bit more afterwards

iii) Summarising
Summarising what patients have just told you reassures them that you have been listening. It gives patients an opportunity to correct any misunderstandings (Maguire & Pitceathly 2002) and also ensures a shared understanding of the problem (Rollnick et al 1999).

B) Paralinguistic Communication
Paralanguage is a mixture of vocal and non-verbal communication that increases the impact of verbal messages. One's tone of voice, silent pauses and vocal segregates such as 'uh-huh' or 'mm-mmm' can encourage patients to continue speaking which may provide a greater understanding of their point of view. The use of silence is especially powerful. A colleague who was a self-confessed silence-phobe now appreciates that a relaxed silence during an encounter gives the patients time and space to think. However, she was initially intimidated by silences and found it difficult not to talk through them.

C) Non-Verbal Communication
Non-verbal communication can have both a positive and negative effect on how effectively a person gets their messages across. When the non-verbal conflicts with the verbal message, we will probably not believe what is being said (Waddell 2004). Non-verbal cues such as eye contact, smiling and touching are important in building a relationship (Rungapadiachy 1999). Within physiotherapy, the 'laying on of hands' has always been a powerful means of communication. Other forms of non-verbal communication include the use of facial expression, gestures, posture and general appearance. These can all convey subtle messages to patients, like how interested we are in them.

We can obtain valuable information about a patient's emotions and beliefs through observing their posture and how they behave, e.g. guarded movements, fidgeting, grimaces, rubbing their back, the use of walking aids and duration of down-time. Thus within a therapeutic encounter HCPs can analyse and utilise body language to their advantage.

Interpersonal communication however, is not just about the messages we exchange via verbal and non-verbal behaviours. The meaning of any message to patients, or how they interpret that message, will be influenced by their past communication with HCPs, or by patients' own expectations and experiences.

Messages we receive from patients

Patients may be selective in the messages they choose to give us. Maguire et al (1996) found that patients frequently withhold important information from doctors. This may be due to patients' beliefs that nothing can be done, a reluctance to burden the doctor, a desire not to seem pathetic or ungrateful or worry that their fears of what is wrong with them will be confirmed. Expressing empathy is fundamental to helping patients feel understood. One way we can facilitate a shared understanding of the patient's problem is through our listening skills.

Active listening within a therapeutic encounter can be defined as the art of capturing the essence of the message patients want us to receive and understand. It involves searching for an understanding of the underlying meaning behind the words used by the patient (Rollnick et al 1999). Giving attention to what the patient is saying also creates a climate of empathy and trust (Salkovskis, personal communication). In this way, we can access patients' beliefs, expectations and concerns and better understand their perspective of their problem.

Typical barriers to effective listening are external distractions (e.g. noise), lack of interest, interpreting and fact-hunting. It is the latter that may be of particular relevance to physiotherapy, especially when instead of listening to the meaning of the patients' pain experience, we may concentrate on the detailed facts within our subjective assessments. When studying manipulative therapy I remember being rewarded if I completed my subjective assessments in 20 minutes – I wonder now how much listening I actually managed between firing questions at my patients and also how many important message I missed.

Patients often use medical language during the therapeutic encounter. They use words like 'discs', inflamed muscles', arthritis' or as one of my patients used to say 'arthur-itis'. This is a form of speech convergence, where patients attempt to adopt the speech pattern of HCPs. This can promote mutual understanding between them and reduce the uncertainty that often characterises first encounters between strangers. However, patients' definition of medical terms may differ from ours. A shared term does not imply a shared meaning so there is a need to explore the patients' perspective.

Patients give us underlying messages through the words that they use. An example of this is when patients rate their pain as 10 out of 10, or 15 out of 10. High ratings of pain is a psychosocial yellow flag (Kendall et al 1997) that indicates a risk of developing persisting pain which could potentially lead to work loss and long term incapacity. The quote below is by a Senior II physiotherapist and reflects how her own beliefs about how patients with certain pain scores 'should' behave causes suspicion, which may be reflected in her communication.

"I suspect if her pain was a lot of the time 10 out of 10, which she was implying at times, I can't imagine many people living on Panadol if the pain was 10 out of 10...If she's only using Panadol, and if she's only using it very rarely when she feels she needs to, that sorts of backs up what I said earlier about pain being useful" (Daykin 2002)

Therefore, instead of assessing the truth of her patient's pain rating perhaps this physiotherapist should have listened to the underlying message her patient was giving her.

Messages patients receive from us

The explanations and advice we give to our patients can have a profound effect on their beliefs (Waddell 2004). Providing a diagnosis for our patients is an example of this. The labelling of back pain is important in signifying to the patient and their significant others that someone is taking their pain problem seriously (Stone et al 2002) and that someone knows what is wrong (Bogduk 2000). However, for patients with LBP a specific diagnosis can be incorrect or counterproductive and over-diagnosis may lead to over-treatment that can be associated with a passive attitude towards their own management and expectations of a cure.

Health care professionals continue to seek a term for LBP that is taxonomically correct, would encourage active participation in their management and dispel fears regarding the resumption of normal activity (Bogduk 2000). In an amusing study Stone et al (2002) explored the differing connotations and potential offensiveness of 10 different medical labels for the symptom of weakness e.g. hysterical weakness, medically unexplained weakness and functional weakness. It was the latter label which was the least likely to offend and avoided the 'non-diagnosis' of 'medically unexplained'. It also provides a rationale for managements aimed at restoring function.

Daykin and Richardson (2004) noted the explanations physiotherapists gave to patients (Table 2). Being told that one has 'wear and tear' in your spine has negative connotations of serious deterioration that is irreversible. Those labels do nothing to enable patients to be pro-active in their management (Hamonet et al 2001). Waddell (2004) goes as far as to say that the diagnosis may make the patients ill thus contributing to iatrogenic incapacity.

95

Mary's explanation to Mr G	The bottom of your back is stiff, bone number 3 is not as stiff, bones 4 and 5 are not doing their job so number 3 is doing too much. It suggests wear and tear nothing sinister or nasty.
Mr G's reaction to the explanation	Well hopefully you know from what Mary says if it's just those ones not working properly if they can be loosened up and everything and em it might make it you know it might improve it...Is it? I can't remember what she said. Wear and tear or er how do you improve that? I mean if it's something that's worn you know I mean how do you actually make that how can you improve it without actually doing something to it? That's what I was wondering. I mean does it always stay like this now?...Obviously if it loosens up em then that might make things better (29-37, 47)
Treatment given	Spinal joint mobilisation techniques, spinal manipulation and home exercises
Outcome of treatment according to Mr G	I wish I had have sort of made the arrangements to come along a while ago, but I think it's doing or has done some good for sure (6-7)

Table 2: An outline of the explanation given by Mary (Senior I) to her patient Mr G and his reaction to the explanation, details of the treatment given and the outcome of treatment (line numbers of transcripts within parentheses)

A meaningful explanation to the patient is one of the key factors that contributes to a perceived good treatment outcome and enables patients to have active participation in, and shared decision making with, the management of their chronic pain (Pendleton et al 2003). By contrast, a limited explanation or none at all leaves many questions unanswered in the patient's mind and seldom convinces the patient of the harmlessness of their symptoms (Tuckett et al 1985).

As can be seen from the narrative example in Table 2, explanations for chronic LBP are often based on a structural-pathology model. This model largely ignores the cognitive, social and behavioural aspects of pain.

Moseley et al (2004) point out that a focus on a structural label for LBP may heighten attention on the pain. In addition, emphasising the vulnerability of the spine to damage may increase patients' health care utilisation. It is not surprising that concentrating on structure or pathology fails to reduce the impact of psychosocial barriers to recovery (Moseley et al 2004), which are of primary importance in the development of chronicity (Burton et al 1999, Kendall et al 1997).

In a series of studies Moseley and colleagues (Moseley 2003, Moseley 2003a, Moseley 2004, Moseley et al 2004, Moseley 2005) have explored the efficacy of neurophysiology education. The teaching material was based on knowledge of the neurophysiology of pain according to the relevant sections of 'The Textbook of Pain' (Wall & Melzack 1999) which included:

The nervous system – basic structures, pain pathways
Synapses – how nerves 'talk to each other', neurotransmitters, postsynaptic modulation and second order nociceptive neurons
Plasticity of the nervous system – adaptability of nervous system, sensitisation, axonial sprouting.

In summary, Moseley and colleagues suggest that:

- Data from a single patient with chronic disabling LBP indicates that neurophysiology education contributes to a distinct reduction in cortical activation during performance of a voluntary abdominal muscle task (Moseley 2005).
- Education about pain neurophysiology changes patients' pain beliefs and physical performance but is insufficient by itself to obtain a change in perceived disability (Moseley et al 2004).
- Conventional education involving the anatomy and physiology of the bones and joints of the lumbar spine, intervertebral disc, normal spinal curves, posture, lifting techniques and ergonomic advice should be questioned (Moseley et al 2004).
- In the chronic LBP patients studied by Moseley (2004) there is a strong association between change in pain-related attitudes and beliefs, and some physical performance measures. In other words, straight leg raise and forward bending range is directly limited by unhelpful pain cognitions.
- A one-to-one neurophysiology education programme when combined with specific trunk muscle training á la Richardson and Jull (1995) in association with mental rehearsal of movements which induced fear of pain such as forward bending, is more effective than group education, but it may not be as cost-effective (Moseley 2003a).
- Health care professionals and patients can understand the neurophysiology of pain but HCPs underestimate patients' ability to understand which may be a primary barrier to reconceptualisation of the problem of chronic pain (Moseley 2003).

Moseley's work and book 'Explain Pain' (Butler & Moseley 2003) suggests that neurophysiology can be fun – something I would never have believed when training! The provision of specific pain knowledge to patients is an effective evidence based management tool. In a recent review of 'Explain pain' (McLennan 2005) it was thought that the book would benefit clinicians' understanding and may be valuable to selected patients, depending presumably on their level of understanding and the meaningfulness of the explanations to their own belief systems.

Moseley's work is very exciting, especially the potential for neurophysiology education to decrease cortical activity. It identifies the messages we should be giving patients in order to affect their beliefs and behaviour. However, we should not forget the evidence-base for other advice interventions such as the 'Back Book' that is based on biopsychosocial principles which also has been shown to produce a positive shift in beliefs and self-reported disability in some patients (Symonds et al 1995, Burton et al 1999). For a good review of biopsychosocial information and advice see Waddell (2004, page 328). In addition, recently it was suggested that the Back Book, when combined with a one-off assessment by a physiotherapist seemed as effective as 'routine' physiotherapy (Frost et al 2004). It is probable that both types of education would complement each other because neurophysiology provides the theoretical rationale underlying the Back Book messages however, this has yet to be formally tested.

When reading patient information regarding back pain it always surprises me how some are still giving inappropriate messages. These are a couple of examples of published patient information:

"The back is a remarkable and highly efficient structure. Yet things can go wrong with it…All you have to do is avoid the sort of stresses that modern-day civilisation puts on your spine and maintain muscular fitness"

"Some people suffer persistent or chronic back pain, and need careful investigation to find out why. Once the cause is identified, a proper treatment programme can be planned."

The former example may encourage fear-avoidance and the latter creates an expectation of investigations identifying a 'cause' and it is only after this 'cause' has been found that treatments can proceed. We are in danger of inducing iatrogenic incapacity via some of the messages we give patients – so please check your written information and make it evidence-based.

Reassurance is a common message we may give patients. Within the therapeutic encounter patients seek reassurance regarding their pain, whether overtly (have I got cancer?) or more subtly (my pain is a little worse). However, giving patients bland reassurance, although sometimes beneficial, may increase doubt and anxiety and cause more alarm to patients. We may explain that they do not have A, B or C – but the patient is then left thinking and worrying "so what have I got?" (Salkovskis, personal communication). This emphasises the need to explore patients' beliefs about their sensations in order to understand their pain experience. It is only then that patients' beliefs can be incorporated within bespoke, evidence-based explanations.

Barriers to Effective Communication

When HCPs use communication skills effectively, both they and their patients benefit. It is to the physiotherapy profession's advantage that communication skills have now acquired a prominent position within undergraduate curricula. However, some experienced physiotherapists are still loath to enquire about the psychosocial impact of patients' problems lest they 'open a can of worms' and unleash distress that they cannot handle. This is despite established evidence citing psychosocial issues as being more important to the development of persistent pain than physical factors. Main and Watson (1999) agree that physiotherapists need to work within the limits of their psychological training, nevertheless, managing psychosocial factors that are primarily related to a patient's pain and functional incapacity should be part of the physiotherapist's responsibility to the patient.

Some physiotherapists have a perception that seeking a shared understanding regarding the patients' problem is time consuming and most physiotherapy outpatient departments are constrained by strict 20 to 30 minute treatment slots. Consequently physiotherapists may respond to emotional cues with strategies that block further disclosure such as, offering advice and reassurance before the main problems have been identified, explaining away distress as normal and attending to physical aspects only (Maguire & Pitceathly 2002). Being creative with the time available, for example seeing patients for one hour every two weeks instead of 30 minutes a week or making use of the benefits of group-work would overcome some of the time constraints. In addition, fostering an atmosphere of practical and emotional support for colleagues within physiotherapy departments may help reduce the instinct for blocking techniques.

Health care professionals' perception of patients can affect communication. Some physiotherapists have patient stereotypes such as 'difficult' patients to treat (Daykin & Richardson 2004). Physiotherapists described how 'difficult' patients presented with "unrealistic expectations" were seen as passive within treatment, were difficult to interact with and usually had multiple areas of pain. Daykin & Richardson (2004) showed how physiotherapists' beliefs regarding 'difficult' patients had negative and unhelpful consequences to the therapeutic encounter. Because of the perceived poor outcome expectancy, the treatment of 'difficult' patients could be cut short and the patient referred to the back pain service or their general practitioner. Conversely, some physiotherapists continued treating for many weeks, even months, in the hope that the patient would eventually improve. This implies that this group of patients experienced treatment inequalities. It is possible that physiotherapists' poor expectations of treatment could be communicated to patients via explanations or advice given, or by non-verbal behaviour, and this may be perpetuating or reinforcing the stereotype and thus a poor outcome.

In addition, treating 'difficult' patients was thought to be disheartening and frustrating, and this may have affected the physiotherapists' attitude (being less sympathetic) and behaviour (switching off) to the patient. This would then create a barrier to communication within the encounter, and the optimal management of the pain problem may not have been achieved. The potential consequences of this is that a waiting list may increase or the patient returns to their general practitioner, seeking alternative treatments and investigations, which can reinforce their back pain-related incapacity (Daykin & Richardson 2004).

The mood of HCPs, whether affected by 'frustrating' or 'difficult' patients, home life or whatever, has an influence on the consultation. Those who are experiencing strongly negative moods may concentrate on just getting through the day, cutting responses to a minimum and avoiding involvement (Pendleton et al 2003). Thus the greatest barrier to active listening and communication is the HCP him or herself.

It is therefore recommended that HCPs reflect on their own beliefs about pain in order to overcome these barriers to communication. Having an awareness of our pain beliefs and their potential influences would help us to identify those that pose as potential barriers to communication with patients with pain.

Other barriers to effective communication include differing cultural beliefs of patients regarding health and pain, differences in ability of patients to deal with abstract concepts and differences in patients' vocabulary and reading ability that are based on educational and social factors (Scott & Weiner 1984). Again, this emphasises the importance of explicitly exploring patients' beliefs to gain a shared-understanding of their problem. It is only then that HCPs can provide bespoke evidence-based and meaningful explanations to patients.

The potential consequences of poor and effective communication

Being unable to overcome the barriers to communication could potentially result in patients being passive recipients of care, being non-adherent or self-terminating their treatment (Daykin & Richardson 2004). Poor communication does nothing to allay the fears of patients and can even increase anxiety and perpetuate unhelpful beliefs about their pain. This may lead to detrimental health behaviours and patients may continue to doctor-shop until they obtain an explanation that they believe is relevant to them (Ley 1988). This may involve many clinical visits and investigations, which creates an economic burden on the NHS. Patients may continue to receive inappropriate treatment that may not only be ineffective for the physical disorder, but also make the psychosocial aspects worse and cause iatrogenic incapacity.

In an atmosphere of effective communication patients improve faster, cope better with their pain, require less medication and experience numerous other health benefits. Good communication encourages patients' active participation in the management of their pain, which is more likely to lead to helpful behaviour change. Eliciting and dealing with patients' concerns reduces anxiety. Finally, there is plenty of experimental and correlational evidence to show that informed patients are more satisfied (Ley 1988).

Summary

In the context of the therapeutic encounter, the primary function of communication is to establish a shared understanding between patients and HCPs. Figure 1 summarises the process of communication between patients and HCPs within therapeutic encounters. It can be seen that effective communication is based upon the influences of beliefs, attitudes, behaviours, past experiences, expectations and understanding of both parties and HCPs need to seek an awareness of these. It is also beneficial to be aware of the potential barriers to effective communication so we can use this knowledge to our advantage within clinical situations. There are many potential health outcomes, both positive and negative, that are dependent on communication. Achieving successful communication enables patients, and leads to significantly higher standards of care. These health outcomes then act as a feedback loop on the original influences, emphasising the cyclic effect of past experiences and beliefs on communication within therapeutic encounters.

Figure 1: The process of communication within therapeutic encounters

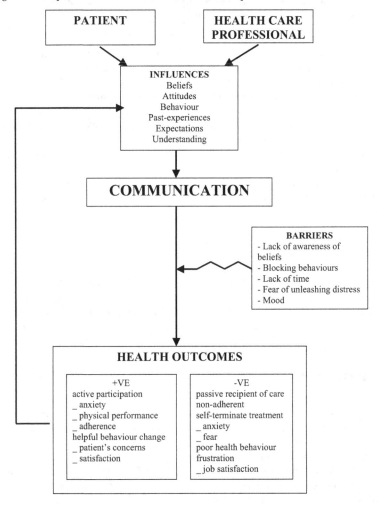

Conclusion

Communication is a skill - and like all skills it requires practice to be performed well. Take every opportunity to practice these skills, observe colleagues in action and even tape record your own interactions. By investing a little time reflecting on our own and our patients' beliefs about pain, the payback in terms of more effective communication can be considerable. We can then be confident that the message has indeed been received and understood by both parties.

References

Bogduk N 2000 What's in a name? The labelling of back pain. Medical Journal of Australia 173:400-401

Butler DS, Moseley GL 2003 Explain Pain. NOI Group Publications, Adelaide

Burton AK, Waddell G, Tillotson KM, Summerton N 1999 Information and advice to patients with back pain can have a positive effect: a randomized controlled trial of a novel education booklet in primary care. Spine 24:2484-2491

Chartered Society of Physiotherapy 2005 Core Standards of Physiotherapy Practice

Daykin AR 2002 A mixed methods study regarding physiotherapists' pain beliefs and their influence on the therapeutic encounter. Unpublished PhD Thesis. University of East Anglia, Norwich

Daykin AR, Richardson B 2004 Physiotherapists' pain beliefs and their influence on the management of patients with chronic low back pain. Spine 29:783-795

Frost H, Lamb SE, Doll HA, Carver PT, Stewart-Brown S 2004 Randomised controlled trial of physiotherapy compared with advice for low back pain. British Medical Journal 329:708-713

Hamonet C, Boulay C, Heiat A, Saraoui H, Boulongne D, Chignon J-C, Wackenheim P, Mace Y, Rigal C, Staub H 2001 Les mots qui font mal (Words that harm). Douleurs 2:29-33

Kendall NAS, Linton SJ, Main CJ 1997 Guide to Assessing Psychosocial Yellow Flags in Acute Low Back Pain. Accident Rehabilitation and Compensation Insurance Corporation and National Advisory Committee on Health and Disability. Wellington, New Zealand

Ley P 1988 Communicating with patients. Improving Communication, Satisfaction and Compliance. Chapman & Hall, London

Maguire P, Faulkner A, Booth K, Elliott C, Hillier V 1996 Helping cancer patients to disclose their concerns. European Journal of Cancer 32a:78-91

Maguire P, Pitceathly C 2002 Key communication skills and how to acquire them. British Medical Journal 325:697-700

Main CJ, Watson PJ 1999 Psychological aspects of pain. Manual Therapy 4:203-215

Main CJ, Watson PJ 2002 The distressed and angry low back pain patient. In: Gifford L (Ed). Topical Issues in Pain 3. CNS Press, Falmouth 175-200

McLennan J 2005 Book Review: 'Explain Pain'. Physiotherapy 91:65

Moseley GL 2003 Unraveling the barriers to reconceptualisation of the problem in chronic pain: The actual and perceived ability of patients and health professionals to understand the neurophysiology. The Journal of Pain 4:184-189

Moseley GL 2003a Joining forces – combining cognition-targeted motor control training with group or individual pain physiology education: A successful treatment for chronic low back pain. Journal of Manual and Manipulative Therapy 11:88-94

Moseley GL 2004 Evidence for a direct relationship between cognitive and physical change during an education intervention in people with chronic low back pain. European Journal of Pain 8:39-45

Moseley GL 2005 Widespread brain activity during an abdominal task markedly reduced after pain physiology education: fMRI evaluation of a single patient with chronic low back pain. Australian Journal of Physiotherapy 51:49-52

Moseley GL, Nicholas MK, Hodges PW 2004 A randomized controlled trial of intensive neurophysiology education in chronic low back pain. Clinical Journal of Pain 20:324-330

Pendleton D, Schofield T, Tate P, Havelock P 2003 The New Consultation: Developing Doctor-Patient Communication. Oxford University Press, Oxford

Richardson CA, Jull GA 1995 Muscle control – pain control. What exercises would you prescribe? Manual Therapy 1:2-10

Rollnick S, Mason P, Butler C 1999 Health Behaviour Change: A Guide for Practitioners. Churchill Livingstone, Edinburgh

Rungapadiachy DM 1999 Interpersonal Communication and Psychology for health Care Professionals. Oxford, Butterworth Heinemann

Scott N, Weiner MF 1984 'Patientspeak': An exercise in communication. Journal of Medical Education 59:890-893

Stone J, Wojcik W, Durrance D, Carson A, Lewis S, MacKenzie L, Warlow CP, Sharpe M 2002 What should we say to patients with symptoms unexplained by disease? The "number needed to offend". British Medical Journal 325:1449-1450

Symmonds TL, Burton AK, Tillotson KM, Main CJ 1995 Absence resulting from low back trouble can be reduced by psychosocial intervention at the work place. Spine 20:2738-2745

Tuckett D, Boulton M, Olson C, Williams A 1985 Meetings Between Experts. London, Tavistock

Waddell G 2004 The Back Pain Revolution (2nd Edition). Churchill Livingstone, Edinburgh

Wall PD, Melzack R (Eds) 1999 Textbook of Pain (4th Edition). Churchill Livingstone, Edinburgh

6

Words that help, Words that harm

JENNIFER KLABER MOFFETT, ANGELA GREEN
AND DAVID JACKSON

The power of words has been understood since Old Testament times. They have the power to make a difference and to change us. So why is it that health professionals pay so little attention to words? In the 21st century people have come to expect that any medical problem can be cured by technology. However, these high expectations are not always realistic. For example, a chronic pain patient may need to come to terms with their problem and learn to live with it as well as possible. Self-management will entail a clear understanding of the condition and how the individual can deal with it. Also if it is to be successful, it will require the person's full engagement or involvement. There are a great many traps that an unwary clinician may fall into when trying to encourage self-management. A high level of communication skill, with an especial awareness of the impact of words, is an essential requirement underpinning any successful encounter.

This chapter relates particularly to physiotherapists who deal with patients with back pain but it is hoped that much of it will also have a wider relevance. It aims to raise awareness of a range of issues, make some practical recommendations but does not always provide the answers! The use of words and the art of communication are complex skills. The benefits of good communication skills are discussed first, and then their key components are considered. Different styles of consultation and their advantages and disadvantages are described next. Words that can be used to inform and influence practice are discussed and then techniques which can be used to ensure a common understanding are described. The chapter ends with an examination of issues around teaching communication skills to health professionals and particularly physiotherapists.

The benefits of good communication

A recent review of the literature has shown that there are positive correlations between effective clinician-patient communication and important health outcomes (Stewart 1995). Positive benefits of good communication skills include an increase in patient's knowledge and improvement in beliefs about medication (Bultman & Svarstad 2000), and improved adherence to treatment regimes (Ong et al 1995, Bultman & Svarstad 2000, DiMatteo 2004). Patients also exhibit better recall and understanding of information given to them in the clinical consultation (Ong et al 1995). There are many other benefits, such as improved data collecting, which enables the clinician to make a more accurate diagnosis and formulate a more effective treatment plan (Fallowfield & Jenkins 1999), improved patient and clinician satisfaction and also reduced incidence of emotional burnout in clinicians (Ong et al 1995, Fallowfield & Jenkins 1999). The most useful information for clinicians diagnosing a clinical problem is elicited not from physical examination or clinical tests, but from listening to, and questioning the patient (Deyo et al 1992). Studies have also noted the influence of clinicians' non-verbal communication on the outcomes of intervention (Fallowfield & Jenkins 1999). So whilst words are important clinicians need also to be aware that messages they transmit in other ways including eye contact and body language can also have impact.

When people with musculoskeletal problems, such as back pain, visit their practitioner they hope to get advice and reassurance and they hope to be told what their problem is and how they can deal with it (Turner & Whitfield 1997, Turner & Whitfield 1999). To do this in an optimal way can be a challenge for the clinician.

Much of the literature relating to communication skills in the clinical setting is focussed on the medical and nursing professions. However, a recent systematic review has examined the impact of physiotherapists' communication styles on patients' perceptions of pain (Jeffels & Foster 2003). It supported general findings within the literature that physiotherapist's communication skills were important in influencing patients' perceptions of their pain. It is important to realise that this influence can be both positive and negative. In particular, it was found that increased attention to the pain (giving detailed descriptions of the pain quality, location, etc.) increases the perception of pain, whilst suggesting coping strategies can increase pain tolerance. Also reinforcement can influence pain perception both positively and negatively. Patients' beliefs and expectations are also important. If they believe that the pain signifies a serious problem then they will tend to experience more pain. It is therefore important for physiotherapists to elicit patients' expectations, beliefs and any fears about their situation and deal with these appropriately. Giving good information and teaching them that 'hurt does not mean harm' may help the patient to cope better. However, the physiotherapist's own beliefs will influence what, and how they transmit the information to the patient and therefore need consideration.

Clinicians probably spend more time listening and talking to patients than carrying out any clinical interventions (Fallowfield & Jenkins 1999) therefore there is a clear need to make sure that communication skills are optimal. This may mean investing time and other resources in training staff in this area (Walker 1996).

Maguire (Maguire & Pitceathly 2002) has outlined in some detail how these skills can be taught to doctors, and has highlighted both the key components required to be taught and the techniques found to be effective in improving doctors' communication skills. Evidence from two randomised controlled trials have demonstrated that it is possible to achieve good results using these and similar methods (Fallowfield et al 2002. Maguire & Pitceathly 2002).

Key Components of Good Communication Skills

Maguire (Maguire & Pitceathly 2002) has identified some key areas of importance regarding communicating with patients. These are briefly summarised below:
- *Elicit* the patient's *main problems* and his/her perception of these and the impact (social and emotional) on the patient and their family.
- Give the patient *appropriate information*, i.e. what is needed and what the patient wants to know. Also, it is important to check that the patient has understood the information.
- Check *patient's reaction to the information and address any concerns* they may have.
- Determine how much the *patient wants to be involved in making decisions* about their situation, especially when options are available.
- *Treatment options need to be discussed* to ensure that patients understand the implications.
- Come to *agreed decisions* about treatment and maximise the likelihood that the patient will adhere to treatment decisions and advice given.

Just how the above might be achieved in physiotherapy practice is the main issue at hand. Treatment options, such as finding out if the patient would prefer to have a one-off intervention, which would aim to help them cope on their own at home, rather than attend regularly for treatment, may need discussing.

Some patients when asked this question prefer to have a less intensive intervention that might require between one and three sessions of attendance rather than a more lengthy and intensive period of treatment. It is important therefore to offer them this choice (Klaber Moffett et al 2005).

A great deal can be accomplished by teaching specific interview skills that encourage the development of a good relationship between the clinician and patient which then enables the patient to disclose the relevant information, and helps them to understand and remember important issues about their situation. In short, an adult-to-adult relationship is established where the patient is on an equal footing to the clinician and feels more in control of the management of their condition.

Klein (Klein et al 1999) has outlined key interview skills that are aimed at establishing empathy and rapport with the patients, and help to empower them both during the interview and afterwards when they are encouraged to take control of self management, insofar as this is possible. These skills are directed towards the clinician developing good listening skills, using a negotiating style and encouraging them to elicit precise information from the patient. This is done by paying close attention to body language (e.g. eye contact and leaning towards the patient when appropriate) and taking great care over language used. This not only means avoiding jargon, but also involves a very careful use of words. Labels are avoided, (or used with care) as these often carry unhelpful meanings to the patient. Questions are used appropriately, for example, it is considered helpful to invite the patient to 'tell their story' early on in the interview by using an open question. However, at some stage during the interview it may be important to ask closed questions in order to elicit the precise information that may be necessary to clarify a diagnosis or help with formulating a treatment plan (screening questions, for example). The common courtesies of any 'good' exchange between two people are emphasised. For example, welcoming the patient, using their name, shaking hands with them (if appropriate) and making sure they are comfortable, etc. An important tactic to avoid is that of 'blocking', where the clinician avoids dealing with the 'real' problem by giving premature advice, not addressing the patient's emotional problems, switching the topic or concentrating on physical problems only (Maguire & Pitceathly 2002). Finding out what really concerns the patient is important. A silence can sometimes be helpful to give the patient time to reflect on what has been said, to express their viewpoint and to ask questions.

Techniques of communication

Therapeutic relationship

A patient is more likely to develop a therapeutic relationship with their physiotherapist if the physiotherapist uses words which convey empathy and respect (Swain 1997). Empathic comments demonstrate that the listener recognises the worry and concern, or the difficulties that the patient has experienced. However, whilst empathy, and a positive attitude can be conducive to the therapeutic relationship (Edwards et al 2001), comments which are perceived as flippant or patronising, can inhibit the patient from sharing any more information (Edwards et al 2001, Little et al 2001). A great deal of sensitivity is required here, and a very careful choice of words may be important. It may be easy to say to a patient in chronic pain, *I know exactly how you feel*, but be prepared that the patient might retort "you don't know because you don't have to live with it" (Potter & Grove 1999)

Structured versus informal

The physiotherapist needs to be willing to devote time to elicit the patient's concerns, by putting the patient at ease, explaining the proposed structure of the forthcoming assessment and using open questions to encourage the patient to tell their story (Martin et al 2003). However, there is also a place for the use of closed questions depending on the information that is sought. For example, when enquiring about which medication the patient has been prescribed or whether the patient has found a particular treatment helpful, a carefully worded closed question may be needed to obtain the information that is required. In a traditional physiotherapy consultation closed questions predominate and tend to comprise the basis of proformas often used during assessment. They should however be used sensitively in conjunction with open questions. A consultation that is primarily based on a check list has the advantage of controlling its structure more easily and making sure that key factors are checked (for example red flags) but it also has many disadvantages. It is likely to omit the consequences of pain and disability for the patient and in any case inhibit a discussion which allows the patient to contribute their views fully.

Authoritarian versus egalitarian

In general, people want medical consultations to address their concerns, and they wish to be involved in decisions which influence the interventions that they receive (Office for Public Management 2000, Entwistle et al 2002). This is particularly true for those with chronic conditions. An in-depth qualitative study of patients with rheumatoid arthritis demonstrated the advantages of a consultation that involve the patient. It found that patients who felt actively involved in the consultation with the rheumatologist, and were given the opportunity to explore feelings and share emotions, subsequently felt in better control of their health (Ryan et al 2003).

From the start of the initial assessment, our choice of words, tone of voice and body language inform the patient of the role that we wish them to adopt during the course of the consultation (Waterworth & Luker 1990, Williams & Harrison 1999). A qualitative study of physiotherapists' initial encounters with patients illustrated that some physiotherapists invite the patient to participate in dialogue in order to achieve an understanding of the patient's perception of their problem, while others view themselves as the authority and use directive questions to elicit the information that they consider to be relevant from the patient (Kumlin & Kroksmark 1992). Such differences in consultation style may be due to many factors, including inexperience (Jensen et al 1990), a desire to retain control or power within the consultation (Williams & Harrison 1999, Swain 2004) or insufficient skill to conduct a biopsychosocial consultation (Barry et al 2001). The use of an authoritarian consultation style can result in a patient failing to voice particular concerns and beliefs (Stewart et al 1979). It can also result in misunderstanding (Barry et al 2000), and failure to meet the patient's needs (Kersten et al 2000). It is often associated with patient dissatisfaction with the outcome of the consultation (Little et al 2001) and a failure to follow advice or treatment recommendations (Barry et al 2000).

In order to effectively involve patients in the consultation, the physiotherapist needs to recognise the value of the information that the patient can provide. This is not necessarily medical knowledge, but is information regarding their own experience of their usually chronic, condition in relation to previous interventions or coping strategies, and the emotional, psychological and functional manifestations of that condition (Stacey & Spencer 1999).

In a study of co-operative language used by GPs, (Skelton & Hobbs 1999) found that question tags such as, *isn't it?*; *don't you?* were often used effectively to invite patients to contribute their views in a non threatening manner. This type of language is characteristic of an egalitarian approach encouraging an adult-to-adult relationship.

Words used to inform and influence

The aim of providing patients with information is arguably to allow them firstly to have a better understanding of their condition and secondly to be better able to cope with it. The latter is especially important. The physiotherapist in the course of a consultation has many opportunities to influence the beliefs, attitude and behaviour of the patient.

Suggestion

We know from our own day-to-day experience that the people around us and their choice of language can influence the way we feel. This is certainly true of our perception of pain and has been demonstrated in a number of experiments carried out in laboratory and clinical settings. For example, if the patient is given 'verbal expectancy' of pain relief the level of pain reporting is reduced (Austen et al 1997, Staats et al 1998, Pascalis et al 2002). Suggestion can have a powerful placebo effect but it can also work in reverse and increase the perception of pain.

Words and the way they are used by physiotherapists not only influence the way the patient feels about their condition, they also influence the likely outcome of the treatment. The practitioner may not always appreciate how emotive a word may be. The same word for one individual may have quite a different meaning for another. This is evident with the dilemma that faces the practitioner when providing the patient with a label as discussed in the section below.

Once an individual becomes aware of a bodily sensation, selective monitoring can occur (Skelton & Pennebaker 1982). Most are then likely to try to provide an explanatory hypothesis for that symptom based on past experience or knowledge. It may often be possible for therapists to influence the patient's hypotheses as they will be seeking some form of verification of their understanding. However, some patients may have a firmly established mind set, or 'cognitve schemata' about their problem that can be difficult to alter (Flor et al 1990). The individual needs to not only alter their hypothesis, but also encode the new information to integrate it into their revised hypothesis (Massad et al 1979). Suggestion and faith which are often enmeshed can play a crucial role in pain relief (Langley et al 1984, Plotkin 1985). Simple experiments can provide insight into this phenomenon. One small 'experiment' which helps to illustrate how easily we are influenced by suggestion and by words is described in the appendix.

Choosing words

Helpful words
In the field of pain management and physiotherapy the issues relate to wellbeing and quality of life. The issue is, do the words we use help that person to come to terms with their pain and get on with their life or do they have the reverse effect?
Metaphors can be a very useful way of explaining what is going on but they need to be used with care. Words and the images they evoke can be emotive. Great sensitivity therefore, needs to be used in their selection. It is important for the health professional to be in the habit of checking with the patient that they have understood the idea that was trying to be conveyed. The use of everyday words, when explaining the problem to the patient is important. For example, clearly explaining that chronic musculoskeletal pain is usually *not a sign of on-going tissue damage*, but may instead be due to *faulty processing in the brain and nerves* can be helpful. Particular *patterns of pain become ingrained* and are further reinforced

111

through habitual stimulation. *Expectation of pain becomes a habit. Patterns of avoidance behaviour become part of the person's life* and may actually be making matters worse. The suggestion that *there are many strategies that can be adopted to take control of the problem* may be of some help. For the chronic ache of arthritic condition the metaphor of a joint being *rusty* can be useful. This then allows the person to understand how gentle movement can be important and that rest and inactivity may make things worse. The concept of improving *lubrication* to the joint through movement can also be helpful and is supported by our knowledge of the secretion of synovial fluid during movements.

Harmful words

It is clear that language is not neutral. Health professionals often use words that are enshrined in idiosyncratic jargon. These words can create fear and can frequently be the source of misunderstandings as noted by Bedell et al (2004). These are words that harm. It seems that harmful language is very common and Bedell (Bedell et al 2004) cites an example from her own experience in the field of cardiology. She refers to a person who has just had a heart attack and finds himself in a coronary care unit. He is having to face mortality, noting every beep on a heart monitor, wondering if it might be his last and then the doctor comes in and announces *you have the type of lesion we call a widow maker!* Or another patient is told *you are living on borrowed time.* Then some of these patients are informed that they need cardiac surgery to see if *the dangerous anatomy* can be corrected.

Phrases that are poorly chosen can have a harmful effect on the patient, will not be forgotten and may be difficult to erase from that person's mind. Helpful words can allow that person to get on with their lives. A person who is concerned about their chronic musculoskeletal condition and its consequences may develop selective attention to words he hears. He may then misconstrue words which would under different circumstances seem quite harmless, to now convey a threatening message.

Techniques for ensuring common understanding

Any form of communication relies on a 'transmitter', a 'receiver' and the 'ether' between the two. The quality of the communication will depend on how the message is transmitted, how the ether interferes with the message and how 'tuned in' the receiver is. So the message may become distorted for a number of reasons often unbeknown to the transmitter. See figure 1.

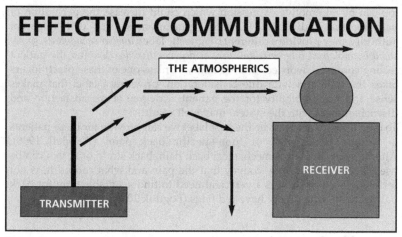

Figure 1

Using Labels effectively

People expect a health professional such as a physiotherapist to provide a diagnosis or a label to explain their pain. However, in musculoskeletal pain this can be a minefield with different practitioners using different labels. It is widely accepted that 90% or more of back pain is best described as non-specific low back pain which can be further sub-divided into acute, sub-acute and chronic back pain. Many other attempts have been made to classify back pain into more specific homogenous groups. Individual practitioners have their own system of classifying and labelling problems such as back pain. This in itself is probably one of the reasons why back pain has continued to result in so much disability. Although usually a self-limiting problem, it is acknowledged that its course is very variable and that recurrences are frequent (Croft et al 1998). However, there seems to be a lack of any consensus on diagnostic terms to describe patients who do not have any serious pathology especially for a patient with 'non-specific low back pain (Bogduk 2000).

Commonly used terms to describe back pain may cause distress. If a patient is told they have *wear and tear* it may be interpreted by some as a problem that needs to be very carefully looked after and that any unnecessary physical activity certainly needs to be avoided. Any movement that is associated with pain may be perceived as adding to the wear and tear. Similarly, the term *arthritis* may be misunderstood and confused with a progressive inflammatory condition such as rheumatoid arthritis. It is therefore incumbent on the practitioner to carefully explain what these terms mean. Equally the label *slipped disc* can conjure up a frightening picture. The individual may believe that if they make the wrong movement the disc will slip out. What about the term *trapped nerve*? It seems that this too can be an emotive expression which could increase the perception of pain for that individual. Different practitioners, each with apparent authority, may provide a different diagnostic label: *lumbar spondylosis, spinal stenosis, prolapsed intervertebral disc, or degenerative disc* leaving the patient feeling confused, worried and/or angry. Unless one of these practitioners takes the time and with due consideration, provides a label that makes sense and has credibility for the patient, a degree of dissatisfaction and disenchantment with the system may well result.

To date it seems that maybe the best label we can provide for these patients is 'simple back pain', or 'non-specific back pain' (Waddell 1998). Alternatively, the terms mechanical back pain, back strain or sprain can be used since (at least) they convey that the pain and what caused it, is not serious. It seems there is a very real need to find a suitable term for back pain patients who do not have red flags (Bogduk 2000).

Shared Understanding

One important challenge of an effective consultation is to achieve a shared understanding of beliefs regarding the nature and cause of the presenting problem, the reason for the patient to attend the consultation, a form of intervention that is acceptable to both physiotherapist and patient, expectations regarding prognosis, desired goals and need for follow up. Such congruence appears to influence the rehabilitation of patients with back pain by helping them to accept their condition, reducing perceived disability, and increasing the likelihood of returning to work (Cedraschi et al 1996, Peebles & Moore 2000).

Shared understanding can be harder to achieve in pain-based assessments, possibly due to the inherent differences in professional and patient's estimation of pain intensity (Solomon 2001). This is due to differences in attitude and beliefs (Daykin 2002). As values and beliefs can be subtly communicated to the patient through the words that we use (Klaber Moffett & Richardson 1997), it is important to recognise how detrimental it can be to a patient's recovery if they perceive that their physiotherapist is underestimating their symptom burden.

It has been suggested that by using words which reflect the patient's illness schemata or visual image of their problem, the health professional is more likely to achieve a situation in which both patient and professional share an understanding (Peebles & Moore 2000). Words that detract from this goal need to be avoided. These could be words which might inhibit the patient's narrative, those which lack attention to cues and clues, and those which emphasise any differences in understanding of the cause of the problem (Zoppi & Epstein 2002).

Patients want health professionals to listen attentively to what they have to say. A physiotherapist spends approximately one quarter of the working day listening to patients, however Conine (Conine 1976) suggests that unless we are trained, it is only possible to concentrate for 25% of that time. It seems that the distinguishing factor in expert physical therapy practice is the use of active listening skills to derive knowledge from patients (Jensen et al 2000; Resnik & Jensen 2003).

Active listening can include a number of techniques that need to be practised. These are repeating key phrases or expressions from the patient's testimony or forming questions based on patient's comments to elicit more information or to clarify a point. This needs to be done sensitively to avoid an impression of patronisation.

During the course of a consultation, assumptions tend to be made by both patient and professional regarding the interpretation of the information provided (Entwistle et al 1998). Understanding is subjective, and depends upon personal feelings, past experience and habits. There are few words which carry a common meaning even within the same culture (Conine 1976). A study carried out in a rheumatology clinic showed that patients who had just left the doctor's office often had an understanding of the explanation that they had just received that differed markedly from what the doctor thought he had said (Daltroy et al 1993). It is therefore important to ensure that we check our interpretation of the patient's story, and, following discussions of treatment plans, invite the patient to share their understanding of the advice, which we have proffered.

Shared treatment goals and plans:

In order to satisfy patients' desire for more information and greater involvement in healthcare decisions, physiotherapists need to offer honest, unbiased information regarding the existence of legitimate choices and relative risks and benefits of the different interventions that are available (Richards 1999, Elwyn et al 2000). However, whilst some patients wish to have control over their healthcare we need to respect the fact that others will prefer the physiotherapist to make decisions on their behalf (Payton et al 1998). It requires skill to determine whether a patient wishes to be involved in decisions, without coercing them against their will (Waterworth & Luker 1990). Patients may have unrealistic expectations and goals (McGregor & Hughes 2002, Arntz & Claassens 2004). Negotiating with the patient in order to agree upon mutually acceptable treatment plans and goals is another skill which includes the careful choice of words. Studies by Payton and colleagues (Payton & Nelson 1996; Payton et al 1998) have highlighted the fact that physiotherapists are not always consistent in their attempts to reflect the patient's views when setting treatment goals.

The judicious use of open questions followed up where necessary with specific questions can help patients to elicit their expectations of physiotherapy. This then provides a basis for the physiotherapist to discuss what would form achievable treatment goals.

Teaching Good Communication Skills

The question has sometimes been asked: "Is it possible to teach communication skills?" (Walker 1996, Skelton & Hobbs 1999). In the clinical situation, good communication skills are known to have positive benefits for both clinicians and patients (Walker 1996, Fallowfield et al 2002, Maguire & Pitceathly 2002, Fallowfield et al 2003).

Maguire (Maguire & Pitceathly 2002) also highlights well used and tested teaching methods that can improve clinician's communication skills. These are noted below:
- The clinician needs to be provided with evidence of current deficits in their communication skills, reasons for these and consequences for both patients and clinicians.
- They require evidence-based information regarding the skills needed to overcome these deficits.
- It is helpful to demonstrate the skills required and elicit clinician's reactions to these.
- Enable them to practice these skills under controlled and safe conditions.
- Give constructive feedback on their performance with reflections about any deficits.

Maguire (Maguire & Pitceathly 2002) suggests that these methods can be effectively implemented by ensuring that training programmes include three main areas of activity: Cognitive input, detailed handouts and/or short lectures regarding evidence-based information on effective communication skills and how to remedy deficiencies.

Modelling
Skills should be demonstrated in action. Audio/videotapes of real consultations should be used. A 'simulated' patient can be used with a trainer to demonstrate key skills. This is done in conjunction with the trainees who offer suggestions regarding strategies to use, etc. The 'patient' can also give feedback to confirm or refute the trainee's views.

Practicing Key Skills
Trainees need to practice the skills and receive constructive feedback. Using simulated patients, or actors, has the advantage of enabling a certain

simulate typical patients that they know. It is very helpful to give feedback by audio/video tape, as this enables detailed comments to be made about each part of the interview, which is accurately reproduced.

Teaching physiotherapists communication skills

Other health professionals such as doctors, nurses and clinical psychologists are taught and spend considerable time practising learnt communication skills. They regularly use role-play and videotapes of role-play to allow feedback to help them rapidly improve these skills during their training. In fact for medical students this is now a core part of the curriculum and they cannot qualify without passing assessments in consultation skills. Why is it that physiotherapists do not also get taught these skills during their undergraduate training? It may be that physiotherapists see themselves as reliant more on physical tests and techniques. Also it may be that they consider themselves good communicators. This may well be true, however, the issue for each of us is can we improve this very complex skill in order to become more effective practitioners. 'Can good interview skills be taught?' Two randomised controlled trials have sought to answer this question (Fallowfield et al 2002, Maguire & Piceathly 2002), largely incorporating the methods and contents described above. They encouragingly found that training could be effective in improving doctors' communication skills. All the issues discussed here apply equally to all clinicians and their interactions with patients and there is every reason to expect that these same strategies will be effective in the training of physiotherapists. This is especially the case as physiotherapists, over recent years, have become much more aware of the need for a biopsychosocial approach to clinical practice.

In a recent randomised controlled trial, evaluating the effectiveness of a brief physiotherapy intervention based on a cognitive-behavioural approach compared to 'usual' physiotherapy (Klaber Moffett et al 2005), physiotherapists were trained to use enhanced communication skills for delivery of the brief intervention arm of the study. Many of the techniques discussed above were employed to deliver an intensive one-day communication training programme. This involved giving evidence-based information on the importance of good communication skills and interview technique and the use of role-play, where trainees interviewed other trainees who simulated patient behaviour (vignettes provided). Video presentations of simulated interviews were used and, after presentation of these, the group were encouraged to discuss their views on problems they identified and possible solutions.

As the physiotherapists were obliged to deliver two different interventions for the study, Usual Physiotherapy (UP) and a Brief Intervention (BI), a monitoring exercise was carried out to attempt to evaluate the effectiveness of this training programme. This was to establish if the training actually caused them to behave differently when using the BI approach compared to their usual UP approach and also to determine if there was any 'contamination' effect over a period of time, i.e. as the physiotherapists used both techniques, did the UP approach gradually include more of the techniques incorporated into the BI approach as time passed?

The monitoring exercise indicated that physiotherapists delivering the BI appeared to include more components of the cognitive-behavioural approach compared with when they delivered the UP approach. They also appeared to be able to switch from one treatment approach to the other whilst maintaining the difference. This was maintained even twelve months after training.

This exercise suggests that a one-day interactive training package designed to help physiotherapists deliver a Brief Intervention based on cognitive-behavioural principles by improving their communication skills can be effective. The training was delivered within the context of a clinical trial, and the exercise was limited to observing only a few physiotherapists (n = 8), therefore these findings may only be cautiously generalised to the normal clinical situation.

However, these results support the findings of the literature discussed above and should encourage physiotherapists to seriously consider making it a priority to improve their own communication skills. This can be achieved and, as discussed, will not only contribute to improving the effectiveness of physiotherapy intervention, but will also benefit the physiotherapist with increased job satisfaction and decreased tendency to emotional burnout.

Conclusions

The use of advanced communication skills by health professionals in consultations with patients with pain, is one that deserves much more attention. It is an art which like playing the violin can only be improved with practice. Most physiotherapists have good communication skills but might be more effective in their daily practice if they were trained and practised using enhanced techniques. Research is needed to help physiotherapists find suitable labels to provide to patients with non-specific low back pain. Also research is needed to find out how communication skills can be effectively taught to physiotherapists. To date we know that some words can help whereas others can harm.

References

Arntz A, Claassens L 2004 The meaning of pain influences its experienced intensity. Pain 109:20-25

Austen F, Polise M et al 1997 The use of verbal expectancy in reducing pain associated with arterotomies. American Journal of Clinical Hypnosis 39:182-186

Barry CA, Bradley CP et al 2000 Patients' unvoiced agendas in general practice consultations: qualitative study. BMJ 320(7244):1246-1250

Barry CA, Stevenson FA et al 2001 Giving voice to the lifeworld. More humane, more effective medical care? A qualitative study of doctor-patient communication in general practice. Soc Sci Med 53(4):487-505

Bedell SE, Graboys TB et al 2004 Words that harm, words that heal. Arch Intern Med 164(13):1365-1368

Bogduk N 2000 What's in a name? The labelling of back pain. Australian Journal of Medicine 173:400-401

Bultman DC, Svarstad BL 2000 Effects of physician communication style on client medication beliefs and adherence with antidepressant treatment. Patient Educ Couns 40(2):173-185

Cedraschi CJ Robert et al 1996 The role of congruence between patient and therapist in chronic low back pain. Journal of manipulative and physiological therapeutics 19(4):244-249

Conine TA 1976 Listening in the helping relationship. Physical Therapy 56(2):159-162

Croft P, Macfarlane G et al 1998 Outcome of low back pain in general practice: a propective study. British Medical Journal 316:1356-1359

Daltroy L, Iversen M et al 1993 Teaching and Social Support: Effects on Knowledge, Attitudes, and Behaviours to Prevent Low Back Injuries in Industry. Health Education Quarterly 20(1):43-62

Daykin AR 2002 A mixed methods study regarding Physiotherapist's pain beliefs and their influence on the therapeutic encounter. PhD thesis. Norwich, University of East Anglia: 333

Deyo RA, Rainville J et al 1992 What can the history and physical examination tell us about low back pain? JAMA 268(6):760-765

DiMatteo MR 2004 The role of effective communication with children and their families in fostering adherence to pediatric regimens. Patient Educ Couns 55(3): 339-344

Edwards A, Elwyn G et al 2001 Consumers' views of quality in the consultation and their relevance to 'shared decision-making' approaches. Health Expect 4 (3):151-161

Elwyn G, Edwards A et al 2000 Shared decision making and the concept of equipoise: the competences of involving patients in healthcare choices. Br J Gen Pract 50(460):892-899

Entwistle V, Sowden AJ et al 1998 Evaluating interventions to promote patient involvement in decision-making: by what criteria should effectiveness be judged? Journal of health service research and policy 3(2):100-107

Entwistle V, Watt I et al 2002 Exploring patient participation in decision-making. Health in Partnership. Aberdeen, University of Aberdeen

Health in Partnership. Aberdeen, University of Aberdeen

Fallowfield L, Jenkins V 1999 Effective communication skills are the key to good cancer care. Eur J Cancer 35(11):1592-1597

Fallowfield L, Jenkins V et al 2002 Efficacy of a Cancer Research UK communication skills training model for oncologists: a randomised controlled trial. Lancet 359(9307):650-656

Fallowfield L, Jenkins V et al 2003 Enduring impact of communication skills training: results of a 12-month follow-up. Br J Cancer 89(8):1445-1449

Flor H, Birbaumer N et al 1990 The Psychobiology of Chronic Pain. Adv Behav Res Ther 12:47-84

Jeffels K, Foster N 2003 Can aspects of physiotherapist communication influence patients' pain experiences? A systematic review. Physical Therapy Reviews 8: 197-210

Jensen GM, Shepard KF et al 1990 The novice versus the experienced clinician: insights into the work of the physical therapist. Phys Ther 70(5):314-323

Jensen GM, Gwyer J et al 2000 Expert practice in physical therapy. Physical Therapy 80:28-52

Kersten P, George S et al 2000 Disabled people and professionals differ in their perceptions of rehabilitation needs. J Public Health Med 22(3):393-399

Klaber Moffett J, Richardson P 1997 The influence of the physiotherapist-patient relationship on pain and disability. Physiotherapy Theory & Practice 13:89-96

Klaber Moffett JA, Jackson DA et al 2005 Randomised Trial of a brief physiotherapy intervention compared with usual physiotherapy for neck pain patients: outcomes and patient preference. British Medical Journal 330(Jan 2005):75

Klein S, Tracy D et al 1999 The effects of the participation of patients with cancer in teaching communication skills to medical undergraduates: a randomised study with follow-up after 2 years. Eur J Cancer 35(10):1448-1456

Kumlin IW, Kroksmark T 1992 The first encounter. Physiotherapists' conceptions of establishing therapeutic relationships. Scand J Caring Sci 6(1):37-44

Langley G, Sheppeard H et al 1984 The analgesic effects of transcutaneous electrical nerve stimulation and placebo in chronic pain patients. Rheumatol Int 4:119-123

Little P, Everitt H et al 2001 Observational study of effect of patient centredness and positive approach on outcomes of general practice consultations. BMJ 323(7318): 908-911

Maguire P, Pitceathly C 2002 Key communication skills and how to acquire them. BMJ 325(7366):697-700

Martin LR, Jahng KH et al 2003 Physician facilitation of patient involvement in care: Correspondence between patient and observer reports. Behavioural medicine 28(4):159-164

Massad C, Hubbard M et al 1979 Selective perception of events. Journal of Experimental Social Psychology 15:513-532

McGregor A, Hughes S 2002 The Evaluation of the Surgical Management of Nerve Root Compression in Patients with Low Back Pain Part 1: The Assessment of Outcome. Spine 27(13):1465-1470

Office for Public Management 2000 "Shifting Gears" Towards a 21st Century NHS. Office for Public Management, London:66

Ong LM, de Haes JC et al 1995 Doctor-patient communication: a review of the literature. Soc Sci Med 40(7):903-918

Pascalis Vd, Chiaradia C et al 2002 The contribution of suggestibility and expectation to placebo analgesia phenomenon in an experimental setting. Pain 96:393-402

Payton OD, Nelson CE 1996 A preliminary study of patients' perceptions of certain aspects of their physical therapy experience. Physiotherapy theory and practice 12:27-38

Payton OD, Nelson CE et al 1998 Physical therapy patients' perceptions of their relationships with health care professionals. Physiotherapy theory and practice 14:211-221

Peebles JE Moore RJ 2000 Illness schemata in patients with low back pain: predictions of rehabilitation success. Pain clinic 12(3):237-246

Pennebaker J 1982 The Psychology of Physical Symptoms. Springer-Verlag, New York

Plotkin W 1985 A psychological approach to placebo: the role of faith in therapy and treatment. In: White L, Tursky B, Schwartz G (Eds). Placebo. Theory, research, and mechanisms. Guildford Press: 237-254

Potter M, Grove J 1999 Mental skills training during rehabilitation case studies of injured athletes. New Zealand Journal of Physiotherapy 27:24-31

Resnik L, Jensen GM 2003 Using clinical outcomes to explore the theory of expert practice in physical therapy. Phys Ther 83(12):1090-1106

Richards T 1999 Patients priorities. British Medical Journal 318:277

Ryan S, Hassell A et al 2003 Control perceptions in patients with rheumatoid arthritis: the impact of the medical consultation. Rheumatology (Oxford) 42(1):135-140

Skelton J, Pennebaker J 1982 The psychology of physical symptoms and sensations. In: Sanders G, Suls J (Eds) Social Psychology of Health and Illness. Lawrence Erlbaum Associates, New Jersey

Skelton JR, Hobbs FD 1999 Descriptive study of cooperative language in primary care consultations by male and female doctors. BMJ 318(7183):576-579

Solomon P 2001 Congruence between health professionals' and patients' pain ratings: a review of the literature. Scand J Caring Sci 15(2):174-180

Staats P, Hekmat H et al 1998 Suggestion/placebo effects on pain:negative as well as positive. Journal of Pain and Symptom Mangement 15:235-243

Stacey R, Spencer J 1999 Patients as teachers ;a qualitative study of patients' views on their role in a community-based undergraduate project. Medical education 33: 688-694

Stewart MA 1995 Effective physician-patient communication and health outcomes: a review. Cmaj 152(9):1423-1433

Stewart MA, McWhinney IR et al 1979 The doctor/patient relationship and its effect upon outcome. Journal of the Royal College of General Practitioners 29(199):77-81

Swain J 1997 Counselling and the use of counselling skills. In: French S (Ed) Physiotherapy. A psychosocial approach.. Butterworth Heinemann, Oxford

Swain J 2004 Interpersonal communication. In: French S, Sim J (Eds) Physiotherapy: A psychosocial approach. Butterworth Heinemann, Edinburgh

121

Turner P, Whitfield T 1997 Physiotherapists' use of evidence based practice: a cross-national study. Physiotherapy Research International 2(1):17-29

Turner P, Whitfield T 1999 Physiotherapists' report for selection of treatment techniques: A cross-national survey. Physiotherapy Theory and Practice 15:235-246

Waddell G 1998 The Back Pain Revolution. Churchill Livingstone, Edinburgh

Walker LG 1996 Communication skills: when, not if, to teach. Eur J Cancer 32A(9):1457-1459

Waterworth S Luker KA 1990 Reluctant collaborators: do patients want to be involved in decisions concerning care? J Adv Nurs 15(8):971-976

Williams S, Harrison K 1999 Physiotherapeutic interactions: A review of the power dynamic. Physical Therapy Reviews 4:37-50

Zoppi K, Epstein RM 2002 Is communication a skill? Communication behaviors and being in relation. Fam Med 34(5):319-324

Appendix

Pennebaker, (Pennebaker 1982) in a series of experiments, investigated psychological factors that influence the reporting of physical symptoms. He invited a series of subjects to run on a treadmill for 5 minutes and asked them afterwards to report in detail on any physical symptoms that they experienced. Subjects in the experimental group were told by the researcher, in an apparently a casual comment, that *there are currently a lot of flu bugs around and that lots of people had mentioned that they thought they were getting flu.* The outcome of the study was that students in the control group, that is those who had not heard any mention of flu bugs, said that they found the exercise made them warm, made their heart beat more rapidly, and made their legs feel slightly tired. The experimental group, however, thought that these sensations or physical symptoms were probably due to the fact that they were probably coming down with a flu bug.

With this experiment in mind we decided to try out a similar procedure on physiotherapists to see whether suggestion could have an impact on our own colleagues. The idea behind this was that our selection of words as physiotherapists might have a considerable impact on our patients and we thought that a simple experiment might go some way to testing this hypothesis.

More specifically our hypothesis was that:
- Subjects in Group B, who had been told that the activity might result in some unpleasant symptoms, would report these symptoms, while subjects in Group A would not report such symptoms.
- Subjects in Group B would be less likely to complete the 2 minutes running on the spot without stopping, compared to Group A.

We invited a group of physiotherapists (n=34) attending a study day on chronic pain to participate in a small experiment. We explained what would be expected of them so that anyone who did not wish to take part could decline to participate. We gave them all the following instructions:

Run as hard you can, trying to get your knees up to waist level for 2 minutes.

We will time you by calling out every 15 seconds that pass. If you have to stop please make a note of the time called out immediately before you stop.

You will be split up into 2 groups called A and B.
It is important you remember which you are allocated to.

Once they were in their separate rooms, Group A and Group B were given a set of written instructions, which differed slightly.

Running experiment: Instructions to GROUP A

Try to keep running as hard you can for 2 minutes.

You will probably not find this too difficult. Just do the best you can.

You may feel your heart beating more strongly and may feel quite warm.

It is possible that your legs may begin to ache by the end but this is not surprising if you have not been exercising regularly. In the unlikely event that you have to stop before the 2 minutes has ended please note the time called out immediately before you stopped.

Running experiment: Instructions to GROUP B

Try to keep running as hard you can for 2 minutes.

You may find this more difficult than you thought. Two minutes is in fact quite a long time to keep going without a stop.

You may feel your heart racing and you may feel you are overheating.

It is possible that your legs may begin to ache so you may feel the need to stop before the end of the 2 minutes. If you do please note the time that was called out immediately before you stopped.

At the end of this intervention they were all asked to complete the following questionnaire.

We would like to know how you coped with the experience.
Please circle the **relevant response.**

Did you keep running for the whole 2 minutes?   YES / NO
If NO how long did you keep running for ? ....

Physical sensations to report:

1   Breathing: Was it comfortable or uncomfortable?

2   Heart rate: faster but not unexpected or faster than I would have liked?

3   Legs : Healthy ache or unpleasant ache?

4   Overall difficulty: Not very difficult or rather difficult?

5   Overall discomfort: not comfortable or rather uncomfortable?

The results of the study

No participants in Group A (n=13) reported any concerns/difficulty or discomfort related to any symptoms on the checklist. In Group B (n=23) where the potential difficulty of the intervention was emphasised prior to it being carried out, 15 out of 23 participants afterwards reported physical symptoms as concern/difficulty associated with carrying it out. Most of these were related to breathing and heart rate. 11 out of 23 reported concern at the discomfort/overall difficulty of the exercise.

Although we did not carry out any statistical analysis on this data, the findings seem to clearly support our first hypothesis that Group B would be more likely to report symptoms/difficulties than Group A.

However, our results do not support our second hypothesis, since all our participants continued to run for the full 2 minutes although they might have chosen to stop. There are at least two possible confounding factors here. One is that it may have simply been such an easy task that even the most unfit physiotherapist could manage it relatively easily. Secondly, possibly peer pressure, that is carrying out the exercise in a group situation, may have encouraged participants to keep going even if they would have preferred to stop.

7

Do investigations reassure patients and health professionals?

PENNY MORTIMER

Over recent years health professionals have become familiar with the concept of the biopsychosocial approach to the management of pain, with its encouragement to move away from the uni-dimensional medical model. However, we live in a technological world, and recognise that investigations will continue to play their part in pain management. Indeed, physiotherapists, in their rapidly developing extended roles, are now often responsible for requesting such investigations. This chapter, using low back pain (LBP) as an example, explores the guidelines for investigations, and the clinical dilemmas that may exist. It goes on to consider the difficulties in formulating an acceptable explanation for the cause of LBP, and finally suggests how decisions about investigations, and results of investigations, may be best handled with patients, in order to address their concerns, and encourage rehabilitation.

Guidelines for investigations

The Clinical Guidelines for the Management of Acute Low Back Pain from the Royal College of General Practitioners (RCGP 1996, 1999), provide clear evidence based guidance on management. They suggest that early management should take place within primary care, for the majority of acute LBP patients. Initially, this should involve reassurance and judicious administration of medication by the GP, coupled with advice on activity modification. Physiotherapy should be considered for further help with rehabilitation, if progress is not being made after a few weeks.

During this time, secondary referral is only recommended where there are particular concerns that the clinical signs and symptoms may be indicative of serious spinal pathology, or severe nerve root problems. If after three months, however, symptoms are still not settling, and improvement in function is not being made, secondary referral is then encouraged.

The Clinical Standards Advisory Group (CSAG 1994) on Back Pain suggested that secondary referral may be made to a doctor, or a specialist physiotherapist, and states that the role of this intervention is to provide a full biopsychosocial assessment. It goes on to say that if serious spinal pathology is clinically suspected from the presence of "red flags", then blood-screening tests and diagnostic imaging, using x-rays and magnetic resonance imaging (MRI) scans will be important. In cases where no serious spinal pathology is suspected, but clinical examination reveals objective signs of nerve root compression, then it is suggested that MRI scans can provide useful information to aid surgical decisions. The guidance is clear, however, that for simple LBP, where "red flags" or signs of nerve root compression are not present, such investigations are specifically **not** recommended.

This guidance is based on the fact that the Royal College of Radiologists (RCR) have stated that LBP, without corresponding clinical indicators, correlates poorly with the degenerative change routinely found on x-rays and scans, and that such findings should be seen as normal age related changes rather than as relevant pathology. (RCR 1993,1999). The CSAG report goes on to say that these high false positive rates, due to normal age related changes, mean that patients with simple LBP are not suitable for diagnostic imaging since these findings are likely to confuse, rather than clarify, the situation for them. This is supported by the work of Jensen et al (1994) who showed that, of 98 people **without** LBP who volunteered to have an MRI scan, only 36% had so-called normal discs at every level, with about half having at least one bulging disc, and about a quarter having at least one disc protrusion.

Dilemmas about investigations

Therefore the guidelines on the use of investigations appear clear. In the clinical setting, however, other pressures exist that may make it more difficult to follow these guidelines. Health professionals, particularly in this age of litigation, perhaps feel the need for the reassurance of investigation, rather than relying solely on their clinical skills. While it is known that findings from MRI scans may not be clear about the cause of simple LBP, they are considered to be one of the most sensitive tests for identifying serious spinal pathology, such as cancer and infection.

Therefore their use, as shown by a review of the diagnostic accuracy of imaging (Jarvik & Deyo 2002), may reassure clinicians that they will be seen as having done all they can to exclude these conditions.

Patients and their families may also have concerns about serious spinal pathology, and want this reassurance. In addition, they are likely to want a clear explanation for the cause of the pain, and believe that tests, such as MRI scans, will show this. This demand may have been fuelled, historically, by the way the medical management of LBP has developed, with its emphasis on the identification of a structural fault, which Waddell (1995, p595) described as part of "the twentieth century health care disaster".

However, a definitive treatable cause for LBP, such as a herniated disc, metastatic cancer or infection, frequently does not exist. It is known that, for an estimated 85% of cases, the symptoms cannot be explained by findings of a specific, anatomical or physiological nature (Spitzer et al 1987). Therefore the most medically accurate diagnostic label that can be assigned, following an MRI scan, may be non-specific LBP (Fordyce 1995), but this may be an extremely difficult concept for a clinician to convey in an acceptable way to a patient, who is distressed by continuing pain, and whose work and home life is severely disrupted.

In the broader context of social theory, Mechanic (1977) observed that humans dislike uncertainty and will constantly strive to make sense of information in order to achieve a feeling of control. Therefore, when patients believe something is wrong, and feel there is a lack of an acceptable explanation, it is likely this inconsistency will result in a sense of dissatisfaction. Thus it is necessary to provide a satisfying explanation in order to resolve this conflict in thinking. This is particularly so because it has been recorded that patients, who are not satisfied with the explanation for their pain, may find it difficult to enter wholeheartedly into the rehabilitation process. (Burton et al 1995). Physiotherapists understand more than most, therefore, how crucial it is that this issue is successfully addressed.

Explaining the cause of LBP

The Clinical Standards Advisory Group (CSAG 1994) suggests that:

> *"information should be designed to reduce apprehension, and encourage progressive mobilisation and rehabilitation" p58*

It recommends that explanations should be given to patients about the structure and function of the back, to provide understanding and reassurance. Care should be taken that, while acknowledging the difficulties the patient is experiencing, descriptions are given in a reassuring form that satisfy the patient's need for information, but do not provoke unhelpful, inappropriate fears that may hinder successful rehabilitation. However, qualitative studies of patient satisfaction have continued to record significant dissatisfaction levels specifically with the explanation given to patients for their LBP (Skelton et al 1996). This dissatisfaction has been shown to be associated with a wish for more diagnostic tests to provide reassurance and validation of their experience of pain (Osborn & Smith 1998).

Validation has been cited as an intrinsic part of patient reassurance, but uncertainty of medical findings may prevent this from occurring (Donovan & Blake 2000). Rhodes et al (1999) recognised the potential *"power of the visible"* in achieving this. In their study they illustrate the validation felt by one patient:

> *"They ran some tests and that's when they realised that my whole spine was kitty catty womper"* (Rhodes et al 1999, p1194)

On the face of it, therefore, it may seem a helpful outcome if the patient feels validated by the findings on an MRI scan, but physiotherapists may feel concerned that the apparent validation may also have left this patient with unhelpful beliefs about the integrity of his spine, and that this could result in fearful avoidance of activity when it comes to rehabilitation.

Clinicians may intuitively feel that giving patients a diagnostic test will provide reassurance, with a resultant improvement in satisfaction with explanation, and ultimately, with outcome. Nevertheless, randomised controlled trials using interventions of x-ray and MRI scans, have demonstrated only small signs of increased satisfaction with care, with no associated improvements in psychosocial and physical outcome measures (Jarvik et al 1997, Kendrick et al 2001, Kerry et al 2000). Rhodes et al (1999) point out that failure of tests to identify a clear cause may result in patients feeling anxious, and the apparent lack of validation of their pain may provoke dissatisfaction and indeed, alienation in certain individuals, who may feel they are not believed.

With these conflicting findings in mind, a local study (Mortimer 2001) collected retrospective, quantitative and qualitative data, from 61 patients on their views about MRI scans. All the subjects had attended a joint rheumatology and orthopaedic back clinic run by a physiotherapist, working as an extended scope practitioner (ESP). It was hoped that this knowledge would help to develop ways of achieving best practice in terms of decision-making and explanations for LBP.

Of these 61 patients, 37 had been scanned, and the decisions for this had been in strict accordance with the criteria of the Royal College of Radiologists (RCR 1993, 1999). It happened that none of the patients exhibited any "red flags" for possible serious spinal pathology, but those scanned all had **non improving** signs and symptoms of nerve root compression, at least three months after onset. i.e. patients described symptoms extending below the knee, and objective tests revealed neural deficit. All scanned patients were shown their scans and given explanations that, it was hoped, would both reassure them, and satisfy their need for information.

The results showed that the recorded level of patient concern that serious spinal pathology might be present was higher than expected, with 29 (47.5%) of patients indicating some concern about the possibility of a life threatening condition before the clinic, and 18 (31.6%) still recording some concern following the clinic. It had been anticipated that the patients who had received an MRI scan would be significantly more reassured than those who did not, but this was **not** found to be the case.

The findings perhaps show that such concern could be greater amongst patients than clinicians generally perceive or expect. It may be that clinicians' own low concern about the possibility of life threatening pathology due to the lack of "red flags", and their trust in the findings of MRI scans, leads to an under-estimation of the fears patients may have, and consequently of the measures that may be needed to address those fears (McDonald et al 1996).

The patients who had received an MRI scan did record a significantly higher level of satisfaction with the decisions made about investigations needed, but receiving an MRI scan was **not** found to be significantly associated with being satisfied with explanations for LBP. Therefore, the findings of this study would appear to support those of the previous randomised controlled trials which failed to find high levels of satisfaction with care, or improvements in outcome, associated with the receipt of an MRI scan.

In order to gain more insight into the reasons behind the findings, the qualitative section of the study asked patients to comment on aspects of their care that had particularly satisfied or dissatisfied them. In some cases the findings of the MRI scans did appear to give reassurance and validation.

> *"The thorough examination and having the MRI scan."*
> *"The MRI offered concrete proof something was wrong."*

However, in other cases the failure of an MRI scan to identify a recognised cause for the pain appeared to result in some patients feeling embarrassed or alienated.

"I feel almost guilty that nothing was found on my scan."
"As far as you are concerned there is nothing wrong."

From further review of the quantitative data it seemed that the patients expressing such views about the lack of conclusiveness of the scan were also likely to be recording that their symptoms were still not improving, and therefore the lack of validation from the scan results was particularly upsetting.

Although the 24 patients who did **not** receive an MRI scan were **not** significantly less satisfied with the explanations for their LBP, they were less satisfied with the decisions made about the investigations needed. However, only two of them commented on the wish for further tests in the qualitative sections.

"I would have liked an x-ray or scan to put my mind at rest."
"Find the cause with a scan."

Perhaps these comments reflect the faith that people have in the power of technology. Yet in the field of cardiology, a study of patients with heart murmurs, who were all shown on echocardiography (ECG) to have a normal heart, showed that 50% had residual anxiety following the test (McDonald et al 1996). So again, the failure of technology to explain and validate the clinical findings caused problems of its own. In the discussion it was noted that cardiology consultants had the skills to make a clinical judgement about an innocent murmur, without recourse to further diagnostic investigations, and it was suggested that this expert decision, coupled with an appropriate explanation, may be more reassuring for patients than having to cope with the confusion that may be provoked by a normal test result.

In summary then it may be said that:

- Investigations for LBP are recommended in specific clinical situations.
- Investigations are not recommended for simple LBP.
- In this age of litigation, clinicians may wish for reassurance about serious pathology, and may feel that MRI scans can provide them with this reassurance.

- Patients may wish for reassurance about serious pathology but perhaps are not as reassured as the clinicians by the results of the investigation.
- Patients who are content with explanations for their pain may feel validated in terms of the cause, but may also be fearful of activity because of the perceived seriousness of the cause.
- Patients who are not content with explanations for their pain may also be fearful of activity, but may also feel embarrassed or alienated.
- Good clinical and communication skills may provide better reassurance than tests.

Clearly patients with specific clinical presentations will continue to have investigations, and need sensitive interpretation of clinically significant and clinically insignificant findings. Patients without these specific clinical presentations will not need investigations, but will need acceptable explanations for their pain, and for the decision not to arrange further tests. It has been said that the ability to satisfy and reassure a patient depends on first knowing what concerns they may have, and being sure to address those directly, e.g. fears about life threatening conditions (Donovan & Blake, 2000).

So how do we ensure that we are giving the patient the best chance of being reassured, whether or not investigations are part of their care?

- By discussing with patients the reasoning behind decisions about investigations.
- By discussing the likely findings **prior** to investigations so that descriptions like "degenerative changes" will not be worrying.
- By recognising that there is no clear evidence that doing more investigations necessarily results in greater reassurance for the patient.
- By instilling the patient with confidence in our expertise and explanations.
- By instilling the patient with confidence that we appreciate the degree of their problem, even when investigation results are inconclusive.
- By giving explanations that resonate with the patient.
- By giving explanations that are designed to reduce apprehension and encourage rehabilitation.

And how do we know if patients feel reassured?

We cannot be perfect, but hopefully bearing these ideas in mind will help. However it may still be useful to ask patients if there are any outstanding concerns, rather than just assuming that what we have said has hit the mark.

And how can health professionals feel reassured?

By ensuring that we gain the clinical skills to be confident in our own judgement.

References

Burton A, Tillotson KM, Main CJ, Hollis S 1995 Psychosocial predictors of outcome in acute and subchronic low back trouble. Spine 20:722-8

Clinical Standards Advisory Group 1994 Back Pain. London:HMSO

Donovan JL, Blake DR 2000 Qualitative study of interpretation of reassurance among patients attending rheumatology clinics: "just a touch of arthritis, doctor?" British Medical Journal 320:541-544

Fordyce WE (Ed) 1995 Back Pain in the Workplace: Management of Disability in Nonspecific Conditions. IASP Press, Seattle

Jarvik JG, Deyo RA 2002 Diagnostic evaluation of low back pain with emphasis on imaging. Annals of Internal Medicine 137:586-97

Jarvik JG, Maravilla KR, Haynor DR, Levitz M, Deyo RA 1997 Rapid MR imaging versus plain radiography in patients with low back pain: initial results of a randomised study. Radiology 204:447-54

Jensen MC, Brant-Zawadzki MN, Obuchowski N, Modic MT, Malkasian D, Ross JS 1994 Magnetic resonance imaging of the lumbar spine in people without back pain. The New England Journal of Medicine 331:69-73

Kendrick D, Fielding K, Bentley E, Kerslake R, Miller P, Pringle M 2001 Radiography of the lumbar spine in primary care patients with low back pain: randomised controlled trial. British Medical Journal 322:400-405

Kerry S, Hilton S, Patel S, Dundas D, Rink E, Lord J 2000 Routine referral for radiography of patients presenting with low back pain: is patients' outcome influenced by GP's referral for plain radiography? Health Technology Assessment. NCCHTA, 13665278, Vol 4: No20:110

McDonald IG, Daly J, Jelinek VM, Panetta F, Gutman JM 1996 Opening Pandora's box: the unpredictability of reassurance by a normal test result. British Medical Journal 313:329-332

Mechanic D 1977 Illness behaviour, social adaptation and the management of illness. Journal of Nervous and Mental Disorders 165:79-87

Mortimer PA 2001 What are the factors influencing patient satisfaction with explanations for low back pain? MSc Health Sciences, St George's Hospital Medical School, London University

Osborn M, Smith JA 1998 The personal experience of chronic benign lower back pain: An interpretative phenomenological analysis. British Journal of Health Psychology 3: 65-83

Rhodes LA, McPhillips-Tangum CA, Markham C, Klenk R 1999 The power of the visible: the meaning of diagnostic tests in chronic back pain. Social Science and Medicine 48:1189-1203

Royal College of General Practitioners 1996, 1999 Clinical Guidelines for the Management of Acute Low Back Pain. RCGP, London

Royal College of Radiologists 1993, 1999 Making the Best use of a Department of Radiology: Guidelines for Doctors. RCR, London

Skelton AM, Murphy EA, Murphy RJL, O'Dowd TC 1996 Patients' views of low back pain and its management in general practice. British Journal of General Practice 46:153-156

Spitzer W, LeBlanc F, Depuis M 1987 Scientific approach to the assessment and management of activity-related spinal disorders. Report of the Quebec Task Force on Spinal disorders, Spine 12:7S (European ed, Supplement 1)S1-S59

Waddell G 1995 Modern management of spinal disorders. Journal of Manipulative and Physiological Therapeutics 18:590-596

3

Return to Work

The subject of this section is vocational rehabilitation. The chapters primarily focus on the following aspects:

a) Returning people to work who are not working due to sickness, ill health or disability. These people may be employed, unemployed or may never have worked. The principles and practices discussed also apply to maintaining and helping people who are struggling in work.

b) Returning people to paid employment or self-employment. It is acknowledged that paid employment is not the only option and that it is not necessarily desirable or appropriate for everyone. Financial and social support is essential for those who can't work. The benefits system is discussed at length (chapter 11).

c) People who have non-cancer pain, low back pain and low back pain related disability. Much of the information is equally applicable to people with other physical or mental health conditions.

8

The Epidemiology and Costs of Sickness Absence and Unemployment

GAIL SOWDEN

This chapter will consider the epidemiology and costs of sickness absence and unemployment. Particular reference has been made to sickness absence and unemployment attributed to low back pain related disability. It will outline the size of the problem and the importance of addressing it.

Low back pain and sickness absence

At any given time, between 4.4% and 33.0% of the adult population suffers from low back pain (LBP) (Dionne 1999). Low back pain is the second most common medical reason for work loss in the United Kingdom (UK) (DWP 2002) and is responsible for about 12% of all sick days (CSAG 1994, CIPD 2004). Within four weeks after the onset of an acute pain episode, 74% of patients with LBP have resumed work and are no longer seeking health care (Spitzer et al 1987, Anderson 1999). Many, however, continue to experience symptoms, although, little is known about those who remain at work and who do not utilise health care services or seek financial compensation (Anderson 1999).

More problematic are the minority of patients who remain out of work after four weeks and who go on to have long-term pain and pain related disability (Waddell et al 2003). Between 10% and 27% of the total sickness absence (all causes) is accounted for by absences of more than 4 weeks (CIPD, 2004).

LBP is often recurrent (Von Korff 1994). Data on initial periods of sickness absence can therefore underestimate total work disability (Waddell 2004). A study involving United States workers discovered that over 60% had more then one episode of work loss and that approximately a third made one or more unsuccessful attempts to return to work (RTW) before being successful. A small proportion went onto receive early medical retirement, often having had repeated episodes of sickness absence (Waddell 2004).

'Presenteeism', sickness absence and unemployment attributed to LBP related disability have major financial implications, particularly as the majority of LBP episodes occur during the most productive years (Bigos et al 1986).

Costs associated with low back pain, 'presenteeism', sickness absence and unemployment

The Confederation of British Industry and Chartered Institute for Personnel and Development estimate that chronic LBP related disability costs £434/yr per employee (CBI & CIPD 2001). Indirect costs from chronic LBP related disability can be up to 1-2 times the direct costs (CBI & CIPD 2001), these include: medical bills, overtime, agency staff, recruitment and training of replacements, income protection premiums, medical retirement premiums and costs associated with litigation.

Sickness absence (all causes) results in significant costs to society (Dionne 1999). It cost the economy £11.6 billion in 2002 (NAO 2003, CBI 2003, CBI 2001, CIPD 2004). Approximately 40% of these costs are attributable to the long term sick (NAO 2003, CBI 2003, CBI 2001). Costs associated with decreased performance and productivity cannot just be attributed to sickness absence. According to the American Productivity Audit most of the pain-related lost productive time occurs while employees are at work and is in the form of reduced performance (Stewart et al 2003). 'Presenteeism' is increasingly being recognised as a significant problem, for individuals, employers and society (Aronsson et al 2000, Pickavance 2004, TUC 2004, Beatty & Fothergill 2004).

There are many non-financial costs associated with sickness absence. Remaining staff may have increased workloads, which can result in overtime, decreased productivity, poorer customer service and higher staff turnover (www.hse.gov.uk). Being short staffed can have a negative impact on morale. Employers can also suffer the loss or absence of qualified, skilled, experienced and job knowledgeable staff.

It is widely acknowledged that the probability of RTW diminishes with duration of time off work (Waddell 2004). Once a worker is off work for 4 to 12 weeks, they have a 10-40% (depending on the setting) risk of still being off work at one year. (Waddell & Burton 2000). Many people on long-term sick leave are at risk of losing their job, either on a voluntary or compulsory basis (James et al 2003). There is only a 50% chance of a person retaining his or her work after 6 months of sickness absence from back pain (BSRM 2000). Thirteen per cent of people not employed cited LBP as their reason for not working (ONS 1999).

Individuals on long-term sick leave and those who are unemployed due to LBP related disability experience financial costs in terms of loss of earnings and healthcare related costs. There are also less obvious personal costs. Sickness absence and work loss are associated with poor physical and mental health (Janlert 1997, Acheson, 1998). These in turn, can affect levels of function, quality of life, family and other relationships (Mayer et al 1986). Unemployment is associated with greater morbidity and mortality (Janlert 1997, Martikainen & Valkonen 1996).

Contrary to popular belief, work is generally good for us (Waddell & Burton 2004). "There is a clear need for training of all health professionals in understanding the importance of work to health, and the interrelationships between employment and health" (BSRM, 2003). In addition to a salary, employment can provide routine, structure, challenge and reward. It can also provide opportunities for the development of skills, self-esteem and social networks.

Health care costs

There are significant health care costs associated with LBP. Low back pain sufferers can undergo multiple surgical procedures and utilise the health care system repeatedly (Mayer et al 1986). Approximately 2% of adults with LBP are referred to a NHS physiotherapist and another 2.7% will consult privately with a physiotherapist, an osteopath or a chiropractor (Croft 1996, CSAG, 1994). £141 million is spent each year on General Practitioner (GP) consultations for back pain and £512 million for hospital care (inpatient, outpatient and emergency) (Maniadakis & Gray 2000). The direct annual healthcare costs for back pain are over £1.6 billion. This includes £1 billion spent every year on National Health Service (NHS) and community care services for LBP and the £565 million spent on private services (Maniadakis & Gray 2000).

Recent trends in Incapacity Benefits in the United Kingdom

Incapacity Benefit (IB) accounts for the majority of disability benefit claimants and overall expenditure in the United Kingdom (UK). Incapacity Benefit figures have illustrated some interesting trends over time, the number of people claiming IB for LBP as well as for all conditions has changed, as have the primary reasons cited for claiming it.

It is important to remember however; that IB figures reflect benefits paid rather then work loss per se. Most people who are off work with back pain do not receive IB while most of those on IB are not employed (Watson et al 1997).

In Britain, the income replacement benefit for many sick and disabled people of working age is IB. Incapacity Benefit is a non-means tested benefit paid to people who are incapable of work. For the first 28 weeks of sickness absence a claimant's General Practitioner will certify whether someone is capable of performing his or her own occupation. During this time most individuals will be in receipt of Statutory Sick Pay (SSP). After 28 weeks most claimants are required to undergo a strict medical test, the personal capability assessment, which is administered by Department for Works and Pensions (DWP) doctors. Providing they meet the qualifying conditions, Incapacity Benefit is paid once SSP has ended or if the individual is unable to get SSP in the first instance. Some people may fulfil therapeutic earnings criteria and receive IB whilst working (www.jobcentreplus.gov.uk). There are now a number of benefit rules, which protect benefits on RTW, are designed to support RTW, or to facilitate return to benefits should RTW be unsuccessful (Waddell et al 2002).

Benefits terminology is complex. In addition to the benefit known as Incapacity Benefit (IB), Severe Disablement Allowance and Income Support with a disability premium are frequently referred to as 'incapacity benefits' (IB's) (TUC, 2005). Many individuals receive more then one benefit, only 40% of sick and disabled claimants of working age receive a single benefit and over 59% receive two or more benefits (Waddell et al 2002). The following is therefore not intended to be an expert discussion of the subject but should give the reader a general overview of the trends over time.

Invalidity Benefit (IVB) was replaced by IB in 1995. In terms of the total numbers claiming IVB/IB there has been an upward trend over the last 30 years (McVicar 2004). There was particularly rapid growth between the mid 1980s and mid 1990s, with the number of claimants increasing from around 1.1m in 1985 to around 2.4m in 1995 (McVicar 2004). The primary reason cited for claiming IB was LBP. LBP claims also increased most markedly during this time, although this could not be explained by changes in health. The overall growth in IB was probably due to a combination of two things, labour market factors together with benefit characteristics (e.g. in terms of generosity and screening intensity).

The first of these, labour market factors, included the loss of many mining and heavy industry jobs that were experienced in some parts of the UK in the 1980s and 1990s (McVicar 2004). In these jobs, levels of in-work ill health were comparatively high (McVicar 2004) and individuals who lost their jobs tended to receive IBs rather then unemployment benefits. The decline in jobs in heavy industry made it difficult for manual workers to find secure work that paid a wage at a higher rate then benefits (McCormick 2000). There is also a suggestion that growing female participation in the UK labour market may have led indirectly to the rapid growth in the number of female disability benefit claimants (McVicar 2004).

The second cause of overall IB growth was benefit characteristics. Benefit characteristics are multifactorial (McVicar 2004). The nature of the United Kingdom (UK) pension system meant that there could be incentives to use disability benefits as an "early retirement vehicle", particularly for low earners. It has been suggested that, at certain times, the employment services may have directed those of the long term unemployed with disabilities off unemployment benefit and onto IVB /IB (McVicar, 2004; Beatty & Fothergill 2004). In Scotland, for example, the unemployment benefit form introduced in 1985 specifically signposted claimants towards sickness benefits (McCormick 2000). GP's in the north of Glasgow became aware in the mid-1980s of an explicit policy of the Employment Services advising claimants to see their doctors and sign off sick rather then register as unemployed (McCormick 2000). There is also some suggestion that governments encouraged the move onto sickness benefits as a way of reducing the numbers on the unemployment register (McCormick 2000). Eligibility criteria for unemployment benefits were made progressively tighter throughout the 1980s and 1990s and individuals on long term IB generally received more money than those on basic unemployment benefit (Job Seekers Allowance). Taken together this created a clear incentive to claim disability benefits in preference to unemployment benefits in the UK.

The rise in the number receiving the long-term invalidity benefits was partly due to an increase in the duration of claims rather than an increase in new claims (ONS 2000). Once people started receiving benefits, they did not tend to come off them. Those who are on IB's for 12 months stay on them for an average of eight years, and are more likely to die or retire than leave for any other reason (Frank & Maddison 2004). In other words, the total number of claimants in any year was added to the previous years figures, and so on, cumulatively.

However, following the publication of a number of UK guidelines, more active clinical management of back pain and changes to social security policy the management of LBP improved. Waddell (2004) has suggested that there were wider changes in social attitudes and practices towards back pain. The change from IVB to IB also resulted in fewer claimants, because people who were in receipt of IVB when they reached state pension age were allowed to carry on receiving the benefit for five more years, whereas with IB the benefit is stopped when the recipient reaches pension age (ONS 2000, Waddell et al 2002). As a result of these various factors, the trend reversed, the number of new awards for back pain fell by 42% between 1994-1995 and 2000, compared with a 25% decrease for all conditions (Waddell 2004). The number of people continuing to receive benefits for back pain fell by 13%, while the total number on benefits remained the same.

Following this, whilst the overall number of people claiming IB for back pain continued to fall between 2000 and 2003, the total number of claimants of IB for all conditions grew back to the 1995 levels. The growth in the numbers claiming benefits has now stabilised, at under 1 percent a year (DWP 2004). There were 2.7 million people claiming IB for all conditions in 2004 (DWP, 2004), in fact, every year since 1995, the number of people claiming IB has exceeded the number of people claiming unemployment benefits (McVicar 2004). Most recently, the beginnings of a new trend may be emerging, the number of new claims has fallen and it appears that the numbers in the caseload may have peaked.

Mental ill-health, rather than musculoskeletal problems, is now the primary reason cited for claiming IB, and the number of new awards for mental ill-health is continuing to grow. This trend is more marked in the southeast of the UK and the midlands and is moving northwards. This may be the result of wider recognition and reporting of such conditions and a growth in disability related to these conditions rather than an actual increase in their incidence (McVicar 2004). Waddell and Aylward (2002) concur with this view, they believe that the reduction in people claiming benefits for musculoskeletal problems and the increase in people claiming for mental ill-health problems is probably due more to social, cultural and social security changes then any biological or treatment variation.

The demand for vocational rehabilitation services

The majority of people who first move onto IB expect to return to work (RTW) in the near future, most of them have manageable health conditions where the outlook should be good. However, without intervention, only 2% of people on IB move into work within two years (Burchardt 2000). The current system is clearly failing them.

Despite the decrease in the number and proportion of new IB claims for LBP, there are still a significant number of people with LBP who remain on benefits long term. Those claiming IB are usually not active in the labour market and might therefore be viewed as a wasted potential labour force (McVicar 2004). They also place a large financial burden upon the state. Sickness absence and unemployment leaves the recipients at increased risk from poverty of wealth and health and from social exclusion (McVicar 2004). Often people are unaware of the full range of options open to them and many are frightened of anything that they perceive may put their benefits at risk, both in terms of losing their money and their status as 'unfit for work' (McCormick 2000). More needs to be done to help people with long-term disabilities and incapacity (Waddell & Burton 2004).

People's situations are complex and many people may be hard to help. They may have a more severe health problem, although many feel that non-health related obstacles to work are more important (a lack of suitable jobs, difficulty obtaining them, financial uncertainty about the transition into work) (Waddell & Burton 2004). Many on IB have no formal qualifications, some have basic numeracy and literacy problems, half are over 50 years old, and many face discrimination and disadvantage in employment on the grounds of disability and age (Waddell & Burton 2004). Approximately 60% of disability and IB claimants have had no recent contact with the labour market (Waddell & Burton 2004). We need to develop strategies that help them into work, perhaps for the first time (Waddell & Burton, 2004).

It will take many years before there are significant inroads into the number of people on IB. At the same time, we need to assess and address the needs of people who are off work but who do not receive IB's and those who are at work but struggling. Consequently, the challenges of assessing and addressing the needs of individuals with health and work related problems are significant. There is clearly an urgent need for appropriate vocational rehabilitation services in the UK.

References

Acheson D 1998 Independent inquiry into inequalities in health: report. Stationery Office, London

Anderson GBJ 1999 Epidemiological features of chronic low-back pain. Lancet 354:581-585

Aronsson G, Gustafsson K, Dallner M 2000 'Sick but yet at work: an empirical study of sickness presenteeism'. Journal of Epidemiological and Community Health. 54:502-9

Beatty C, Fothergill S 2004 The Diversion from 'Unemployment' to 'Sickness' Across British Regions and Districts. Nottinghamshire Research Observatory

Bigos S, Splenger D, Martin N et al 1986 Back injuries in industry. A retrospective study. Employee related factors. Spine11:252-256

British Society of Rehabilitation Medicine 2000 Vocational rehabilitation: the way forward. BSRM, London

British Society of Rehabilitation Medicine 2003 Vocational rehabilitation - the way forward (2nd edn.). Report of a working party BSRM, London

Burchardt T 2000 Enduring economic exclusion: Disabled people, income and work. York Publishing Services

CBI 2001 Business and Health Care for the 21st Century. Confederation of British Industry, London

CBI 2003 Confederation of British Industry Absence and labour turnover survey 2003. The lost billions: addressing the cost of absence. CBI, London

CBI and CIPD 2001 Pulling Together - Absence and labour Survey. Confederation of British Industry Absence and Chartered Institute of Personnel and Development. CBI, London

CIPD 2004 Employee absence 2004: a survey of management policy and practice. Chartered Institute of Personnel and Development, London

Croft P 1996 The epidemiology of pain: the more you have, the more you get, Ann Rheum Dis 55:859-860

CSAG 1994 Back Pain: Report of a Clinical Standards Advisory Committee on Back Pain HMSO

Dionne CE 1999 Low back pain. In: Crombie IK (ed) Epidemiology of pain. IASP Press, Seattle

DWP 2002 Pathways to work: helping people into employment. Department for Work and Pensions CM 5690:1-65

DWP 2004 Building capacity for work: A UK Framework for Vocational Rehabilitation. The framework work document. Department for Works and Pensions

Frank AO, Maddison P 2004 Work and the musculoskeletal conditions. Clinical Medicine 4(4):362-365

James P, Cunningham I, Dibben P 2003 Job retention and vocational rehabilitation: The development and evaluation of a conceptual framework. HSE books

Janlert U 1997 Unemployment as a disease and diseases of the unemployed. Scandinavian Journal of Work and Environmental Health. 23(3):79-83

Maniadakis N, Gray A 2000 The economic burden of back pain in the UK. Pain 84(1):95-103

Martikainen P, Valkonen T 1996 Excess mortality of unemployed men and women during a period of rapidly increasing unemployment. Lancet 348:208-213

Mayer TG, Gatchel RJ, Kishino N., Keeley J, Mayer H, Capra P, Mooney V 1986 A prospective short-term study of chronic low-back-pain patients utilizing novel objective functional measurement. Pain 25:53-68

McCormick J 2000 On the sick: incapacity and Inclusion. Paper number 17 The Scottish Council Foundation

McVicar D 2004 Why have UK disability benefit rolls grown so much? School of Management and Economics, Belfast

NAO 2003 A Safer Place to Work. National Audit Office

ONS 1999 The prevalence of back pain in Great Britain in 1998 Office of National Statistics

ONS 2000 Recipients of benefits for sick and disabled people 1981-2000: Office for National Statistics Social Trends 31

Pickavance S 2004 "In Sickness and in Work". Hazards 85:4–5

Spitzer WO, LeBlanc FE, Dupuis M 1987 Scientific approach to the assessment and management of activity-related spinal disorders: report of the Quebec Task Force on Spinal Disorders. Spine12 (Suppl. 7):S1-S59

Stewart WF, Ricci JA, Chee,E , Morganstein D, Lipton R 2003 Lost productive time and cost due to common pain conditions in the US workforce. JAMA 290:2443-2454

TUC 2004 "Attack of the Mucus Troopers!" workSMART newsletter no 19

TUC 2005 Sicknote Britain? Countering an urban legend. Trades Union Congress Von Korff M 1994 Studying the natural history of back pain. Spine19 (suppl):2041-2046

Watson PJ, Main CJ, Waddell G, Gales TF, Purcell-Jones G 1997 Medically certified work loss, recurrence and costs of wage compensation for back pain: A follow –up study of the working population of Jersey. British journal of Rheumatology 36:1-5

Waddell G 2004 The Back pain Revolution. 2nd ed. Churchill Livingstone, London

Waddell G, Burton AK 2000 Occupational Health Guidelines for the management of low back pain at work. Evidence review and recommendations. Faculty of Occupational Medicine, London

Waddell G, Aylward M 2002 Pathways to work: helping people into employment. Department for Work and Pensions CM 5690

Waddell G, Aylward M, Sawney P 2002 Back pain, incapacity for work and social security benefits: An international literature review and analysis. The Royal Society of Medicine Press, London

Waddell G, Burton AK, Main CJ 2003 Screening to identify people at risk of long-term incapacity for work. A conceptual and scientific review. Royal Society of Medicine Press Ltd, London

Waddell G, Burton AK 2004 Concepts of rehabilitation for the management of common health problems: Evidence base. The stationery Office

Web sites

www.hse.gov.uk
www.jobcentreplus.gov.uk

9

Vocational Rehabilitation

GAIL SOWDEN

Introduction

This chapter provides an introduction to vocational rehabilitation. It introduces occupational obstacles to return to work in the form of "blue" and "black flags" and briefly explores some of the recent strategies to address sickness absence and unemployment attributed to ill health and disability in the United Kingdom. Finally it considers the future direction of vocational rehabilitation in the United Kingdom and the role of physiotherapists in it.

The appendix outlines some current and planned strategies to address sickness absence and unemployment attributed to ill health and disability in the United Kingdom.

The National Health Service and vocational rehabilitation

"At present, most health professionals regard their job as health care. We assume if we make patients better, they will automatically return to normal activity and work. As a result we pay little direct attention to work issues" (Waddell 2004).

The health care we deliver aims to achieve maximum medical recovery (MMR) and it is only once MMR has been achieved or treatment has failed to 'cure', that rehabilitation is considered (Waddell & Burton 2004). Delays in providing medical consultations, investigations and treatments by the

National Health Service (NHS) mean that the opportunity of early intervention to address rehabilitation and occupational needs is often missed (BSRM 2000). We cannot afford to defer rehabilitation until health care has failed (Waddell & Burton 2004). In fact, MMR need not have been achieved before rehabilitation and return to work (RTW) are considered and in some cases MMR may never be achieved.

The NHS 'rehabilitation services' are limited and they are primarily directed at activities of daily living and independence, they lack any focus on urgent work related problems (Gibson 2000). Often, workers have lost their jobs before they receive any active rehabilitation (Waddell et al 2002). Vocational rehabilitation is rarely considered or provided by the NHS (Waddell & Burton 2004). As a result, it is almost a lost skill within the NHS (BSRM 2000). Whenever it is considered it is usually added on after treatment and medical rehabilitation have been completed, even though best practice demands that the two processes are simultaneous (BSRM, 2000, Chamberlain & Frank 2004).

Within the NHS, there is limited awareness and consideration of work issues. This is despite the fact that work is of paramount importance (Waddell 2004). It is an essential part of normal function for many people and central to the way they think of themselves (Waddell & Burton 2004). According to Hazard, et al (1996), RTW should be the major goal of rehabilitation. Return to work is more than a goal; work is therapeutic and aids recovery, it restores physical and mental capacity and improves self-esteem and confidence (Waddell & Burton 2004).

Health care professionals need to be interested in and take responsibility for rehabilitation and occupational outcomes (Waddell & Burton 2004). "..we have not fulfilled our professional responsibilities until we get our patients back to work" (Waddell 2004).

We need to change our understanding and management of health and work issues. Most sickness absence, long-term incapacity for work and premature retirement on medical grounds is no longer caused by severe conditions with objective evidence of disease or permanent impairment (Waddell & Burton 2004). They are caused by less severe 'common' health problems such as musculoskeletal, mental health and cardiovascular conditions. In these 'common' health problems there is often limited evidence of objective disease or impairment. Many of them are potentially remediable and long-term incapacity is not inevitable (Waddell & Burton 2004).

Occupational obstacles to return to work

In common health problems, such as non-specific LBP, the obstacles to RTW are predominantly psychosocial in nature rather than due to the severity of pathology or impairment (Waddell & Burton 2004). These health, personal/psychological, and social/occupational obstacles to RTW need to be assessed and addressed (Waddell & Burton 2004). We need to develop the necessary skills, knowledge and expertise to be able to do this.

Many health care professionals are already familiar with assessing and addressing health related obstacles to recovery. Enlightened professionals will also pay attention to psychosocial obstacles to recovery. Psychosocial factors include attitudes and beliefs, psychological distress, illness behaviour and the social environment. Unfortunately, however few professionals pay any attention to health, personal/psychological, and social/occupational obstacles to RTW. Those that do, seldom consider occupational obstacles to RTW, and yet RTW is not simply about health or health care, it also depends on the workplace and the employer (Waddell & Burton 2004). Organisational policy, process and practice as well as the workers and employers perceptions and attitudes are important (Waddell & Burton 2004). Environmental and workplace obstacles also need to be considered.

Occupational obstacles to RTW are symbolised by blue and black coloured flags. The distinction between the flags is not absolute and there are relevant factors that are not necessarily currently encapsulated by the coloured flags system. It is important to be aware that the factors that influence why individuals stop work, may be different from those that influence why they stay off work and different again from those that influence RTW (Waddell et al 2002).

Occupationally focused blue flags are a subdivision of the original acute LBP 'psychosocial yellow flags' (Kendall et al 1997, Mayou et al). They originate from the occupational stress literature and are perceived features of work or social environment that are associated with higher rates of symptoms, ill-health and work loss. They may delay recovery or be a major obstacle to it. They include perceptions of job characteristics such as job demand as well as perceptions about social interactions (management or fellow workers) (Mayou et al 2004).

BLUE FLAGS

High Demand / Low Control
- E.g. perceived physical psychological demand of job, capabilities and perceptions of control.

Unhelpful management style
- E.g. negative experience of workplace management of health conditions.

Poor social support from colleagues
- E.g. Poor relationship with colleagues, interpersonal conflict, suspicion that colleagues don't believe the person is genuine.

Perceived time pressures

Low job satisfaction
- **E.g. Perceptions about monotony, unrewarding,** repetitive, boring or unpleasant work.

Source
Bold   **- Mayou et al 2004**
Non Bold   - Authors own words

There are labour market and social security obstacles to coming off benefits and (re) entering work. The pervasive nature and detrimental effects of these obstacles has lead to them being described as 'black flags' (Waddell & Burton 2004). Whereas blue flags are concerned with perceptions of work, black flags are more to do with objective work characteristics (Mayou et al 2004). Black flags affect all workers equally; they include working conditions specific to a particular organisation as well as nationally established employment and sickness policies (Mayou et al 2004). The evidence suggests that certain working conditions and adverse work characteristics are risk factors for ill health and associated sickness absence. They may delay recovery and RTW after an injury (Mayou et al 2004).

BLACK FLAGS

Company policy on rehabilitation
- E.g. Absence of a reporting system; lack of occupational health provision, minimal or no availability of selected duties or opportunities for graded return to work; limited/no job availability or retraining opportunities; **an all or nothing return to work policy, rigidity of rules of employment.**

Threats to financial security
- E.g. Lack of financial incentive to RTW **or presence of financial disincentives to RTW. (income protection policies, 12 months full pay, loan and mortgage protection policies, final salary pension schemes,** benefits trap)

Litigation
- **E.g. Adversarial litigation system - can be prolonged and distressing process**

Qualification criteria for compensation
- E.g.having to prove that you are injured, disabled or unable to work and your ability to do this being rewarded. benefits system in which you are deemed either disabled or fit to work.

Lack of contact with work

Source
Bold   **- Mayou et al 2004**

How to assess blue and black flags

Blue and black flags can be assessed via interviews. Simple open-ended questions can facilitate discussion about RTW (Waddell & Burton 2004). More specific questions can then explore the perceived physical and mental demands of the job, the support available to RTW, motivation to RTW, and the obstacles to RTW (Waddell & Burton 2004). Appropriate self-report questionnaires may be an efficient means of collecting background information and may inform subsequent dialogue (Waddell & Burton 2004). It may be necessary to speak to the other relevant parties (occupational health, personnel, General Practitioner etc) and to conduct one or more workplace visits as part of the assessment.

How to address obstacles to return to work

Obstacles to RTW are multifactorial, a purely healthcare or a purely occupational approach cannot therefore appropriately assess or address them. Health and occupational approaches need to be combined (Main & Spanswick 2000). There are unacceptable gaps between the health service and employment in the United Kingdom (UK) - a treatment paradigm shift is therefore required (Main & Spanswick 2000). There is no integration or clear pathway between treatment, rehabilitation and vocational rehabilitation (Waddell & Burton 2004). Optimum clinical management, rehabilitation and organisational interventions should be integrated (Waddell & Burton 2004). This will require radical changes in NHS and health professionals' thinking (Waddell & Burton 2004).

In the case of back pain, there is extensive evidence that multi-dimensional biopsychosocial interventions are most effective for occupational outcomes (Waddell & Burton 2004). Waddell and Burton (2004) suggest that successful interventions need to incorporate:
1. A physical conditioning programme designed to restore the individual's systemic, neurological, musculoskeletal or cardio-respiratory function.
2. Significant cognitive behavioral components (e.g. correcting dysfunctional beliefs and behaviors).
3. Close association with the workplace, with work-related goals and outcomes.

Reassurance, advice and education should be designed to overcome fear avoidance beliefs and behaviours (Waddell & Burton 2004). Return to normal activities, including work, as soon as possible, should be encouraged. Goal setting, graded activity and a graded RTW will help give the worker evidence of and confidence in their abilities. Collaborative problem solving can help overcome specific obstacles to RTW and can help empower the worker. Communication, co-operation and agreed goals between the worker with LBP, the occupational health team, supervisors, management and health care professionals is fundamental for improving clinical and occupational health management and outcome (Waddell & Burton 2000). The aim of RTW in priority order is: same job/same employer; different job/ same employer; same job/different employer, different job/different employer. Temporary, time limited, and clearly defined lighter or modified duties may facilitate RTW and reduce time off work (Waddell & Burton 2000). Permanent modifications may be required (hours, roles, responsibilities, physical demands etc), but only in a minority of cases. The Disability Discrimination Acts require reasonable adjustments in order to meet the needs of individuals to enable them to overcome their disabilities (Waddell et al 2002).

The current state of vocational rehabilitation in the United Kingdom

It is apparent, that, compared to other countries, the UK is woefully behind in the provision of rehabilitation and vocational rehabilitation services (ABI 1999). In fact, Britain has the worst record in Europe for getting people back to work following illness or injury; only 15% of British workers RTW after serious illness, compared with 50% of Swedish employees (TUC 2005). The escalation in disability benefits in the UK could reflect the decline in its rehabilitation services (Grahame 2002).

"There is now broad agreement on the importance of rehabilitation and the need to improve occupational health and vocational rehabilitation in the UK " (Waddell & Burton 2004).

Definition of vocational rehabilitation
Vocational rehabilitation is a process to overcome the barriers an individual faces when accessing, remaining or returning to work following injury, illness or impairment (DWP, 2004).

There is growing social, political and economic interest in sickness absence, rehabilitation and vocational rehabilitation issues. In the UK, this interest has come from a variety of sources, including the private, public and voluntary sectors.

One example of this is the Health and Safety Commission and Health and Safety Executive targets for 2010 (HSE 2004). These include:

- Everyone currently in employment but off work due to ill health or disability to be, where necessary and appropriate, made aware of opportunities for rehabilitation back into work as early as possible.
- Everyone currently not in employment due to ill health or disability to be, where necessary and appropriate, made aware of opportunities to prepare and find work.

Vocational rehabilitation is being placed at the centre of the UK government's health, workplace and social security agenda. The government have committed themselves to a 'welfare to work' strategy, 'work for those who can, security for those who cannot' (DWP 2003, Waddell & Burton 2004).

A number of recent initiatives have aimed to help economically inactive people back into work both in government schemes, including the Access to Work programmes and those devised by voluntary organisations, such as MIND and the Royal National Institute for the Blind (Thornton & Howard 2000). Some of the strategies that are applicable to musculoskeletal conditions are mentioned below.

Working Backs Scotland. The Health Education Board for Scotland (HEBS) (www.healthscotland.com) and the Health and Safety Executive (HSE) (www.hse.gov.uk) launched Working Backs Scotland in October 2000. This major public education campaign aims to ensure that patients with back pain are provided with consistent advice and management. Twenty organizations representing health professionals, employers and unions were initially involved. Thirty-five thousand information packs were distributed, a radio campaign broadcast almost 2000 advertisements and there was extensive media coverage. Population surveys showed a 60% penetration and a 20% positive shift in public beliefs. The campaign is continuing to develop. (www.workingbacksscotland.com)

Work focused rehabilitation projects were conducted in Salford and Bristol for people out of work long term due to LBP. A multidisciplinary team of employment advisors, psychologists and physiotherapists tackled physical, psychological and vocational obstacles to RTW. At 6- months follow up, 39.5% were employed and another 23% were in education, training or voluntary work (www.le.ac.uk/anaesthesia/lc85/NATDISRE.pdf, Waddell & Burton 2004).

Job Retention and Rehabilitation Pilot's (JRRP's) were part of a randomized controlled trial designed to study the effectiveness of services aimed at getting people back into work after sick leave of between 6 and 26 weeks. The participants were off sick but still employed and the interventions involved multidisciplinary teams of providers. The goal was to stop people moving onto Incapacity Benefit. The research was conducted in six regions under the names of Workcare, Healthy return and Routeback, for a limited length of time. The JRRP's were jointly funded by the Department of Work and Pensions (DWP) and the Department of Health. The results will be published in the winter of 2005 (www.natcen.ac.uk/jrrp, Waddell & Burton 2004).

In an effort to address the needs of the sickness absent and unemployed due to disability or ill-health in the UK, a number of additional strategies are currently under way or are planned. These initiatives focus on different issues, e.g. benefit system reform; sickness absence management; occupational health or rehabilitation services. These initiatives have been outlined in the appendix to this chapter.

Vocational rehabilitation in the UK is starting from a low baseline; as a result, there is considerable room for improvement. Rehabilitation depends on commitment, motivation and effort. Consequently, engagement, recruitment, and retention in vocational rehabilitation and RTW schemes are major issues (Waddell & Burton 2004). Many vocational rehabilitation pilots only manage to enrol 3-6% of the potential clients and these clients are highly self-selecting and may be those who would have RTW anyway (Waddell & Burton 2004).

Most projects to date have had limited availability, both in terms of numbers of eligible and participating individuals, their geographical location and in terms of their duration. There are clearly challenges involved in the early identification and referral of those at risk and in the development of appropriate screening tools (Waddell et al 2003). Projects have also tended to have a narrow focus, for example, on benefits, litigation or occupational health and have largely been under-resourced and poorly integrated. International studies have underlined the importance of 'joined-up' approaches in order to achieve effective vocational rehabilitation services (Riddell 2002).

According to Chamberlain and Frank (2004), despite all the resolutions, good intentions, conferences and new groups of interested professionals, there has been little actual change in the area of vocational rehabilitation in the UK. We still don't really know what vocational rehabilitation services are required as no budget for research has been established, no resources have been specifically allocated and there have been no new models of service delivery apart from those being piloted by the DWP (Chamberlain & Frank 2004). There are no plans to develop the expertise needed by the NHS and by the mushrooming private sector (Chamberlain & Frank 2004). There is also no system to facilitate links between employers, healthcare providers, vocational therapists and the employment services (Chamberlain & Frank 2004).

The future of vocational rehabilitation in the United Kingdom

As well as ensuring greater alignment between existing pilots, we need to conduct further research and development into new cost effective and innovative approaches (Waddell & Burton 2004). It is not perhaps until the results of these endeavours are known that a standardised national system can be implemented (Waddell & Burton 2004).

The NHS needs to be able to respond quickly to healthcare and rehabilitation needs. Legislation, benefits and the insurance industry must be so structured as to encourage rehabilitation and vocational rehabilitation at an early stage (Bloch & Prins 1997).

Standards, guidelines and frameworks need to be established, in order to:
* Improve health at work
* Improve the management of sickness absence
* Provide vocational rehabilitation
* Help people to maintain, return or enter employment

When it comes to employment, attention needs to be paid to assessing and addressing the needs of those who:

- Are currently in employment, but experiencing difficulty in retaining employment because of a health condition or impairment.
- Are temporarily absent from work because of a health condition or impairment.
- Have a health condition or impairment that has resulted in longer-term absence, which may lead to unemployment.
- Have not worked for some time, or never worked, because of a health condition or impairment.

Awareness of obstacles to RTW needs to increase. Effective national vocational rehabilitation services need to be established. These services will need to be staffed by people who have developed the necessary expertise to be able to assess and address health, personal/psychological, and social/occupational obstacles to recovery and to RTW (Waddell & Burton 2004). Systems will need to be able to facilitate and support much closer dialogue between employers, Disability Employment Advisors and health care professionals.

The role of physiotherapists in vocational rehabilitation

There are debates about whether the locus of responsibility for vocational rehabilitation should lie within health, education, employment, economic development, social security or community care (Riddell 2002). The many challenges ahead will require the combined efforts of all stakeholders, government, insurers, employers organizations, trade unions and other trade associations, health care organizations, the Health and Safety Executive and many more. All stakeholders need to take an interest and responsibility for occupational outcomes.

Physiotherapists have a pivotal role to play in researching and developing the future of vocational rehabilitation services in the UK. Few people in the UK will have the necessary knowledge, skills or expertise to deliver these services. Consequently, there is going to be increasing demand for people who can. Physiotherapists are well placed to develop this expertise.

References

ABI 1999 Second UK bodily injury awards study. International Underwriters Association of London, Association of British Insurers. ABI, London

Beaumont D 2002 Rehabilitation and retention in the workplace - the interaction between GPs and occupational health professionals. A consensus statement. Occup Med 53:254-255

Bloch F, Prins R 1997 Work incapacity and reintegration—theory and design of a cross-national study. Int Soc Sec Rev 2:3–23

BSRM 2000 Vocational Rehabilitation: The Way Forward. British Society of Rehabilitation Medicine, London

Chamberlain MA, Frank AO 2004 Congratulations but no congratulations: should physicians do more to support their patients at work? Clinical Medicine. 4:102-104

CIPD 2004 Employee absence 2004: a survey of management policy and practice. Chartered Institute of Personnel and Development, London

DCA 2004 Tackling the "Compensation Culture". Government Response to the Better Regulation Task Force Report: 'Better Routes to Redress'. 10 November 2004, Department for Constitutional Affairs (www.dca.gov.uk/majrep/bettertaskforce/better-task-force.pdf)

DWP 2002 Pathways to work - Helping people into employment. The Stationary Office

DWP 2003 Opportunity for All. Department for Works and Pensions 5th Annual Report

DWP 2003a. Review of employers' liability compulsory insurance. First stage report. Department of Work & Pension, June

DWP 2004 Building capacity for work: A UK Framework for Vocational Rehabilitation. The framework work document. Department for Works and Pensions

DWP 2004a 'Jobcentre advisers help double the number of IB claimants getting back to work in reform pilot areas', Press Release 30th November. Department for Works and Pensions

DWP 2004b "IB Reforms –helping people back to work". Department for Works and Pensions, Touchbase 34

DWP 2005 Five Year Strategy Opportunity and security throughout life. Department for Work and Pensions

Gibson A (Chair) 2000 Getting better at getting back: TUC consultation document on rehabilitation. TUC, London

Grahame R 2002 The decline of rehabilitation services and its impact on disability benefits. J R Soc Med 95:114-117

Greenstreet Berman Ltd in association with Callund Consulting Ltd for the Association of British Insurers 2003 Costing of a UK no fault compensation scheme.

Hazard RG, Haugh LD, Reid S, Preble BP, Macdonald L 1996 Early prediction of chronic disability after occupational low back injury. Spine 21(8):945-951

HSE 2002 Survey of use of Occupational Health Support. Health & Safety Executive, Contract Research Report 445/2002

HSE 2004 A strategy for workplace health and safety in Great Britain to 2010 and beyond. Printed and published by the Health and Safety Executive (www.hse.gov.uk/aboutus/hsc/strategy2010.pdf)

Hussey S, Hoddinott P, Wilson P, Dowell J, Barbour R 2004 Sickness certification system in the United Kingdom: qualitative study of views of general practitioners in Scotland. British Medical Journal 328:88-91

IRS 2002 A case for management. IRS Employment Review. Issue 747

IRS and EEF 2004 Absence culture needs urgent reform. IRS Employment Review

IUA and ABI 2003 Third UK bodily injury awards study. International Underwriting Association of London, London

Kendall NAS, Linton SJ, Main CJ 1997 Guide to assessing psychosocial yellow flags in acute low back pain: risk factors for long term disability and work loss. Accident Rehabilitation and Compensation Corporation of New Zealand and the National Health Committee (www.nzgg.org.nz)

Main CJ, Spanswick CC (Eds) 2000 Pain management: An interdisciplinary approach. Churchill Livingstone, Edinburgh

Mayou R, Main CJ, Auty A 2004 In: Psychology, Personal Injury and rehabilitation. The IUA/ABI Rehabilitation Working Party: Evidence based guidelines Royal College of General Practitioners (www.rcgp.org.uk)

Pilkington A, Graham MK, Cowie HA et al 2002 Survey of Use of Occupational Health Support. Health and Safety Executive Contract Research Report 445/2002

Riddell S 2002 Work Preparation and Vocational Rehabilitation: A Literature Review. Strathclyde Centre for Disability Research. University of Glasgow, NDDI

Roberts P 2004 Stemming absence (www.hi-mag.com/healthinsurance/article.jsp?articleid=1084814611200)

Sawney P 2002 Current issues in fitness for work certification. Br J Gen Pract 52:217-222

Thornton P, Howard M 2000 Possible interventions for job retention. In Lewis J (ed.) Job Retention in the Context of Long-term Illness, The proceedings of a seminar organised on 1 March 2000, DfEE Research Report, Department for Education and Employment: London (www.dfee.gov.uk/nddp/retention2.htm)

TUC 2002 Rehabilitation and retention: what matters is what works. Trade Union Congress 2002 survey

TUC 2005 Sicknote Britain? Countering an urban legend. Trades Union Congress

Waddell G 2004 The Back pain Revolution (2nd edn). Churchill Livingstone, Edinburgh

Waddell G, Burton AK 2000 Occupational Health Guidelines for the management of low back pain at work. Evidence review and recommendations. Faculty of Occupational Medicine. London

Waddell G, Burton AK 2004 Concepts of rehabilitation for the management of common health problems: The stationery Office

Waddell G, Aylward M, Sawney, P 2002 Back pain, incapacity for work and social security benefits: An international literature review and analysis. The Royal Society of Medicine Press, London

Web pages cited in this chapter:

www.bicma.org.uk/cobp.php
www.cmsuk.org
www.dca.gov.uk/majrep/bettertaskforce/better-task-force.pdf
www.dfee.gov.uk/nddp/retention2.htm
www.dpp.org.uk
www.dwp.gov.uk
www.hse.gov.uk/aboutus/hsc/strategy2010.pdf
www.healthscotland.com
www.hi-mag.com/healthinsurance/article.jsp?articleid=1084814611200
www.hse.gov.uk
www.hse.gov.uk/aboutus/hsc/strategy2010.pdf
www.jobcentreplus.gov.uk
www.le.ac.uk/anaesthesia/lc85/NATDISRE.pdf
www.natcen.ac.uk/jrrp
www.nzgg.org.nz
www.rcgp.org.uk
www.workingbacksscotland.com

Appendix

CURRENT AND PLANNED VOCATIONAL REHABILITATION INITIATIVES IN THE UNITED KINGDOM

Pathways to work are DWP led pilot schemes for Incapacity Benefit reforms involving Jobcentre Plus, the NHS and voluntary sector. **They** incorporate work-focused interviews for all new claimants, earlier intervention with dedicated personal advisers, immediate access to Job Centre Plus New Deals and financial incentives (return to work credits, discretion funds, job grants, permitted working). In January 2005 the DWP announced the expansion of the scheme to cover about one third of the country so that by October 2006 it would cover nearly one million people. According to the government, in the pathways areas, the improvement in the number of recorded job entries has been approximately double that of other areas (DWP 2004a, DWP 2004b).

Condition Management Programmes are creating new local partnerships between employment and NHS health services (Waddell & Burton 2004). These multidisciplinary rehabilitation programmes aim to teach people to understand and better manage their health condition, and refocus them on their potential for work (Waddell & Burton 2004). They are aimed primarily at people with musculoskeletal conditions, moderate cardio-respiratory conditions and mild to moderate mental health conditions. They have incorporated elements of the expert patient programme and last between 6 and 13 weeks. They can be individually or group–based and they use 'cognitive behavioural therapy' based interventions and other validated techniques. Participation in the Condition Management Programmes is entirely voluntary and does not affect benefit entitlement (www.dwp.gov.uk).

New deal for disabled people (NDDP) provides case management via a personal advisor. It draws in a number of employment-related services to improve employability and to help place people into employment. It provides information on work, benefits and other government services. NDDP is a voluntary scheme and anyone on Incapacity Benefit is eligible (www.dwp.gov.uk).

Job centre plus has brought job centres and benefits offices together in integrated offices. This new approach to dealing with benefit customers is still being rolled out (www.dwp.gov.uk).

Incapacity Benefit reforms. In February 2005 the government announced that all initial applicants for Incapacity Benefit will be put on a "holding allowance" before medical assessment. Following medical assessment they will be divided into those receiving a "disability and sickness allowance" or a "rehabilitation support allowance". The "disability and sickness allowance" will be an increased allowance for the permanently disabled or sick. Access to the higher rates of the "rehabilitation support allowance" will be conditional on attending-focused interviews and taking steps to get back into the labour market. Recipients who refuse to cooperate with job and medical assessment will be kept on a "holding" allowance at the level of the jobseekers' allowance. The Government are not intending to introduce the system until 2008 (DWP 2005).

Insurance
There are many different types of insurance e.g. Critical Illness, Mortgage or Loan Protection Insurance, Personal Injury Insurance (PII), Employers Liability Compulsory Insurance (ELCI) and Income protection insurance (IPP). Work status following injury or illness has relevance either directly or indirectly to these insurance policies. Early intervention, better rehabilitation and RTW as soon as possible, rather than financial compensation for remedial harm, should be at the heart of the response to injury and the insurance system (Waddell & Burton 2004). This may require a major cultural shift in the insurance industry processes and procedures and a radical change towards early intervention (Waddell & Burton 2004). Some insurance companies and solicitors are being proactive and are issuing joint instructions for rehabilitation. The government will be reviewing the cost incentives on insurers and business in relation to the provision of occupational health and vocational services (Waddell & Burton 2004). The cost of a no-fault compensation system has been explored (Greenstreet Berman 2003).

The Rehabilitation Code, Early Intervention And Medical Treatment In Personal Injury Claims. Significant increases in the cost of both Employers' Liability Compulsory Insurance (DWPa 2003) and personal injury claims has resulted in increasing interest in the role of early intervention and vocational rehabilitation. The Association of British insurers and the International Underwriters Association introduced the rehabilitation code, covering early intervention and medical treatment in personal injury claims. The code aims to ensure that claimant's solicitors and the insurers (and the insurer's solicitor or handling agent) both actively consider assessment of health and employment issues and active intervention in the form of rehabilitation at the earliest practical stage, when it is most effective. This is a voluntary code and has replaced the Code of best practice on Rehabilitation, Early Intervention and Medical treatment in Personal Injury Claims, which was first published in 1999 as part of the Second UK Bodily Injury Study published (IUA/ABI). The Post Magazine Rehabilitation First Campaign aims to win widespread acceptance of the rehabilitation code. (www.bicma.org.uk/cobp.php).

Occupational Health Provision. Stakeholder's views of occupational health services are that some of them are reactionary (Roberts, 2004) and fail to seek or adopt best practice in sickness absence/attendance management or in the clinical management of common health problems. Only a small percentage of employees have access to an occupational health service (Pilkington et al 2002, TUC 2002, HSE 2002, Sawney 2002). Consequently, the Health and Safety executive (HSE) will be trialling Workplace Health Direct. This provides independent occupational health advice and support for small to medium enterprises (SMEs). It will primarily be a telephone based helpline and website. In addition however, up to six separate pilots will be established in regions across England and Wales in order to provide a problem-solving occupational health, safety, and RTW service to employers and workers in SMEs. NHS Plus is also operating as an occupational health service (www.hse.gov.uk/workplacehealth).

The Sickness Certification Scheme. Various issues around sickness certification and the role of General Practitioner's (GP's) in sickness certification have been discussed (Beaumont 2002, Sawney 2002). General Practitioner's currently provide the majority of sickness certifications in the UK but some organisations believe they have insufficient knowledge on basic fitness for work issues, place insufficient emphasis on work retention and rehabilitation, issue sickness certificates too easily (CIPD 2004) and don't always seek to find out what patients do at work. Communication between doctors and employers is also poor. GPs, in turn, are not happy with the current system, as many feel that if they challenge or confront patients about sickness absence, they risk endangering their relationship with them (Hussey et al 2004). GP's have unmet training needs and the lack of NHS vocational rehabilitation services means that they have limited management options (IRS and EEF, 2004). In its 2002 green paper, Pathways to Work, the Department for Work and Pensions, announced an investigation looking at the feasibility of alternatives to the current arrangements of sickness certification and whether sickness certification duties could be extended to other healthcare workers (DWP 2002). A UK charity, The Developing Patient Partnership (DPP), is using a number of pilot sites to explore the role of occupational health professionals in sick certification and sickness management, instead of GP's. An interim report is expected in June 2005 (www.dpp.org.uk).

The role of case management. There may be up to 30 medical and non-medical agencies and professionals involved in a typical rehabilitation case and there is usually a lack of co-ordination between these different agencies. Consequently, interest has grown in an approach used in Australia and the United States, where a case manager liases with all the parties involved in a sick or injured worker's care. They co-ordinate and oversee the overall programme of rehabilitation and RTW (BSRM 2000, IRS 2002).

The Bodily Injuries Claim Management Association (www.bicma.org.uk), have facilitated the creation of the Case Management Society of the UK (www.cmsuk.org). Their primary focus to date has been on case managing health and social care.

Vocational rehabilitation standards of practice. The National Vocational Rehabilitation Association (NVRA) is developing Standards for accreditation in vocational rehabilitation.

"A UK Framework for Vocational Rehabilitation" This document was produced by the DWP in the summer of 2004 following responses to the discussion document :- 'Developing a framework for Vocational Rehabilitation- A discussion Paper' (DWP 2004). This document fulfils the Government's commitment to produce a Framework for Vocational Rehabilitation, given in the Second Stage Report into the Review of Employers' Liability Compulsory Insurance (ELCI) in December 2003 (DWP 2003). It sought to establish a definition, focus and range of work for vocational rehabilitation and to provide a framework for effective intervention and management by adopting a flexible and diverse range of provision. It emphasises delivery as a shared effort (business, insurers and unions). The document helps stakeholders who are considering introducing vocational rehabilitation. It highlights the key messages in research and allows stakeholders to influence current practice and encourage the development of good practice. (www.dwp.gov.uk/publication)

The Chief Medical Officer (CMO) has commissioned a scoping study of current provision of NHS and social care rehabilitation services. The Department of Health is working with other government departments to improve access to vocational rehabilitation (DCA 2004).

10

Obstacles to return to Work: Beliefs and Behaviours

GAIL SOWDEN

Current approaches to the management of musculoskeletal problems in the workplace, focus on identifying and addressing obstacles to recovery and return to work (RTW). It is becoming increasingly recognised that fear avoidance beliefs (fear of pain, fear of hurt and harm) and avoidant behaviours are important mechanisms in low back pain (LBP) and disability (Main & Waddell 2004, Vlaeyen & Linton 2000, Vlaeyen et al 1995). According to Main & Waddell (2004), beliefs regarding pain and its relationship to work are fundamental for rehabilitation and RTW. This includes beliefs held by employers, health care professionals, employment advisors and other stakeholders, as well as beliefs held by workers themselves.

Employer's beliefs and behaviours can be obstacles to workers RTW, for example, they may erroneously belief that hurt always equates with harm or that an individual must be 100% fit before RTW.

Amongst the most important beliefs are the workers / patient's beliefs about their condition, specific fears about work-related injury, and their beliefs about their work and the workplace (Main & Waddell, 2004). Their own expectations have been shown to be the best predictor of RTW after rehabilitation (Main & Waddell 2004). Workers behaviours can also be obstacles to RTW. If they attribute fault or blame for their condition or injury to their employer they are less likely to be co-operative about returning to work and much less likely to RTW (Main & Waddell 2004). Part of our job as health care professionals (HCP), is to assess our patients' beliefs and behaviours and to address them if they are erroneous, inappropriate or unhelpful. This assumes however that our own beliefs and behaviours are not erroneous, inappropriate or unhelpful.

Health care professional's beliefs and behaviours

We all have beliefs about pain and its relationship to activity and work. Whilst our beliefs do not always determine our behaviour, they often influence it. Our behaviours, what we do and do not do, can in turn impact on our beliefs.

As HCP, we are our patient's main source of advice about work (Waddell & Burton 2004). Our perceptions and behaviour can therefore be a powerful influence (Waddell & Burton 2004). Patients may reasonably expect us to provide accurate information and advice. They may ask us questions about the relationship between pain, activity and work, for example:
• Do you think I should RTW? If so, when?
• Do you think I can do my old job again?
• Do you think my job has caused my back problems?
• Does lifting and bending cause back problems?
• Do I need a special chair?

What we say and do in response, can impact on the workers RTW. However, what we say and do may partly depend on what we believe about pain, activity and work ourselves.

As a HCP, a personal concern is that we often assume causal relationships, despite a lack of evidence to support them. For example, where is the rigorous up to date evidence demonstrating causal relationships between the following?
1. Symptoms, "poor" posture and pathology.
2. Symptoms, pathology and manual handling.
3. Symptoms, pathology and work.

What messages do we give patients about these relationships? What evidence are we basing this on? Are we even aware of the impact of erroneous messages?

What are your beliefs and behaviours about pain and its relationship to activity and work? Are they in line with the available evidence and clinical guidelines? Try the following: read the first "possible belief held by a clinician" in the table below and think about what you believe. Then compare that with the evidence statement underneath. Repeat this for the subsequent belief statements. Try the same for the behaviour statements.

168

CLINICIANS BELIEFS, BEHAVIOURS AND THE EVIDENCE BASE
Sources
Some of the clinician's belief and behaviour statements in this table, are from a questionnaire that was used by Linton et al (2002) to assess physical therapists and general practitioners fear avoidance beliefs and behaviours. I have composed the remaining belief and behaviour statements (authors statement); however, they do not reflect my beliefs or my behaviours. The evidence statements are from "Occupational Health Guidelines for the Management of Low Back Pain at Work" (Carter & Birrell 2000).

1. Possible belief held by clinician: The clinical features of low back pain (LBP) are the most important factors in determining disability (authors statement).
   What the evidence indicates: *** Care-seeking and disability due to LBP depends more on complex individual and work-related psychosocial factors than on clinical features or physical demands of work.

2. Possible belief held by clinician: The main cause of LBP in workers is the physical demands of their work (authors statement).
   What the evidence indicates: ***Physical demands of work (manual materials handling, lifting, bending, twisting, and whole body vibration) can be associated with increased reports of back symptoms, aggravation of symptoms and 'injuries'.
***Physical demands of work are a risk factor for the incidence (onset) of LBP, but overall it appears that the size of the effect is less than that of other individual, non-occupational and unidentified factors. (Authors underlining).

3. Possible belief held by clinician: A reduction in pain is a prerequisite for RTW (Statement from Linton et al's study, 2002).
   What the evidence indicates: *** Most workers with LBP are able to continue working or RTW within a few days or weeks, even if they have some residual or recurrent symptoms, and they do not need to wait until they are completely pain free.

4. Possible belief held by clinician: Sick leave is a good treatment for back pain (statement from Linton et al's study, 2002)
   What the evidence indicates: ***The longer a worker is off work with LBP, the lower their chances of ever returning to work. Once a worker is off work for 4 to 12 weeks, they have a 10-40% (depending on the setting) risk of still being off work at one year.

169

5. Possible belief held by clinician: Symptomatic treatment is the best course of action for someone off work because of LBP related disability (authors statement).

What the evidence indicates: ** Changing the focus from purely symptomatic treatments to an 'active rehabilitation programme' can produce faster return to work, less chronic disability and less sickness absence.

6. Possible clinician's behaviour: Would you advise a patient to avoid painful movements? (Statement from Linton et al's study, 2002)

What the evidence indicates: ***Most adults (60-80%) experience LBP at some time.

***Advice to continue ordinary activities of daily living (ADL) as normally as possible despite the pain can give equivalent or faster symptomatic relief, and lead to shorter periods off work loss, fewer recurrences and less work loss over the following year than "traditional medical treatment" (advice to rest and 'let pain be your guide' for return to normal activity)

7. Possible clinician's behaviour: Would you tell your patients whose jobs involve repeated exposure to physical stressors that their jobs caused their LBP? (Authors statement)

What the evidence indicates: *There is limited and contradictory evidence that length of exposure to physical stressors at work (cumulative risk) increases reports of back symptoms or of persistent symptoms. (Authors underlining).

** Physical demands of work play only a minor role in the development of disc degeneration.

The strength of evidence for each statement is classified as follows:

***=**Strong evidence**- provided by generally consistent findings in multiple, high quality scientific studies.

= Moderate evidence- provided by generally consistent findings in fewer, smaller or lower quality scientific studies.

*= **Limited or contradictory evidence**- provided by one scientific study or inconsistent findings in multiple scientific studies.

It is quite obvious that the evidence statements do not support the belief and behaviour statements in the table above. Linton et al (2002) found that physical therapists and general practitioners held some of these beliefs and that these beliefs influenced their (self-reported) treatment practice. Inappropriate treatment practice, particularly if combined with unhelpful advice and information, may not only be ineffective but may block more appropriate management and RTW (Waddell & Burton 2004).

How are health care professionals beliefs and behaviours obstacles to RTW?

Health care professionals may be obstacles to RTW, both by what they say and do as well as by omission. Their beliefs about pain, manual handling, physical demands of work and ergonomics may not only be erroneous but by placing undue emphasis on these factors they may be neglecting more important psychosocial and workplace obstacles to RTW. Health care professionals who hold erroneous beliefs and whose behaviours are unhelpful may be:

a) Failing to address their patient's erroneous beliefs and unhelpful behaviours.
b) Reinforcing their patient's erroneous beliefs and unhelpful behaviours.
c) Adding additional (their own) erroneous beliefs and unhelpful behaviours to those of their patients.
d) Failing to ensure that their patients have accurate beliefs and helpful behaviours
e) Preventing, undermining or failing to facilitate their patient's RTW.

According to Waddell and Burton (2004) HCP's seldom demonstrate an interest or seem to understand occupational issues. They seldom consider obstacles to RTW and as a result they usually fail to assess or address them. Unfortunately, rather then viewing work as the goal or part of the solution, HCP's often see work as the problem, despite the fact that work is generally good for people's physical and mental health (Waddell & Burton 2004).

When they do consider obstacles to RTW, some HCP and patients view symptoms as an obstacle. However, the correlation between symptoms, pathology, impairment or incapacity for work is low (Waddell & Burton 2004). "All stakeholders should start with the basic premise that the individual is employable...the DWP has recognised the importance of changing the culture among health professionals and the need to concentrate on what people can do as opposed to what they cannot while protecting people from harm" (DWP 2004).

In the author's experience, many HCP's do not believe that it is possible for their patient to RTW, particularly if they have a physically demanding job. The advice and information they give is often in line with this belief. However, in reality, few patients with common health problems have any absolute physical or mental barriers to doing most jobs (Waddell & Burton 2004). Many do their job or return to their job despite persisting symptoms.

Approximately half of all men and women who are of working age and report some form of disability are in employment. This includes 25% of those who by self-report are severely disabled (Waddell & Burton 2004). Only 73% of people on disability and incapacity benefits regarded themselves as disabled and one third say that they would like to work, although on further questioning only 6% of these said they would currently be available for work (Waddell & Burton, 2004). Disability isn't and shouldn't be a bar to working.

Significantly more individuals could be helped to RTW by the timely assessment and management of obstacles to RTW. Disability is not a static state. It can be reduced by active rehabilitation, the removal of obstacles to work and appropriate support in the workplace.

What are the consequences of health care professionals' erroneous beliefs and unhelpful behaviours?

Health care professionals need to be aware of the messages (verbal and non-verbal) that they are communicating and be aware of the impact and potential consequences of these messages? Advice to refrain from work may not be the most appropriate clinical management or in the patient's best long-term interests (Waddell & Burton 2004). However, many HCP's seem oblivious to the disastrous impact of prolonged time off work (Waddell & Burton 2004). The longer an individual stays off work, the more likely they are to become disabled and the more likely they are to lose their job. If they are advised not to work again or not to do a particular job, this could have a profound affect on that individual's future life. Perhaps they really enjoy their job; maybe they have worked long and hard to get it. It is worth considering how we would feel if we were advised never to do our jobs again or not to go back to work? What might the consequences be for our finances, physical and mental health, housing, quality of life and relationships?

Exclusion from work is a disabling process. We need to ask our selves - could we be part of the problem? In the first year after becoming disabled one in six workers lose their job. However 60% do not leave of their own accord, they are either dismissed, or advised by health workers or other professionals to leave (Meager et al 1998). Forty percent of economically inactive disabled people who had left work had been advised to do so by a health professional (Meager et al 1998). This advice may not have been appropriate.

What do health care professionals need to do?

Health care professionals need to be discerning, critical consumers of the various theories, techniques, schools of thought, articles and courses available to them. They need to be critical thinkers.

Definition of Critical thinking
Critical thinking is the disciplined ability and willingness to assess evidence and claims, to seek a breadth of contradicting as well as confirming information, to make objective judgements on the basis of well-supported reasons as a guide to belief and action, and to monitor one's thinking while doing so" (www.ltsn.ac.uk).

Health care professionals should question current clinical practice. They need to ensure that it is evidence led and not opinion based. It should be informed by good quality research and not place undue emphasis on individual articles or personalities. In areas where the evidence is lacking, HCP need to be honest about the lack of evidence or the contradictory nature of it.

Fortunately, there are a number of national clinical guidelines available on the assessment and management of health and work problems (Carter & Birrell 2000, Mayou et al 2004, Waddell & Burton 2004, Waddell et al 2004). Unfortunately, there are many obstacles in getting HCP's to alter their behaviour to match the evidence about best practice (Jones 2005). Clinical guidelines are consequently often not implemented. Whilst effective education can change individual's beliefs, attitudes and knowledge, education on its own is insufficient to change behaviour (NHSCRD 1999, Jones 2005). More needs to be done to identify obstacles to HCP's behaviour change and to develop effective strategies to overcome them.

In terms of beliefs and behaviours about health and its relationship to work, health care professionals need to:
1. Be aware of their own beliefs and behaviours
2. Be aware of the available evidence base
3. Examine their beliefs and behaviours in light of the available evidence base
4. Address their beliefs and behaviours if they are not consistent with the available evidence base.
5. Assess and address their patients unhelpful, inaccurate or erroneous beliefs and behaviors

Unless HCP's examine their beliefs and behaviours with regards to health and work, they risk being obstacles to their patients RTW.

References

CarterJT, Birrell LN (Eds) 2000 Occupational health guidelines for the management of low back pain at work-principal recommendations. Faculty of Occupational Medicine, London

DWP 2004 Building capacity for work: A UK Framework for Vocational Rehabilitation. The framework work document. Department for Works and Pensions

Jones D 2005 Attitudes and beliefs about chronic non cancer pain and the role of education in preparing community based health and social care professionals to undertake pain management. Unpublished PhD Thesis. Queen Margaret University College, Edinburgh

Linton SJ, Vlaeyen J, Ostelo R 2002 The back pain beliefs of health care providers: Are we fear avoidant? Journal of Occupational Rehabilitation. 12(4):223-232

Main CJ, Waddell G 2004 Beliefs about Back Pain. In: Waddell G (Ed) The Back Pain revolution. 2nd edition. Churchill Livingstone, Edinburgh

Mayou R, Main CJ, Auty A 2004 Apparently disproportionate injury outcomes and their causes. In. Psychology, Personal Injury and rehabilitation. The IUA/ABI Rehabilitation Working Party: Evidence based guidelines Royal College of General Practitioners (www.rcgp.org.uk)

Meager N, Bates P, Dench S, Honey S, Williams M 1998 Employment of Disabled People: Assessing the extent of participation. DfEE Research Report RR69

NHSCRD 1999 'Getting evidence into practice' Effective Health Care Bulletin. NHS Centre for Reviews and Dissemination The Royal Society of Medicine Press, London 5:1

Vlaeyen JWS, Linton SJ 2000 Fear-avoidance and its consequences in chronic musculoskeletal pain. A state of the art. Pain 85 317-33.

Vlaeyen JWS, Kole-Snijders AMJ, Rotterveel AM, Ruesink R, Heuts PHTG 1995 The role of fear of movement / (re)injury in pain disability. Journal of Occupational Rehabilitation 5(4):235-252

Waddell G, Burton AK 2004 Concepts of rehabilitation for the management of common health problems. (Report prepared for UK Department for Work and Pensions), London , The Stationery Office

Waddell G, Burton AK , Bartys S 2004 Concepts of rehabilitation for the management of common health problems – evidence base. (www.dwp.gov.uk/medical)

Web-sites and web-pages referred to in this chapter:

www.ltsn.ac.uk
www.rcgp.org.uk
www.dwp.gov.uk/medical

11

Chronic Pain and the Benefits System: Obstacles to returning to work for unemployed patients.

PAUL WATSON AND SHILPA PATEL

Introduction

It is the mark of a civilised society that those who are unable to work should not loose their dignity and should be cared for by society. This is, by and large, an accepted fact in modern society. The contentious ground lies in how disabled should a person be before society relieves him or her of the obligation to contribute to society and to then become a recipient of social welfare benefits and in how much that person should receive in relation to those who are working. At the end of the 20th century the amount being paid in supporting those who were unable to work, had come to the end of their working lives, or who were identified as suffering social disadvantage, grew rapidly forcing governments to review how much should be spent in these areas. This led to a reappraisal of the qualifying criteria for receipt of benefits (Bloch & Prins 2001, Waddell et al 2002).

People with chronic pain conditions are well represented in those who are in receipt of social support due to the inability to work. They are in receipt of wage compensation (benefits received in lieu of a wage) and early retirement benefits due to ill health (Waddell 2004, Waddell et al 2003). This had led governments to look to alternative strategies to reduce the costs including: reducing benefit levels, increasing the medical "threshold" for benefit qualification, restricting access to early retirement, the introduction of rehabilitation and re-employment programmes for disabled people and regular reviews of those who remain on benefits.

In the UK the responsibility for assisting people to move off benefits and into work has been undertaken by the employment services, in the past this has been done outside of the healthcare system. More recent "joined up" approaches have been piloted and the government has promoted initiatives to link health and employment services to provide more comprehensive programmes of rehabilitation (Crossman et al 2004, Department of Work and Pensions 2002).

In this chapter we will explore the problems of returning unemployed people dependent on benefits to work. Firstly we will examine the "barriers" involved in returning to employment from the perspective of the claimant. We will also look at how those who have to address return to work see the problems through an analysis of the literature on people working in jobcentres and benefit offices. In this we will hope to cast some light on the so-called "Black Flags" (Main et al 2005) or organisational "systems" problems which can prevent people from returning to work - even if they want to. We will not address the medical and psychosocial issues of return to work as we hope that readers will be familiar with this through previous editions of Topical Issue in Pain (Kendall & Watson 2000, Watson 2000, Watson & Kendall 2000), the companion chapters in this section of the book and other reviews (Waddell et al 2003a). We hope that this will enable the reader to get a different perspective of the return to work literature that is specific to those on long term benefits and which differs from those faced by the employed. This is not to say that the obstacles to return to work for the employed are not faced by the unemployed, but the unemployed face specific, additional problems that are often overlooked.

When writing for a healthcare audience it is difficult to know how to refer to the objects of interest. Health care practitioners refer to people as "patients", people in the benefits agencies used to refer to people as "claimants" and those in job centres called them "clients", but the latter two have been dropped in favour of "customers". For simplicity's sake we will refer to people as "claimants" to distinguish that we are talking about people who are claiming benefits; we hope that this will not upset the politically sensitive among you.

Cost of benefits

Musculoskeletal pain problems have been identified as the commonest cause of certified absence from work for the employed in the UK (Cherry et al 2001) making up nearly half of all reasons for absence from work. Musculoskeletal pain conditions account for at least 20% to 34% of the primary self reported cause of disability for those on Incapacity Benefit (Waddell et al 2003). In a recent analysis of all incapacity benefit recipients in Salford, Greater Manchester (UK) on a single day in February 2004 we found that 22% of claimants reported musculoskeletal pain as the main reason for claiming (Watson and Patel unpublished data).

The costs of chronic pain can be highlighted from research findings presented by Maniadakis and Gray (2000) who reported chronic low back pain alone cost £1,623 million in healthcare costs in 1998, the last year for which accurate data is available. When looking at the wider picture, additional costs incurred due to wage compensation and loss of production accounted for an additional £10,668 million.

In November 2004 8.6% of the working population of the UK was reported as not working due to sickness or disability and 7.7% was in receipt of IB, SDA or IS (Department of Work and Pensions 2004). The trend is currently downwards from the high points in the late 1990s – more people are leaving these benefits than are joining. In the same dataset there were over half a million people claiming IB or SDA for musculoskeletal conditions, this of course does not represent all those with a chronic pain problem which might be classified in other groups. There is also considerable overlap between painful conditions and mental illness such as depression. Whichever way you look at the data we are spending a lot of money on disability due to a condition that is the bread and butter of many physiotherapists' work – musculoskeletal pain.

Relationship between benefits and work loss

It is helpful to recap on what is paid to whom when we talk about wage compensation/benefits. In the UK the first 28 weeks of wage compensation for employed people is normally paid by the employer (sickness benefit) depending on the employee having paid sufficient contributions – normally around 2 years of contributions. The qualification for the benefit is self-certification, valid for the first 7 days, and a medical certificate thereafter. For many employees the rate is paid at the same rate as their usual weekly or monthly wage and many would not loose significantly during this time period. Contractual agreements vary but there would be a reduction in the amount of compensation after a 6 months period. If the person remains off work for longer than the employer compensation arrangements then they will convert to Incapacity Benefit. In the initial phase the employee typically receives about 80-90% of their weekly wage (MISSOC 2000). Those not covered by additional employer agreements might be eligible for basic statutory sick pay which is payable at a much lower rate – around £66 pounds per week at the time of writing (April 2005). If a person remains off work for longer than 6 months they will progress to Incapacity Benefit which is currently £56-£89 per week depending on the level of benefits and the claimant's age (www.dwp.gov). For the first 28 weeks of incapacity, people previously in work are assessed on the 'own occupation' test - the claimant's ability to do their own job. Otherwise incapacity is based on the 'personal capability assessment' (formerly 'all work test') that assesses ability to carry out a range of work-related activities, or their ability to do *any* job. The test applies after 28 weeks of incapacity or from the start of the claim for people who did not previously have a job i.e., the unemployed.

Workers might be eligible for an industrial injury benefit if the health condition was deemed to be caused by an industrial injury. This is paid at a flat rate related to a percentage of the level of previous earnings and is payable in addition to other benefits.

Access to incapacity benefit triggers eligibility to other benefits. The main benefits being Incapacity benefit, Disabled Living and Income Support, few claimants are on a single benefit. Data from the DSS Statistics for 2000 demonstrate that over half receive two or more benefits. In 2000 nearly 79% of IB recipients received Disabled Living Allowance (DLA) and 40% received Income Support (IS). In addition to this claimants might be eligible for other benefits for help with housing and school meals for children or travel.

Whichever arrangement the employee comes under it is evident that their income eventually reduces with prolonged absence and for most this is pronounced once they proceed to claiming State benefits.

Secondary gain

"Malingering" is a word that developed in military service to refer to the shirking of one's own responsibilities. In the context of work it refers to the fabrication of symptoms in order to avoid work. We suggest that wilful fabrication of symptoms or incapacity is relatively rare, most people who report symptoms genuinely have those symptoms. What is often in dispute is the degree of recovery, the level of expected function, the ability to work, level of incapacity and how that persons should be expected to contribute to society with respect to their social role including working (Fishbain et al 1995).

Secondary gain refers to the rewards a person receives economically, emotionally and the responsibilities they are allowed to avoid as a result of their condition. In this respect all illness is associated with some secondary gain in the form of support from health care professionals or family and temporary release from responsibilities. It is also a convenient excuse for healthcare professionals to blame the level of benefit or compensation seeking behaviour for failed treatment or poor compliance on the part of the patient. In the literature there is often a focus on the monetary aspect of secondary gain with an assumption that receipt of benefits is the main reason why people are not in work and a reduction in this benefit will result in an increased rate of return to work. This is simplistic and wrong. Unfortunately for the person with back pain, the cause of which is difficult to determine in most, this has been a particular issue, which is not the case in those with paraplegia or stroke where the cause of the incapacity is more obvious.

Most of the data on secondary gain has come from the Workman's Compensation systems in North America where industrial injury, receipt of wage compensation and access to health care are linked together in a way in which it is not in the UK. The evidence from such a system demonstrates a link between more generous compensation and longer work absences, for those who are employed. If the rate of compensation is increased there is an increase in absence. Likewise schemes that have longer qualification periods (more days without pay), before payment of wage compensation, report lower incidences of work loss. It must be remembered that these data refer to people who are working prior to absence and the injury is sustained at work. These data also better represent blue-collar workers than workers as a whole (Waddell 2004). Nevertheless, most people agree that there is a link between more generous wage replacement and slow return to work in the *employed*. This is often misused and people refer to this data when speaking about the unemployed. In the UK, as reported earlier, the provisions for wage compensation vary, some employers pay only the minimum state sick pay whereas others give generous, often full pay, to absent workers. In this respect financial secondary gain would appear to be more likely in those who are employed and who do not loose out financially when absent from work. It is those of us who are employed who take more time off if we have a more generous wage compensation package. Remember the old adage "when you point your finger three point back at yourself"!

In contradistinction to the concept of secondary gain is the matter of secondary losses, which can be substantial. These include the social benefits of working (social contact, support networks), loss of social status and for many, financial loss in the form of lost wages and increased personal expenditure on health care. Waddell (1998) and Linton (1998) both independently report that those with chronic musculoskeletal pain are financially worse off than those who work. How much financially worse off is difficult to assess. In the UK Erens and Ghate (1993) reported that 50% of people on benefits received only half of their previous income and Burchardt (2000) reported that disabled people had incomes of less than half the national average wage.

Waddell et al (2003) point out, that although people on Incapacity Benefit have modest incomes, many of them are unskilled and would be likely to only access low paid work which would be covered by the minimum wage. Their income on IB would represent 70-90% of what they might expect to earn in a minimum wage employment. Although this is rather a hard analysis of the data one must consider the wage replacement ratio, that is, the proportion of wage that is replaced by wage compensation payments. It might be reasonable to believe that the nearer the wage replacement ratio is to the claimants previous wage the less likely they are to return to work. In this respect a low wage economy might be less likely to attract people back into work.

Other out of pocket expenses are rarely calculated, Goosens et al (1996) reported that of the total cost of healthcare for a group of fibromyalgia patients, 49% was paid for directly by the patient as over the counter medicines, home help and additional professional care. Ferrell (1996) also points to the additional economic cost of chronic pain in people whose income is compromised and the cost of care and additional help is funded from dwindling resources.

Other costs of remaining unemployed

Benefit costs are only part of the cost associated with unemployment; there are social and health costs too. Prolonged unemployment can result in additional healthcare and social costs that are not calculated in the total cost of unemployment. Those who loose their employment are likely to suffer mental health problems (Janlert 1997, Kposowa 2001, Weich & Lewis 1998) and have a lower life expectancy. Unemployed people also consult more often for physical complaints, have a higher incidence of alcohol and drug related problems and are more likely to be admitted to hospital than people who remain in employment. All this represents a cost not only on the individual but also a potential additional cost on society and healthcare supporting the results of unemployment.

Work and motivation

Those who are unemployed, if work plays a key role in their life, are more motivated to retain or return to work than those who place less emphasis on it. Work involvement according to Kanungo (1982) depends on beliefs about the value of work relative to other pursuits (family, leisure etc) and the moral imperative a person feels they have to contribute to rather than receive support *from* society. It is also influenced by the intrinsic needs of work, which relates to an interest in work in itself and the need for achievement and self-fulfilment through work and the extrinsic needs, such as the need for money, status, and acclaim (Riipinen 1996). Involvement in work and the type of work people are prepared to take may be influenced by financial imperatives (extrinsic) and past socialisation (adoption of the work ethic) rather than the need for job satisfaction (intrinsic) (Misra et al 1985). The relative influence of intrinsic and extrinsic needs and the moral imperative differs between individuals (Deci & Ryan 1991). Return to work at any job may require satisfaction of the moral imperative and extrinsic (financial) needs, others may only return to work if the moral imperative, the extrinsic *and* intrinsic (the type of work) needs are met; they are unwilling to take just *any* job (Fishbain et al. 1999). How these factors influence return to work and how they interact with the other factors such as health anxieties is unclear and has not been investigated in the unemployed with pain problems.

Claimants' perceived barriers to employment

In reviewing the literature for this chapter it is very apparent that there is a paucity of material on how unemployed people with chronic pain view the problems associated with returning to work and the possible bridges to successful re-employment. The published research suffers from poor methodology and all those on incapacity benefits are viewed as a homogenous group as if the difficulties are the same for all IB claimants (i.e., the problems are the same for those with mental health conditions as for those with chronic pain). This might be true, but to date this has not received appropriate attention and research, so we simply cannot tell.

Lack of appropriate skills

Some people who are in the IB register have been out of work for many years. In a rapidly changing employment market skills can become out of date very quickly and those not working can have an increasingly difficult job returning to work if they lack the skills employers need (Peters 2003, Thornton 1998, Waddell 1998). A lack of qualifications in the unemployed both with and without disability has been a perennial predictor of a poor rate of return to work. IB claimants in possession of some form of qualifications are usually at an advantage over those with no qualifications but 62% of IB claimants have no qualifications (Dorset et al 1998). This suggests that future interventions for IB claimants should provide these people with opportunities to gain skills and qualifications to maximise their chances of returning to work and at the same time enhance self-esteem and confidence.

Straaton et al (1996) reported that high levels of educational attainment were associated with better rehabilitation outcomes. However Osgood et al (2003) reported return to IB was much higher among those with few or no qualifications suggesting that those with more qualifications were less likely to accept any job. This might be a problem with skilled people in an area where only low status unskilled work is available.

Smith and Crisler (1985) reported that those claimants who had low levels of education usually also had fewer transferable skills. In a world where skills are quickly outdated this has serious implications. Some claimants may have very specific skills that, although well respected in their own field, are not applicable to the wider job market. In some situations, claimants are unable to return to the same type of work they had previously undertaken. In the Pathways to Work report (Goldstone & Douglas 2003) some claimants saw this as a significant setback, in particular, in cases where they felt they had few skills to apply to other areas of work. In situations such as these it was important for employment staff to help clients identify and apply transferable skills as well as training needs.

Health concerns

Dorset et al (1998) studied IB recipients who returned to IB after a period of employment. 47% had musculo-skeletal problems, 16% cardio-vascular problems, and 18% mental health problems, in particular depression. Those who reported a perception that their job was too heavy for them and who insisted on a restriction on the number of hours that could be worked because of their health, were more likely to return to IB and also continued consulting for treatment. These results demonstrate how important preoccupation with health related issues is in militating a successful outcome.

Evaluation of the New Deal for Disabled people pilots (NDDP) (Hills et al 2001) identified how 93% of people who registered reported that their disability or health limited their ability to participate in activities including work. However, in only 38% of cases was this limitation assessed as being greatly limiting. Nearly half of the registrants did not expect any changes in their health condition, whereas a third expected positive change and the rest anticipated deterioration. Attitudes towards the future of their condition played a key role in the action people planned and undertook towards employment, only those who expected to improve had a positive attitude towards work.

Recent research has identified an important relationship between fear of pain or injury and failure to return to work (Fritz & George 2002, Vowles & Gross 2003). Fear avoidance has been covered in previous editions of Topical Issues in Pain (Gifford 1998) so there is no need to cover them in detail again here. Briefly, those who fear that activity will cause them physical damage fail to engage in activities that, they believe, are damaging. This is particularly important in those who were injured at work, as they are more likely to believe that work (sometimes all work), is injurious to their health.

Distorted beliefs about pain and the ability to work can be reinforced by others. This includes family, healthcare professionals and people working in the employment services. Peebles & Moore (2000) found that if a patient's perception of rehabilitation was positive and in line with that of their physician there tended to be a better relationship between the two and often this improved patients' chances of a participating in rehabilitation programmes. If there is a tacit agreement that unless one is 100% fit one should not return to work, there is a poor chance of engagement in any form of rehabilitation. This is particularly problematic in chronic pain patients where the pain is likely to continue indefinitely and where treatment places the emphasis on coping and managing pain rather than expecting a full recovery. Studies like this suggest the strong relationship between the patient and practitioner could be both positive and negative because healthcare practitioners not only provide a means of validation of their condition and treatment but also are very powerful agent for legitimising the condition and providing support for benefit claiming. This can develop to the point that the GP may not challenge the patients perception of illness and unwittingly (or otherwise) colludes in continued incapacity and claiming (Chew & May 1997, Chew-Graham & May 1999). A claimant who perceives his/her GP is of the opinion that work is not appropriate is likely to remain on benefit and it will be very difficult for others to challenge or change this opinion.

Those working in the employment and benefit offices have rarely received training in how to address issues of health. Reassurance about work and the effect it might have on the person's health is an essential starting point for engagement. Those who see the person on IB in the job centre do not have medical training and cannot give advice on these matters, yet it is these people who have the very difficult job of trying to engage claimants in rehabilitation and return to work. Claimants have great difficulty in identifying jobs which they feel are appropriate and within the limitations of their condition (Peters 2003, Thornton 1998; Thornton & Corden 2002) and Job centre staff often feel unable to offer advice in the absence of positive and useful guidance and support from health care practitioners.

Chronic pain is a variable condition characterised by "good" days and "bad" days, which the patient finds difficult to predict. This unpredictability of the condition and the patient's inability to sustain a regular level of activity was reported by Thornton (1998) as a key reason why people would not engage in employment. They felt that there was little point in looking for work when they could not guarantee an employer regular hours of attendance everyday; their perception was that this would eventually lead to their dismissal.

Perceptions of work and employers

Unemployed people report that they are less employable than others. This in itself is a self-fulfilling prophecy. If you believe no one will give you a job you are less likely to apply for one for fear of a set back.

Osgood et al (2003) reported on the association between perceptions of employability and return to work among IB claimants. Those who perceived themselves as employable were more likely to return to and remain in work and have less absence when employed. Rowlingson and Berthoud (1996) ascribed the lack of success among initiatives to move people from benefits, such as IB, into work could be because people have a lack of expectation of working and a lack of expectation that anyone would wish to employ them. Other factors preventing people from trying to return to work are the disabled person's belief that there is a lack of suitable job opportunities and other peoples' attitudes towards their disability. These barriers are not in any particular order of importance but claimants commonly perceive that there is a lack of suitable job opportunity and/or that other people, such as employers and work colleagues, hold negative attitudes towards disabled people or people who have been on benefits for a long time and this is a deterrent from seeking future employment.

Research conducted by Arksey (2003) analysed the People Into Employment (PIE) project. Integrating both qualitative and quantitative research methods they found that claimants perceived a number of barriers to work including their length of time out of work, availability of stable and secure jobs and lack of confidence to hold down a job. All the people questioned referred to more than one barrier to returning to work and many had reported multiple barriers.

The lack of suitable job opportunities refers to the perceived availability of jobs that would be suitable for a person with a disability. Customers cite the need to be able to take regular breaks, to be able to work around a condition that varies in severity and is relatively unpredictable, and the availability of part time jobs. The latter appears to have changed in recent years. In a previous review (Waddell et al 2003a) unemployed disabled people reported that they would not find part-time work acceptable because of the poor pay and job prospects associated with such work. More recent work suggest this has changed (Dickens et al 2004). Whether this is a result of changed perceptions about part-time work or a difference in the groups sampled is not clear. Women were more likely to consider part-time work, but this too appears to have changed and how stable the change is has not been determined. If part-time work is more acceptable, linking this with additional benefits such as work credits might mean that more people would be prepared to consider employment.

Lifestyle substitution

If a person is not working there is often an assumption that they are not engaged in any productive activity. This is not necessarily the case. People can have interests and duties outside work and these can often substitute for work, which can then complicate any return to work. Furthermore, the emphasis on employment as an outcome measure for people with chronic pain can be criticised as too authoritarian and controlling, and that coping with pain in a productive way may not mean a return to paid employment for many people. Andersen (2002) found in a Danish longitudinal study of chronically unemployed people that 58% reported advantages to unemployment. Interviews reported improvements in relationships with children while being unemployed. Involvement in other activities including childcare for own children or grandchildren, home making, training and unpaid work (voluntary work) was seen as a way to fill spare time, provide social interaction, give a sense of reward and even improve job prospects, which in turn helped to counteract the fear of losing skills and experience. Young and Murphy (2000) found 40% of unemployed people who responded to a questionnaire said they were satisfied with being unemployed. Of this 40%, about half were involved in productive behaviour of some sort. Where there are high levels of satisfaction from unemployment a much greater incentive will be required to motivate people to find work or engage in rehabilitation and work seeking. In addition, the role they were fulfilling (childcare for example) has to be provided elsewhere, which might involve additional costs, thus reducing the attractiveness of working especially if the wage available is low. We must also bear in mind the amount of fulfilling work possible in unemployment might be determined by level of disability, and reduced physical ability may prevent people with chronic pain developing fulfilling substitute lifestyles.

Age

People who are approaching retirement age may be unwilling to consider a return to work, they might regard themselves as already retired, or to have contributed sufficiently to the common good and that it is their turn to benefit. Since the 1980s there has been a big increase in the number of people who have retired before the qualifying age (Waddell et al 2002, Waddell et al 2003a) and there is an increasing desire in older workers to retire from full-time work before the retirement age (Scales & Scase 2000). Waddell et al (2002) suggest that in the 1980s and 1990s there was a reduction in the criteria for granting early ill health retirement which fed the expectation of being excused work for relatively minor health problems. It also became accepted that an older worker, once on benefit, would remain there until the retirement age and then proceed onto a retirement pension. In the UK about 28% of men and 33% of women over age 50 are not economically active (not working) (Hotopp 2005).

Goldstone & Douglas (2003) reported that staff felt claimants perceived their age as a barrier to returning to work. In some cases advisors felt older workers were more difficult to place into work or rehabilitation due to the claimants' attitudes and perceptions of their employability or acceptability to employers.

The recent problems with pension funds have brought this into the limelight and early retirement has often been used to address problems of redundancy and workforce downsizing. As a consequence, pension funds have been unable to support large numbers of early retirements and in so doing forced the criteria for qualification to be raised. This may well result in increasing numbers of older people considering themselves unsuitable for work and claiming incapacity benefit.

Need for financial stability

Moving from benefits to a wage can be very daunting for people, particularly if they are not sure that they will be able to sustain the return to work and maintain their income. In the NDDP evaluation (Hills et al 2001) the need for financial stability was rated highly as a precursor to participation. Claimants needed reassurance that their benefits would not be affected by participation in work-based initiatives. Claimants perceive that the transition from benefits to a wage is risky, especially if it is supplemented by other payments (e.g. tax/family credits: - they fear that an increase in number of benefits meant an increased chance of one or all would not be paid.) The ability to return to benefits easily and without delays in payment should a job not work out was considered important.

Many claimants had experienced difficulties in payment of benefits in the past and therefore were wary of any change for fear that payments would not occur on time. Claimants are frequently worried that they would not be able to understand new benefits and payments and consequently reluctant to abandon the familiar IB (Arthur et al 1999, Corden & Sainsbury 2001). From this it is apparent that claimants regard income stability as very important. Thus, fear of financial instability is a significant barrier to engagement in job seeking.

Counter-intuitively the take up of top-up benefits, a key feature of the UK Government's approach to return to work, can be affected by concerns about financial stability. Some schemes allow the claimant to work a set number of hours to earn money in addition to benefits. This is appreciated by claimants, but if it is time-limited, and the claimant feels there is no chance of taking up a full time job at the end, they perceive they will face a fall in income when the scheme terminates and as a result, prefer to keep on their own (lower) benefit. The UK government plans to use top-up incentives as a way of encouraging people to take up rehabilitation and get back into work, but these might do little to encourage some people to take them up because of their temporary nature (Corden & Sainsbury 2001, Dewson et al 2004). Income top ups might only work for those who fully intend to return to work and in this situation the extra payments may smooth their return. Those who are less sure that they will be able to work sufficient hours might take up these temporary benefits.

Ball and Orford (2002) conducted interviews with long term unemployed people in Birmingham and found a reluctance to accept 'any job' that came along. They felt there were 3 main reasons why the long-term unemployed failed to pursue available jobs:

1. Low pay led to concerns related to economic stability.
2. They found it unacceptable that the jobs available to them were of low pay and status.
3. The consequence of accepting a low pay, low status job would make finding a better job more difficult.

The above are important findings but how they relate to disabled people has not been evaluated. Some people with chronic pain problems may have been in relatively well-paid jobs with additional responsibilities and status. To "start at the bottom" as they may see it, could be a considerable disincentive if they felt there would be little prospect of advancement, particularly in view of the considerable personal investment needed. The risks they take in trying to regain employment are not off-set by an increase in income, indeed the perception is that to return to work may consign them to the low wage economy for good.

Staff and process barriers

As we have already indicated, few of the people who are given the responsibility of trying to help those with chronic pain into work have a background in rehabilitation and none will have any previous healthcare experience. As a result they will be unable to specifically advise people on the type of work that is suitable for their disability. For this information the jobcentre staff rely on the opinion of healthcare professionals. Re-organisation within the DWP has meant that many staff have been assigned to advise people on IB with limited experience and little training. Although the Government has invested in training in some areas many feel they have been thrown in at the deep end. Goldstone & Douglas (2003) found a variety of attitudes and perceptions about IB recipients depending on whether the decision to work with IB customers was voluntary or not. Staff reported a number of barriers in their work with IB customers including, lack of knowledge (lack or awareness) of initiatives, organisational barriers (communication problems, in particular in large Jobcentres) and lack of specialist skills. IB recipients themselves felt specialist advisors provided a better range of facilities in comparison to general advisors.

Lack of awareness of initiatives

Any observer of Government policy on benefits and incentives to return to work cannot fail to be astonished by its complexity and fluidity. New initiatives are introduced regularly, some are "piloted" in one area and not another or are implemented differently depending on local needs and availability. It is very difficult to keep abreast of these changes. Some initiatives are only available for short period and staff are often unaware or unsure of the period for which they are available. A lack of awareness of initiatives, or a lack of familiarity with the detail of the initiative and the implication for the IB claimant make staff anxious of offering some benefits. This problem has bedevilled initiatives throughout recent history and led to poor take up (Corden & Sainsbury 2001, Dewson et al 2004, Dickens et al 2004, Gardiner 1997, Lacovou & Berthoud 2000).

Claimants often report that a particular incentive or programme has not been offered to them even when it was available. This may be because of a lack of awareness by staff. Conversely, it is possible that staff may not have offered the prospect of a particular programme or incentive because they could not be sure that it would still be available when the claimant was ready to take it up. It certainly demonstrates that the DWP needs to review its marketing strategy to both staff and claimants.

Health and access to treatment

We have already mentioned that people on IB have considerable concerns about their health status and frequently rely on their general practitioner to advise them on their suitability for work. Benefits staff felt that approaching issues of health were very difficult, particularly where the claimant relied on their GPs report of their readiness to work. Staff felt obliged not to question the claimants' perceptions about this because they felt uninformed and not qualified to do so. They identified some people as more difficult to help than others. For example, they felt it was hard to advise people with mental illness or low back pain who they perceived as difficult to place in programmes or with employers (Berglind & Gerner 2002, Osgood et al 2003). They also reported a lack of support when they felt it might be appropriate to ask for another opinion. Medical reports are criticised as they are only concerned with the fitness to work and do not offer material for an explanation to the claimant. Staff have no access to an independent professional who can examine the claimant and give good advice and an explanation upon which to develop a return to work plan. More recently attempts to integrate medical and vocational rehabilitation has attempted to address this (Department of Work and Pensions 2002, Dickens et al 2004, Watson et al 2004).

Staff working on the recent Incapacity Benefits Personal Advisor trials reported that those who were still awaiting medical referrals, investigations or treatments were particularly difficult to help. They were resistant to help and were unwilling to engage in any programmes to facilitate skill enhancement or job seeking (Dickens et al 2004). Staff reported that they normally deferred these claimants (did not take further action). This experience will be familiar to many physiotherapists and those working in pain management where the patient is unwilling to engage in rehabilitation until medical issues are resolved (Main & Spanswick 2000). If this experience is common inside the healthcare field what chance have those from the DWP of engaging these people?

Resources and targets

In terms of organisational barriers, a lack of resources, money, time, pressures, and other targets inhibited work with IB claimants (Goldstone & Douglas 2003). Where staff had performance targets there was a tendency to "cherry pick" easy claimants such as those who were already looking for work, and those recently out of work, and avoid the difficult cases such as the chronic pain and serious mental illness claimants. They said outcome targets (usually assessed by the number of people in work following intervention) changed how they did their job.

They would not offer interventions, or would offer less help to those who were deemed difficult to help and might concentrate on "easier" clients. At the time of writing there are no specific targets or incentives in place for engaging claimants in the processes of returning to work or entering rehabilitation. But this is intended in the future and is likely to make DWP staff concentrate once more on the "easier" claimants. However, local, office targets still exist and these lead to staff concentrating on "voluntary customers", i.e. : those who are actively seeking help to return to work, who are considered more "job-ready", and who have skills that are in demand locally. Less help is likely to be offered to those who have to attend for interview. Under new guidelines for IB all claimants have to attend for an interview: so called "mandatory customers". These claimants are more likely to be deferred – in effect put back on a review list without being offered assistance. The analogy is similar to the old NHS regime when day case surgery patients were more likely to be offered treatment than more complex surgery to increase the successful through put.

This has had a knock on effect on the new Pathways to Work Condition Management Programmes. Staff are unlikely to refer those they do not consider "job-ready" to local Condition Management Programmes – where pain management might be available, because they feel it will not help the person move forwards towards work. This may be counterproductive because a pain management programme might be the place where health concerns could be addressed (Dickens et al 2004) and where the claimant could be persuaded that they are ready to look at returning to work.

Timing the approach to claimants

On review of a specific initiative where claimants were called to interview for a 'One stop shop' for advice on return to work help (not rehabilitation) and benefits advice (Cotton et al 2000) a number of organisational issues inhibited customers chances of participating. In particular staff reported the inappropriate timing of the initial interviews and this has been reported in other work. Claimants are called up for interview with the prospect of trying to return them to work without consideration of their personal circumstances. For example, claimants may be currently undergoing or waiting to begin treatment or medical investigations. Other factors are cited such as difficulties with housing, marital problems, medico-legal actions and social stresses which make concentrating on rehabilitation and return to work difficult if not impossible (Dickens et al 2004).

In summary

It is all too easy to sit back and say that those who are on Wage compensation benefits and unemployed are either "benefit dependent", institutionalised or simply not motivated to work. One or all of these may be true in specific cases, but we cannot forget that there is a unique set of problems faced by unemployed people when they either try or are encouraged to return to work. What is apparent is that the health care system cannot address all the problems and this is probably why "rehabilitation" programmes and pain management programmes do not return people to work successfully. Without an integrated approach to address these barriers we will not be adequately helping the person in pain from returning to what most of us accept as a normal life – working. Without addressing these barriers and providing meaningful employment we risk leaving a lot of people socially isolated and impoverished. These barriers can only be addressed if a joined up approach is taken and that health care staff understand the barriers to returning to work in the unemployed and work with those in the DWP to help them manage people better.

Glossary

Wage compensation – benefits received in lieu of wages – employers sick pay, statutory sick pay, incapacity benefits

NDDP - New deal for disabled people

PA - personal advisor

DWP Department of work and Pensions

Claimant – a person claiming and receiving state benefits

References:

Andersen GJ 2002 Coping with long-term unemployment: economic security, labour market operation and well being. Results from a Danish parallel study 1994-1999. International Social Welfare, 11:178-190

Arksey H 2003 People into employment; supporting people with disabilities and carers into work., Health and Social Care in the community 11:283-292

Arthur S, Corden A, Green A, Lewis J, Sainsbury R, Stafford B, Thornton P, Walker R 1999 New Deal for Disabled People: Early implementation. DSS Research report No. 106 Leeds

Ball M, Orford J 2002 Meaningful patterns of activity amongst the long term inner city unemployed: A qualitative study. Journal of Community and Applied Psychology 12:377-396

Berglind H, Gerner U 2002 Motivation and return to work among the long-term sicklisted: an action theory perspective. Disabil Rehabil 24:719-726

Bloch FS, Prins R 2001 Who returns to work and why? A six country study on work incapacity and reintegration. Transaction Publishers, London

Burchardt T 2000 Enduring economic exclusion: disabled people, income and work. Findings - Report 60, York

Cherry NM, Meyer JD, Chen Y, Holt DL, McDonald JC 2001 The reported incidence of work related musculoskeletal disease in the UK: MOSS 1997-2000, Occupational Medicine, 51:450-503

Chew CA, May CR 1997 The benefits of back pain Family Practice, 14:461-465

Chew-Graham C, May C 1999 Chronic low back pain in general practice: the challenge of the consultation. Family Practice 16:46-49

Corden A, Sainsbury R 2001 Incapacity benefits and work incentives. Department of Work and Pensions Report No 141, Leeds

Cotton D, Stone V, Thomas A 2000 Why not ONE? Views of no-participants before full participation. Department of Work and Pensions research report No. 127, Leeds

Crossman K, Mahon M, Watson PJ, Oldham JA, Cooper RG 2004 Chronic low back pain-associated paraspinal muscle dysfunction is not the result of a constitutionally determined "adverse" fiber-type composition. Spine 29:628-634

Deci E, Ryan R 1991 Intrinsic motivation and self-determination in human behaviour. In: Steers R, Porter L (Eds), Motivation and work behavior. McGraw-Hill, New York

Deparment of Work and Pensions 2002 Pathways to work: Helping people into employment. The Stationary Office, London

Department of Work and Pensions 2004 Incapacity Benefit and Severe Disablement Allowance Quarterly Summary Statistics. November 2004, London

Dewson, S, Davis S, Loukas G 2004 A Stepping stone to employment? En evaluation of the permitted work rules- Wave 2. Institute for Employment Studies, Brighton

Dickens S, Mowlam A, Woodfield K 2004 Incapacity benefit reforms- the personal adviser role & practices. National Centre for Social Research, York

Dorset R, Finlayson L, Ford R, March A, White M, Zarb G 1998 Leaving incapacity benefit. DSS Research report number 89, Leeds

Erens B, Ghate D 1993 Invalidity benefit: a longitudinal study of new recipients. Department of Social Security Research Reports No.20 HMSO. London.

Ferrell BR 1996 How patients and families pay the price of pain. In: Cohen MM, Campbell JN (Eds), Pain treatment centres at a cross roads: A practical and conceptual reappraisal. IASP Press, Seattle 229-237

Fishbain DA, Rosomoff H, Cutler RB, Rosomoff-Steele R 1995 Secondary gain concept; a review of the scientific evidence. Clinical Journal of Pain 11:6-21

Fishbain DA, Cutler RB, Rosomoff HL, Khalil T, Steele-Rosomoff R 1999 Prediction of "intent", "discrepancy with intent", and "discrepancy with nonintent" for the patient with chronic pain to return to work after treatment at a pain facility. Clinical Journal of Pain, 15:141-50

Fritz MJ, George ZS 2002 Identifying psychosocial variables in patients with acute work-related low back pain: the importance of fear-avoidance beliefs. Physical Therapy 82(10):973-983

Gardiner K 1997 Bridges from benefit to work. Social Policy research report 130. Joseph Roundtree Foundation, York

Gifford LS (ed) 1998 Topical Issues in Pain 1. Whiplash - science and management. Fear-avoidance beliefs and behaviour. CNS Press, Falmouth

Goldstone C, Douglas L 2003 Pathways to Work from Incapacity Benefits. Department of Work and Pensions, London

Goossens ME, Rutten-van Molken MP, Leidl RM, Bos SG, Vlaeyen JW, Teeken-Gruben NJ 1996 Cognitive-educational treatment of fibromyalgia: a randomized clinical trial. II. Economic evaluation, Journal of Rheumatology 23:1246-1254

Hills D, Child C, Blackburn V, Youll P 2001 Evaluation of New Deal for Disabled People innovations scheme pilots. Department of Work and Pensions Research report No 143, Leeds

Hotopp U 2005 The employment rate of older workers: An econometric analysis of the main influences on the growth since 1993. Labour Market Trends 113:73-88

Janlert U 1997 Unemployment as a disease and diseases of the unemployed. Scandinavian Journal of Work, Environment & Health. 23 Suppl 3:79-83

Kanungo R 1982 Measurement of job and work involvement. Journal of Applied Psychology, 67:341-349

Kendall NAS, Watson PJ 2000 Identifying psychosocial yellow flags and modifying management. In: Gifford L (Ed), Topical Issues in Pain Vol 2, CNS Press, Falmouth 131-140

Kposowa AJ 2001 Unemployment and suicide: a cohort analysis of social factors predicting suicide in the US National Longitudinal Mortality Study. Psychological Medicine, 31:127-138

Lacovou, M, Berthoud R 2000 Parents and employment. DSS Research Report No 143, Leeds

Linton SJ 1998 The socioeconomic impact of chronic back pain: is anyone benefiting? Pain 75:163-168

Main CJ, Spanswick CC 2000 Pain Management: An interdisciplinary approach. Churchill-Livingstone, Edinburgh

Main CJ, Phillips CJ, Watson PJ 2005 Secondary prevention in health-care and occupational settings in musculoskeletal conditions, focusing on low back pain. In: Shultz I, Gatchel RJ (Eds), Handbook of complex occupational disability claims: early risk identification, intervention and prevention. Kluwer Academic, New York 387-404

Maniadakis N, Gray A 2000 The economic burden of back pain in the UK. Pain 84:95-103

Misra S, Kanungo R, Rosenstiel L, Stuhler E 1985 The motivational formulation of work and job involvement. Human Relations, 38:501-518

MISSOC 2000 Social protection in the member states of the Union: Situation on July 1st (1995-2000), European Union, Brussels

Osgood J, Stone V, Thomas A, Dampsey S, Jones G, Solon R, 2003 ONE Evaluation: summary of service delivery findings. Department of Work and Pensions in house report No 108, London

Peebles JE, Moore RJ 2000 Illness schemata in patients with low back pain: Prediction of rehabilitation success. The Pain Clinic, 12:237-246

Peters J, Wilford J, MacDonald E, et al 2003 Literature review of risk factors for job loss following sickness absence. Department of Work and Pensions, In-house Report 122

Riipinen M 1996 The relation of work involvement to occupational needs, needs satisfaction, locus of control and affect. The Journal of Social Psychology, 136:269-303

Rowlinson K, Berthoud R 1996 Disability, benefits and employment. Department of Social Security Research Report No 54. The Stationary office, London

Scales J, Scase J 2000 Fit and fifty? A report prepared for the Economic and Social Research Council, University of Essex Institute for Social and Economic Research

Smith JK, Crisler JR 1985 Variables associated with vocational rehabilitation outcome of chronic low back pain individuals. Journal of Applied Rehabilitation Counselling 16:22-24

Straaton KV, Maisiak R, Wrigley JM, White MB, Johnson P, Fine PR 1996 Barriers to Return to Work Among Persons Unemployed due to Arthritis and Musculoskeletal Disorders. Arthritis & Rheumatism, 39:101-109

Thornton P 1998 International research project on job retention and work strategies for disabled workers, Geneva: International Labour Office

Thornton P & Corden A 2002 Evaluating the impact of access to work: a case study approach. Social Policy Research Unit. York.

Vowles K, Gross R 2003 Work related beliefs about injury and physical capability for work in individuals with chronic pain. Pain 101:291-298

Waddell G 1998 The Back Pain Revolution. Churchill Livingstone, Edinburgh

Waddell G 2004 The Back Pain Revolution (2nd Edn). Churchill-Livingstone, Edinburgh

Waddell G, Aylward M, Sawney P 2002 Back Pain, Incapacity for work and social security benefits an international literature review and analysis. Royal Society of Medicine Press Ltd. London

Waddell G, Burton KA, Main JC 2003 Screening People at risk of long-term incapacity: a conceptual and scientific review. Royal Society of Medicine Press Ltd. London

Waddell G, Burton KA, Main JC 2003a Screening People at risk of long-term incapacity: a conceptual and scientific review. Royal Society of Medicine, London

Watson PJ 2000 Psychosocial predictors of outcome from low back pain. In: Gifford L (Ed), Topical Issues in Pain 2. CNS Press, Falmouth 85-110

Watson PJ, Kendall NAS 2000 Assessing psychosocial Yellow Flags. In: Gifford L (Ed), Topical Issues in Pain 2. CNS Press, Falmouth 111-140

Watson PJ, Booker CK, Moores L, Main CJ 2004 Returning the chronically unemployed with low back pain to employment. European Journal of Pain 8:359-369

Weich S, Lewis G 1998 Poverty, unemployment, and common mental disorders: population based cohort study. BMJ 317:115-119

Young E, Murphy C 2000 A social psychology approach to measuring vocational rehabilitation intervention effectiveness. Journal of Occupational Rehabilitation 12:175-189

12

Addressing return to work issues

JACQUELINE ADAMS

Introduction

Why do we need to address return to work issues? Why bother? What fears and beliefs do we hold about health and work and how do these influence our practice and our clients? Should people automatically be helped to return to work as part of treatment under the National Health Service? Is getting an employee back to work solely an employer's problem? Is it the General Practitioner's responsibility to decide when their patient is ready to return to work and do they have the time to understand the complex issues and reach the best long-term decision for the client's health and career? Surely all those client's requests for letters and medical reports for benefits agencies, solicitors and insurers are because someone somewhere does not want to pay an individual what they are due for being unable to work? If we commit ourselves to an opinion about someone's capacity to work will we end up defending our opinion in court? So what if an individual does not want to return to work; surely that is their choice? Can we ever say someone is permanently incapable of working, what psychological affect does such a judgement have? How did an individual come to be unemployed or medically retired in the first place and can we look back and try to understand the process which led to 'not working' as the chosen or only option? What if the employer seems to be being unhelpful? What are an employee's rights under the Disability Discrimination Act and what are 'reasonable adjustments' in the workplace? How do risk assessments work and where do manual handling guidelines fit in with helping a client with back pain return to a heavy lifting job? How can we start to even try to help individuals return to work when the number and range of obstacles seems so huge? On top of all these questions, is there a lack of time to address work issues with clients and/or competing priorities?

This chapter explores some of the issues around facilitating a return to work when a client is off sick from work. Situations where a client is unemployed or at work but struggling are touched upon, although many of the issues discussed are pertinent to all situations. It is written as a starting point for health professionals and taken from personal experience over the last 12 years from working with patients with longstanding pain, researching barriers to work for clients with 'repetitive strain injury' (Adams & Williams 2003) and working in an interdisciplinary team specifically addressing work reintegration issues for clients off sick or unemployed concurrent with a health problem. The topic is huge and experience shows that new issues and potential obstacles to work arise as employment, government, health, legal, financial and social policies change. Although the chapter in this book is in the context of clients with pain problems, from clinical experience many of the issues discussed also arise with clients with other health conditions.

Understanding motivation to return to work

A good place to start is in trying to understand all the potential influences on a client's motivation to work/return to work. Personal experience shows that this should be done with the understanding that it is common for a client to believe that work is not possible and/or that there is no means of help to return to work (Adams & Williams 2003). Mitchell (2000) partly illustrates this in a diagram of elements of work motivation, see Figure 1. The equation incorporates the elements of 'value' (V) and 'costs of work' (C) and shows their interrelation in terms of how they effect an individuals motivation to return to work.

'Value' of work is described in terms of the success a person has achieved at work, the degree of job satisfaction, and the quality of their work. The self-esteem derived from work may be essential to a person, or they may view work solely as a necessity.

Economic 'costs' as well as perceived 'costs', for example in terms of increases in pain and discomfort or stress, are also seen as important by Mitchell (2000). He suggests we consider the impact of health on work in relation to the person's career stage, and reminds us how depression as well as cognitive distortions such as catastrophising and over-generalisation can influence motivation. We already know that increased incidence of depression is related to being unemployed, and likewise, an increase in frequency of negative thinking to increased pain.

$$\text{Motivation} \quad \int \quad \frac{V + Pos}{C}$$

The value or utility of work (V)
The perceived chances of (POS) successfully going back to work
The real and perceived costs of going back to work (C)

Figure 1. Elements of work motivation

When reading a client's notes with the aim of facilitating a return to work, it is important to consider the motivations of all those involved e.g. general practitioner, employer, occupational health, family, insurer, solicitor. Because it is generally not possible to predict whether a client will return to work simply from reading initial notes, assessing a client or even when a client begins rehabilitation, the advice here is that it is best to avoid making any firm judgement on this. The best approach is to be open and willing to discuss the potential motivations of other parties involved with the client who may have many undisclosed concerns and fears in this regard. Unfortunately the growing evidence base that highlights the importance of psychological influences on injury, recovery and rehabilitation is frequently misunderstood and misinterpreted by the client and the parties involved with them. For example, it is often assumed that a client does not want to get better or return to work when this is actually not the case. The client may just lack information or support to help him/her do so. Being able to provide correct, evidence-based information and ongoing (but time-limited) support is the key to being able to help a client to return to or manage work. Ultimately we can only try to facilitate the client in helping themselves to return to work and we must respect that the final decision to return to work or not, rests with the client. Shaw et al (2002) illustrate the various influences on this decision in their excellent paper promoting the importance of individual perceptions of their impairment and the personal relevance of work, see Figure 2.

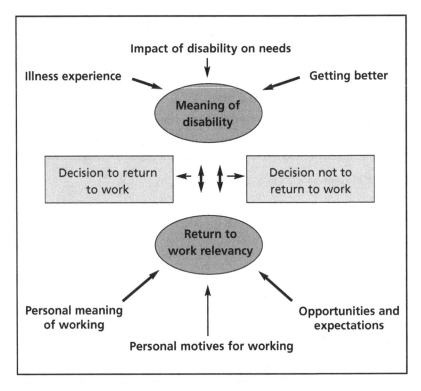

Figure 2. new constructs and categories in the study of return to work (redrawn from Shaw et al 2002)

Assesment

Consider a scenario whereby a client has problems with getting back to work and has been referred to you or you happen to be treating them for a health problem but they are concerned about not managing work. In order to assist with a return to work it can be worthwhile viewing the problem from a different perspective, i.e. put the 'health' issues to one side and assess from a 'not being at work' or 'absence due to sickness' perspective.

Try to be able to stand in the client's shoes in order to build up an understanding of what they think and feel about work and all the obstacles to getting back to work. Then stand in the shoes of all others involved and appreciate their concerns regarding the 'not being at work' problem. This should reveal the individuals' motives and desires with regard to work, see Box 1.

Chapters elsewhere (see chapters 9, 10 and 11) have examined the evidence with respect to the psychosocial variables that are linked to the likelihood of return to work following treatment for people with persistent pain problems. It is imperative to continually keep these potential indicators of a poor outcome in mind during assessment and when making recommendations for management.

Box 1 In relation to the work problem each client presents with a unique combination of some or all of the following:

- Client's own concerns
- Family concerns
- Health care professionals' concerns
- Employer's concerns
- Insurer's concerns
- Solicitor's concerns

As already stated, it is ultimately down to the client to decide their work goal. When appropriate it may be worth pointing out to the client that getting back to work has been shown to be a significant factor in getting better and also that we live longer and more healthily if we are working. Of course there are 'unhealthy workplaces' but often there is a complex interaction between personal and workplace factors that contribute to this 'unhealthiness factor'. With sufficient skills and resources we can help clients to positively influence this broader work environment.

OBTAINING DIFFERENT PERSPECTIVES ON THE PROBLEM

Client's perspective

When a client is off sick from work or unemployed with a health problem, it is important to assess the client's view of obstacles to a return to work, their future plan for work and their ideas about a return. Box 2 outlines the subject areas covered in a vocational assessment. Please note that it is not a physical, psychological, medical or work station assessment. Throughout the assessment with the client it is important to listen carefully, accept their current view of obstacles to return to work and to remain non-judgmental. Each item is discussed in detail below

Box 2 Components of a vocational assessment

- **Current job and role**
- **Previous work history**
- **Sickness absence**
- **Relationships with work**
- **Perceived current obstacles to return to work**
- **Financial situation**
- **Legal situation**
- **Future plans for work**
- **Other issues**
- **Recommendations**

Current job and role:
A starting point can be to try and really understand what the client does for a living, and the minutiae of what their typical day at work is like. By asking the client to tell you about their current job and their skills you can start to get a feel for what they like or dislike about work, whether they enjoy work, what elements of their work give job satisfaction and whether a return to this job is ultimately something they would like or positively want to avoid. Allowing the client to talk about their work can help to build rapport and they often report that it is a relief to be able to air their hidden worries about their job and their working future.

Ask the client to describe their job, try and understand what it involves and show interest in this. Job satisfaction itself is a complex concept and much research has been carried out examining different elements of it and its links with return to work (Linton SJ 1994, Lennon MC 1995, Krause et al 1997). For example: perception of difficult job conditions and demands, e.g. daily hassles; getting along with co-workers; how much the individual likes their job; role conflicts; pre-injury stressors.

Previous work history:
If a client has not been in their current job for very long, if they are unemployed or if they dislike their current job so much that returning to it at all is very unlikely, then asking about previous work history can be useful. For example, it enables us to get a feel for other skills a client may have or other potential work directions. If someone needs to apply for a new job, unexplained gaps in their curriculum vitae may be an issue for potential employers. In framing a relevant line of questioning here it is important to try and gauge the amount of support required to help a person find new work.

Sickness absence:
Clarify the details of the current period of sickness absence: i.e.: the date the client went off work, any attempted returns in the period and the details of the circumstances and events that led up to stopping work. Enquire about previous sickness absence including frequency and duration and try to get a feel for any ongoing procedures relating to this from the client's employer. Some employers' have a policy that non-return to work after one year results in loss of job on the grounds of incapacity to manage. One ironic example of such a policy in the United Kingdom was of a Primary Health Care Trust whose own employees were on a waiting list to see a medical specialist that would take more than one year! Clients are often worried about their sickness absence, its implication for their job and promotion prospects, and any punitive affects it might have in the workplace. These issues are all worth investigating and clarifying.

Relationships with work:
Ask the client about any contact with work since they have been off sick and about relationships at work with line managers and colleagues. Look out for difficult relationships or any new factors that might affect relationships. For example, unhappiness with an appraisal or failure to gain an expected promotion. Contact with work is a two way process so also ask about how the client has maintained their contact with work. From personal experience of interviewing many clients off sick from work it would seem that there is room for improvement in how a relationship with work is maintained when a client is off sick. Employers may strive to follow sickness absence procedures while the client is grudgingly sitting at home wondering why no one has contacted them. They often report feeling unimportant and neglected by work despite years of working hard for their employer. Conversely, but more rarely, clients who may be quite ill wish that their employer would stop turning up unannounced at home, or keep requesting regular meetings. Clearly it is a hard balance for the employer to strike and not easy to please all employees. However, if there were standards set for contact with employees off sick from work then this would negate the need for speculation about why and when the employer should contact the client. It may also help to dispel any worries that their job is safe for the future. It is suggested that if a standard procedure is devised it should always endeavour to link with sickness absence monitoring and occupational health procedures. Clients can get very distressed when sent different information from different branches of their employing company. The experience of workplace management of health problems and its effect on return to work rates and any decision to pursue legal action is worthy of much further study.

Perceived current obstacles to return to work:
In order to identify obstacles to return to work a useful opening question can be:, "What obstacles would there be if I were to say that you were going back to work tomorrow?" Reassurance that this won't actually be recommended is swiftly given of course! When the client's initial list is exhausted, it is worthwhile pressing for the possibility of more:- Clients are quite commonly concerned about mentioning particular obstacles for fear of being considered ridiculous.

Examples of obstacles often given include: travel to work difficulties, poor sleep, current routine, uncertainty about job availability, and any changes at work. Always be open to consider both physical and psychological obstacles that may be present.

Common physical obstacles for pain sufferers include difficulties with prolonged sitting, standing, walking, driving, lifting and bending, low stamina and flare ups of pain or just having pain.

Common psychological obstacles cited and that can be discussed include current mood, poor memory and concentration, the perceived cause of the health problem, confidence in ability to do the job, concern about safety at work, professional advice given to withdraw from work, and stress in the workplace. Employers in the United Kingdom cite stress, anxiety and depression as a more frequently occurring reason for sickness absence (TUC, 2005). The final list of obstacles obtained provides the starting point for helping that client to return to work as these obstacles are easily translatable into rehabilitation goals, should the client so wish.

Financial situation:
Asking about financial factors helps to develop an understanding of the client's current financial position. For example:
Are they receiving any benefits? : Statutory Sick Pay (SSP), Incapacity Benefit, Unemployment Benefit, Income Support, Family Tax Credit, Industrial Injuries payment, Disability Living Allowance, assistance with Council Tax or prescription payments?
Are they receiving any insurance assistance, such as mortgage or credit card payments, or income protection payments? Clients' may have an insurance claim and it is useful to ask what they are expecting from this.

Most clients are very concerned about finances when off work and about the possible short-term effects on income of going back to work. Some employees go onto SSP almost immediately they are off work, though most seem to receive a few weeks full pay followed by half pay and then no pay (see chapters 8 and 11). In some extreme cases employees receive full pay for up to two years of sickness absence, which may provide a significant lack of incentive to return to work. Employees may only be entitled to so many days full pay and half pay when off sick over a set period i.e. over 1-2 years. For example, an employee may have to be back at work for six months without absence before they are entitled to another 6 months full pay if off sick again. Pay bonus schemes can be affected by being off sick, or may be a cause of concern whilst grading back into work. Also, some employers operate pay bonus schemes to reduce incidence of sickness absence and again it is useful to know what schemes are operating and whether they affect the client's return to work plan.

It is important to understand the financial implications of ongoing changes in a client's workplace. For example, impending redundancies may cause financial concern or hopes, as can the prospect or desire for medical retirement. Occasionally the presence of a final salary pension scheme when someone is in receipt of income protection insurance has been a barrier to return to work. This is particularly the case when the job no longer exists or is one of less pay, after a lengthy period of absence.

Legal situation:
It is tempting not to ask about ongoing litigation as it can feel like prying. However, it is necessary to know as the process can be stressful and this in itself can affect rehabilitation efforts. Perhaps the best approach is to accept that claims for accidents and injury are a right of a client, are common practice and can be, and usually are, pursued alongside successful rehabilitation. Good practice is to offer rehabilitation as an integral part of a personal injury claim and to instigate it well before going to court. It is worthwhile setting time frames to speed up the process of litigation, and joint instruction for specialist opinions has been encouraged (BICMA Code of Best Practice on Rehabilitation, Early Intervention and Medical Treatment in Personal Injury Claims 2000). Should a client be expecting a large pay-out for damages it is worth discussing with them whether undergoing rehabilitation to return to work and actually returning to work will adversely affect their claim. A solicitor will point out that a client has a duty to mitigate their losses. Clients are sometimes involved in more than one legal claim, or successful completion of one claim can have a desired effect on another financial situation. For example, admittance of fault of an employer relating to an accident at work claim can result in the increased worth of an early medical retirement scheme. Ongoing divorce proceedings can affect work rehabilitation and expectations may need to be clarified.

Future plans for work:
Intent or anticipation to return to work prior to entering into treatment can be predictive of final work status independent of objective physical impairment (Fishbain et al 1999). Shaw et al (2002) has offered some useful questions for client's about absence from work, decisions made as to whether to return to work or not, experience of length of time off work, and what advice to give others in a similar situation. For example - Ask the client about their thoughts regarding future work. This usually helps to shape a return to work goal. If the client is feeling that a return to work is not possible but from your assessment you feel that they could be helped

to overcome their expressed obstacles, then it may be appropriate, either immediately, or in your recommendations, to raise the hope that return to work may be a possibility.

Other issues:
Enquire whether there are any other issues or worries the client has with regard to work. For example, the journey to work a client will have to undertake may be thought unmanageable because their work place has moved further away from where they live, or their job has excessive travel demands which hugely impact on home life.

Recommendations:
Mitchell (2000) asserts that time with the clinician should be a reminder of positive work expectations. When discussing your recommendations with the client it may be appropriate to raise hope that work is possible by outlining approaches that can be taken. Recommendations usually take the form of a review and an acknowledgement of all the obstacles that will require help and support to overcome plus some kind of graded return to work plan to be negotiated with the employer.

Finding evidence or recommendations in the literature for the optimum length of time required for a graded return to work plan has so far proved fruitless. At least employers seem to be getting more familiar with the concept and benefits of a graded return to work after a period of absence. Unfortunately lack of flexibility in how this is paced may be a problem. For instance, at one extreme there may be an expectation of immediate return to half the usual hours on light duties in the first week with an increase to full hours in the second and then a rapid progression to full-duties. At the other extreme may be a time-unlimited increase in hours and/or tasks, with the result that a client does not progress quickly enough and does not have any clear targets. Many employers now instigate a 3–4 week graded plan themselves. Personal experience is that a graded return to work period of between 6-12 weeks for someone off work between 6 weeks and up to around 4 years can be successful. However this needs to be balanced with helping the client to succeed in getting back to work rather than rushing back to work and failing. In the case of someone being unemployed or not wanting to return to his or her job, it is recommended that a clear work goal be clarified either before any rehabilitation begins or quite soon once it has started.

Family's perspective

The client's family will have their own concerns and beliefs about the client's ability to work, the safety of work, the attitude of the client's employer, the health of the client and the possible impact of work upon this. There may also be advantages or disadvantages to them if the client returns to work, for example, less time for the relationship, or for childcare, household chores and social activities. There may be financial incentives or disincentives. It can be useful to think about your own situation - What does your spouse or 'significant other' advise you to do when you are ill? What do they think about your employer? Or how hard you work? Or feel you are 'owed' from your employer? Are there advantages for them if you do not go to work? Are there disadvantages?

Health care professionals' perspective

The client may be involved in a range of treatments from a variety of health professionals, see Box 3. Each may give different advice regarding health and work and it is not uncommon for a client to have as many as three conflicting medical opinions about their health and whether they can return to work or not.

Pain management alone has been shown not to be sufficient to enable patients to return to work (Scheer at al 1997).

Personal experience shows that GP's are not best placed to discuss how client's overcome obstacles to work. They usually lack time to encourage an early return to work or any in-depth discussions regarding the complexity of issues involved. A common problem is that clients misinterpret the length of a sick note to mean they have to stay off work for the given period.

Many employers do not have an occupational health service, and those that do may have outsourced it. Even though there may be a referral procedure for occupational health it is often the case that the client has been off work a good while before they are referred or seen. Occupational health can be very under-resourced. A recent example was of three full time nurses looking after 12,000 employees. Experience shows that liasing with occupational health and human resources personnel takes up a good deal of time and often the communication links between the parties can be laboriously slow (Beach & Watt 2003).

Box 3 Potential health professionals involved

- **General Practitioner**
- **National Health Service**
- **Occupational health**
- **Private healthcare**
- **Holistic medicine**
- **Medical experts for medico-legal or insurance cases**

Employer's perspective

A great many different personnel (see Box 4) can have an interest in a work absentee. As already discussed, liaison between those involved often leaves much room for improvement.

There can be a great many issues involved for the employer: for example: productivity and lost time, staff replacement, managing the absence itself, absence monitoring, costs of absence, costs of pensioning staff off, increased pressure on workforce, claims against the employer, protection for the employee, and growing costs of insurance.

The motivation of the employer towards the client may depend on their 'ideal scenario for client' (Mitchell 2000). In some instances, and most frequently with income protection cases, the motivation of the employer is harder to determine than that of the client, who is usually much more open. Quite commonly, the employer may act as though the employee has been 'retired' when it is not actually the case. One observation is that employers do not understand persistent pain conditions, are unable to understand why employees do not get better quickly, do not always have access to any medical guidance or information, and do not know what to do to help their employee to return to work. Employers may also have a lot of fears and concerns. For example, they may fear they will need to spend a lot on adaptations, that work might aggravate the health problem, that they will be sued, that if they make changes in the workplace for one employee that precedents will be set for others in the future, or that the absent employee has other motives.

Box 4 Employer personnel whom may have an interest in a client's return to work

> - Personnel /Human Resources
> - Occupational health - role of sickness absence
> - Line manager
> - Colleagues
> - Legal Department
> - Insurance Department
> - Pension Department
> - Union

Insurer's perspective:

Types of insurance are listed in Box.5. An insurer may be keen to provide rehabilitation that leads to a client's return to work especially if this will cut their financial burden. However it is accepted that a client should be given the opportunity to be compensated for any health losses they have sustained. Good practice is that any rehabilitating organisation should be independent of the insurer and it has been suggested that the National Health Service is ideally placed to offer this rehabilitation ('Getting back to work' – A Rehabilitation Discussion Paper 2002)

Box 5 Types of insurance in United Kingdom

> - Employer's liability insurance
> - Motor insurance
> - Income protection or wage replacement insurance
> - Health insurance or Critical illness cover
> - Mortgage payment protection insurance
> - Credit card payment protection insurance

Solicitor's /Union's perspective

Clients often report seeking help from their union with their health and work problem. Commonly they say their union representative has put them in touch with a solicitor to represent their 'grievance' against their employer. This may be to apportion blame for any accident in the workplace or any poor workplace practice.

A solicitor will aim to help a client seek compensation and it can be helpful to understand exactly what the aims of a claim are from both the solicitor and client's perspective as these may differ. Usually solicitors follow the BICMA Code of Best Practice on Rehabilitation, Early Intervention and Medical Treatment in Personal Injury Claims (2000) and will try to speedily resolve the client's issues with the employer. From personal experience, if a solicitor is not adequately helping move the client towards a return to work, it can be useful to change the way the client communicates and handles the solicitor. This will only work if the client wishes to return to work. In the future it would be desirable for union representatives to be able to assist employees in immediately accessing return to work rehabilitation.

Management of return to work issues

Some items that are important to a successful return to work are illustrated in Box 6 and discussed below.

Box 6 What helps successful return to work?

1. A clear work goal and that the client wants to return to work

2. Work preparation and planning as part of the rehabilitation process

3. Discussion of effective communication skills with client, practice to increase confidence in use of these

4. Providing better information about practicalities of return to work, graded exposure and/or refamiliarisation to workplace and personnel. This can change the client's confidence in their ability to return to work

5. Assisting the client to develop their own time-limited graded return to work plan which is then negotiated with the employer

6. A workplace meeting

7. Understanding concerns of all parties involved and supporting them i.e. the individual client, the employer. Include support for an insurer or solicitor in understanding the rehabilitation process

Clear work goal:
It is important to ensure that there is a clear work goal prior to beginning rehabilitation. Personal preference is for a client to pursue a graded return to their original job rather than onto permanently restricted or prolonged light duties options if at all possible. The reason being that it is not uncommon for employers to say that they can no longer offer light duties.

Work preparation and planning as part of rehabilitation process:
The client is the most important person in any rehabilitation and return to work process and therefore a reasonable plan can only be made in collaboration with them. This section discusses the vocational aspects of rehabilitation only, but it would be carried out in the context of help from other professionals who may be working on such areas as health beliefs, functional capacity, and confidence to return to work. An overriding aim is to give unconditional support as the client discusses work problems and issues, sets goals, takes small steps towards a goal, reviews goals, takes on increased personal responsibility for their problem with work, makes his or her own return to work plan, negotiates it with work and carries it out with regular review. A useful starting topic that can assist with motivation is to discuss the advantages and disadvantage of working, and how the client thinks a return to work should be approached.

Communication:
From the start, regular communication and liaison between all involved parties makes all actions transparent. Woods (1987) advises employers to have 'sympathetic communication with the worker and non-adversarial handling of workers compensation claims'. It is also extremely important for the health professional to remain positive and confident about the possibility of a return to work, even if might look doubtful. It is not that uncommon for cases where a successful return to work seems highly unlikely, but when a plan has been drawn up and agreed the client has actually achieved it. Also, there are occasions when an employer has been convinced (or extremely fearful) that a client would be unable to 'manage' their job but has been disproved.
It is important to be aware of what your non-verbal body language may convey about your personal views regarding the work situation. This applies not only to the client, but to their employer or any other involved party.

It is worthwhile discussing effective communication strategies with your client with particular emphasis on competency in presenting a return to work plan and liasing with all parties interested in their return to work.

Assisting the client to develop his or her own time-limited graded return to work plan which is then negotiated with the employer:
The aim is to help the client to develop their own plan. It should be a realistic graded return to work plan based on graded experiments and trials. At this point, further influences of the client's beliefs about health and work may become more apparent and can then be tested. The worksheet shown (see Box 7) is useful to help the client shape up their return to work plan. They can then be encouraged to write the first draft of their provisional return to work plan. It can be useful to show the client other people's plans, and to re-discuss the principles of graded activity.

Useful discussion points can derive from answers to further questioning, for example: 'What do you think will be important for your plan to be successful?'

'What issues are you worried about today in relation to your return to work plan?'

'Can you think of other examples in your life where you have tackled a difficult goal or experience like this?' 'What helped you get through it?'

'Who do you need to tell about your plan?'

'Is the reaction you anticipate from those you tell what you will actually get?'

'Is there anyone you can practice outlining your plan to, in order to gain confidence in presenting it?'

Box 7 Where to start when making a return to work plan

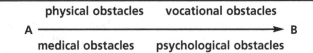

physical obstacles   vocational obstacles

A ————————————————————▶ B

medical obstacles   psychological obstacles

1. Define A, that is what you are doing now with work; be clear exactly what you are doing e.g. what duties and how many hours – if you are currently in work.
2. Define B, that is where you eventually and ideally aim to be with work; be as specific as possible
3. Make a list of all the possible hurdles to overcome
4. Make a list of the tasks you can carry out within work at present
5. Make a list of the tasks you need to be able to do at work that you cannot yet carry out
6. Decide from Question 5's list, which is the easiest task to do, and which is the most difficult. Then number each task starting from 1 'the easiest', progressing to 2 'the next easiest' and so on until you have numbered them all including the 'most difficult.'
7. Decide how you would like to build up the hours doing your original work. Would it be starting with 1 hour twice a week? Would it be increasing by 15 minutes each day? There are many possible combinations of ways to build up – choose the one that you think fits you best.

The initial plan may be the first draft of several versions attempted until the client reaches one he or she is happy with. From experience, as clients discuss work issues, visit the workplace, discuss their plan with work personnel and continue to make physical and psychological improvements, they gain confidence and often shorten their initial plan. However, clients should still be encouraged to stick to their plan for increasing hours and tasks once they actually start back at work.

Workplace meeting:
It is recommended that the rehabilitation specialist attends the initial workplace meeting/s with the client to offer impartial support and to ensure the meeting/s achieves it's aims. The aims for a workplace meeting are outlined in Box .8. A client may have remaining negative thoughts about an aspect of their employer's behaviour or their job and may need to develop a strategy to manage these thoughts during the meeting or to change their thinking style. Graded exposure to the work environment may be required prior to a formal workplace meeting if the client suffers undue anxiety and panic.

Supporting all parties:
Once the client starts their return to work plan, regular review can be very supportive. Most clients usually have a good idea of the regularity of the support they require. Some do well with a weekly review looking back and discussing the previous week and then looking forward over the next week. For others, a couple of meetings, or a well-timed phone call can be enough. How long you offer support will depend on your service; Butler (1995) has warned about anticipating a successful return too soon.

The importance of understanding the concerns of all parties involved with the client has been emphasised. However, in addition to understanding their concerns it is also helpful to be able to give support to these other parties during the client's return to work process. This may include the family, the GP, the employer, the insurer or the solicitor. Sometimes there are competing and conflicting interests and the client will not be able to return to work until these are discussed openly and some kind of resolution reached. Of particular importance is the role in educating those involved about the rehabilitation process. If pressures and priorities of work do not allow much input with these other parties, at the very least you should discuss communication strategies with the client. If at all possible try and find the time to call or write to the employer encouraging an early, graded return to work for the client, or even better, to attend a meeting with relevant work personnel. A visit to the workplace with the client and/or a meeting with work personnel does much to restore the absent client's confidence about possibilities of returning to work and positive attitudes of others to them at work. It also shows the employer that the client is doing all they can to get better and to return to work.

Box 8 Rehabilitation specialist's aims for the workplace meeting:

1. To help the client build confidence through a 'good' experience in the meeting
2. Present idea of a graded return to work; client may have unsuccessfully tried a graded return and this may need discussing first to look at where it failed
3. Check the employer is aware of the difference between acute and chronic pain, and give positive messages about its management. Give information and answer questions about the rehabilitation the client is undergoing.
4. Outline why it is important to aim for return to the original job (if this is medically appropriate and is a shared goal for all involved parties)
5. To allow the client to present their proposed return to work plan and support them whilst they negotiate their plan
6. Observe communication between client and line manager/s. Watch employers' responses - are they overprotective? Observe how the client presents their plan; do they give a clear message of confidence in returning to work?
7. To support the client in trying to resolve any outstanding workplace issues that may affect their long term success in returning to their job
8. Raise sensitive issues if the client cannot e.g. pay during graded return, annual leave or other worries that are hinted at. Suggest compromises on tricky issues e.g. car parking, time in lieu built up before being off sick. As far as possible, ensure client is not 'rewarded' for ill health through advantages over other employees but also ensure they are not disadvantaged.
9. To discuss how the line manager can offer support to the client. Verbally clarify that the client is responsible for their own return to work plan and that they will tell the line manager if at any point they feel they cannot manage it. This is to enable the employer to relax and not feel they have to constantly check that the employee is managing.
10. Clarify changes at work, listen out for work culture issues e.g. redundancy
11. To develop a problem definition from the employer's view; check it matches your client's own.
12. Listen and acknowledge the employer's fears – this can highlight potential problems that may occur during the return to work period. For example, they may have picked up on pain behaviours and wonder how to handle them, they may have a fear of the client reinjuring themselves upon a return to work or fear they may do the wrong thing by asking the client to do a work task. You may also hear of other factors that potentially contributed to the sickness absence e.g. the client was doing two people's work, the client received a written warning
13. Discuss what external help is available to employer if appropriate – e.g. financial support.
14. Look at the work environment with the client; ask them to point out any remaining difficulties
15. Book a review meeting if required

Clients who are working but struggling

Clients who are still at work but struggling to manage with both work and everyday personal and leisure activities can be problematic and challenging. Their situation may be related to the familiar over/under activity cycle common to chronic pain and chronic fatigue conditions. Both they and you may wonder if they can continue working? Here, not assisting the client with tackling relevant work issues may lead to the client dropping out of work altogether in the future. Conversely, taking the client completely out of work for rehabilitation purposes can lead to a magnification of the health problem. They are also in danger of losing the structure and routine of work as well as the opportunity to implement strategies and changes in the workplace and to simultaneously review their effectiveness.

A useful starting point is to ask the client to make a detailed daily timetable of their working week from the point of waking to the point of going to bed. They can do this as their week progresses or write out a plan of a typical week. This can then be reviewed in the light of the client's current physical and psychological capacity and then management strategies discussed and applied. Alternatively, reviewing the day or week ahead with the client and facilitating the setting of goals to make changes or apply other strategies can be helpful. This should also be done in consideration of other personal and work activities the client has planned both on that day and for the week ahead. When the client has tried out their strategies they can be evaluated.

Conclusion

This chapter has aimed to raise confidence in the health professional that working is nearly always a possible option for clients. It has provided some practical tools for assessing the vocational issues and supporting the client in developing their optimum return to health and work goal. It recognises the importance of the health professional raising hope in a client that work is possible and that numerous and varied obstacles can be overcome.

References

Adams JH, Williams A CdeC 2003 What affects return to work for graduates of a pain management programme with chronic upper limb pain? Journal of Occupational Rehabilitation 13(2):91-106

Beach J, Watt D 2003   Editorial: General Practitioners and occupational health professionals Consensus statement to improve interaction is timely and welcome. BMJ 327:302-303

BICMA Code of Best Practice on Rehabilitation, Early Intervention and Medical Treatment in Personal Injury Claims, A Practitioner's Guide to Rehabilitation 2000 Bodily Injury Claims Management Association

Butler 1995 Managing work disability: why first return to work is not a measure of success Industrial and Labor Relations Review 48(3):452-469

Fishbain DA, Cutler RB et al 1999 Prediction of "intent", "discrepancy with intent", and "discrepancy with nonintent" for the patient with chronic pain to return to work after treatment at a pain facility. Clinical Journal of Pain 15:141-150

'Getting back to work' – A Rehabilitation Discussion Paper Submissions of the Association of Personal Injury Lawyers, Association of British Insurers /Trades Union Congress September 2002

Krause N, Lynch J et al 1997 Predictors of disability retirement. Scandinavian Journal of Work Environment and Health 23(6):403-413

Lennon MC 1995 Work conditions as explanations for the relation between socioeconomic status, gender and psychological disorders. Epidemiologic Reviews 17(1):120-127

Linton SJ 1994 The role of psychological factors in back pain and its remediation. Pain Reviews 1: 231-243

Mitchell K 2000 The Dance of the Invisible Impairments: Chronic Pain Syndrome & the Disability Insurer. UNUM, Disability Prevention Partnership. Prepared for American Society of Pain Bulletin 10(4)

Scheer SJ, Watanabe TK, Radack KL 1997 Randomized controlled trials in industrial low back pain. Part 3. Subacute/chronic pain interventions. Archives of Physical Medicine & Rehabilitation 78:414-423

Shaw L, Segal R et al 2002 Understanding return to work behaviours: promoting the importance of individual perceptions in the study of return to work. Disability and Rehabilitation 24(4):185-195

Trades Union Congress January 2005 Countering an urban legend Sicknote Britain?

Woods DJ 1987 Design and evaluation of a back injury prevention program within a geriatric hospital. Spine 12:77-82

13

Evidence based management of low back pain in occupational health.

NICOLA HUNTER

Introduction

The economic impact of muscloskeletal disorders and low back pain to business, the insurance industry and the government has led to several national initiatives to identify better management strategies for these conditions. There is an urgent need for a biopsychosocial approach to management to be widely applied across UK in line with evidence based guidelines. This presents a significant opportunity to physiotherapists to be key players in the provision of an alternative management approach. A barrier is that physiotherapy is still externally perceived (and practiced by many) as a 'mechanistic, tissues targeted and modality dominated therapy' (Thacker & Gifford 2002). To many stakeholders the physiotherapy profession is seen to be part of the problem and not the solution (discussed in detail in chapter 10).

To secure this work, physiotherapists need to be able to demonstrate the service they offer makes good business sense i.e. that it adds value to the organisations bottom line. Employers are looking for a service that helps them comply with their legal obligations under employment law and also to recover more than the cost of the service through reduced absence and associated costs. Insurance companies require a clinically effective service that reduces their claim liability. The government needs an effective rehabilitation service that prevents chronicity and disability resulting in the need to claim incapacity benefit.

This chapter outlines the programme set up in Suffolk in 2000 that is in line with evidence-based guidelines and using a bio-psycho-social approach. I have illustrated the approach with a case study.

The problem with musculoskeletal disorders for UK

In business and industry musculoskeletal disorders (MSD) and low back pain (LBP) are the commonest form of ill health at work. In the UK each person with back pain and related conditions takes an average of 13 days off work each year. This is estimated to cost £6 billion a year, with two thirds of this due to time lost from work (for further details see chapter 9).

Health and Safety Executive (www.hse.gov.uk) research indicates that 9/10 of companies do not know what work related ill health (musculoskeletal disorders) costs them. Only 3% of UK organisations currently use across the board occupational health support to manage work absence. Most UK companies expect the NHS to manage an employee with a musculoskeletal disorder back to health and fitness for work. Medicalisation of the problem and long NHS waiting lists frequently result in the employee developing a chronic problem and prolonged work absence or never returning to their original, or any job.

Rehabilitation has been the 'buzz' word in insurance over the past 4 to 5 years led by the Rehabilitation First campaign by the Insurers POST magazine and driven by economic factors. The IUA/ABI Rehabilitation Working Party Report: Psychology, Personal Injury and Rehabilitation (2004), suggests that the current medical model of management of these conditions rehabilitation is contributing to poor outcomes. Evidence from the insurance industry indicates that 20-30% of cases suffer disability greater than may be expected from the medical history. These cases account for 80% of the cost to the insurers.

The IUA/ABI report (2004) recommends a systematic, stepped approach to prevention, (primary intervention) early advice (psychological first aid) screening tools to identify 'at risk' patients, early treatment (secondary intervention) and a biopsychosocial model (tertiary intervention) for those not responding to early treatment. The report concludes that resources for rehabilitation should be targeted at the 'at risk' group, but that these services are currently not widely available in the UK.

MSD accounts for at least 21% of people receiving incapacity benefits (IB). Back pain is the nation's leading cause of disability and 1 in 8 unemployed people are not working because of back pain. The Department of Work and Pensions have a national strategy to kerb the rising cost of IB to the State.

This includes 3 important initiatives.
1. Securing Health Together An Occupational Health Strategy for Great Britain (2000).
2. The Job Retention and Rehabilitation Pilot (JRRP) (Nice & Thornton 2004).
3. Job Centre Plus and NHS Condition Management. A complete package of support to help people on incapacity benefits get back to work.

The current focus of employers, insurance industry and the Government has evolved because too many people are developing chronic ill health and disability from conditions such as musculoskeletal disorders and low back pain that should not be disabling. Treatment for people of working age should be focused on return to work or to meaningful occupation to ensure the long-term health of the individual. Lack of work, or meaningful occupation, results in low self-esteem and poorer physical and mental health. Those without work show greater use of health services and have increased mortality (McKee-Ryan et al 2005).

Low back pain and musculoskeletal disorders need to be tackled effectively at an early stage to prevent long-term disability. This requires a significant change in current practice to ensure good management and a partnership approach, in which employers, workers and health care providers work together to provide a cohesive programme of workplace interventions, management and treatment.

Evidence Based Guidelines

There are 3 evidence-based guidelines in UK that outline best management for low back pain. These are:
- Clinical Standard Advisory Group: Back Pain (1994)
- Royal College of General Practitioners Guidelines for Management of Acute Low Back Pain (RCGP 1996)
- Faculty of Occupational Medicine Guidelines for Management of Low Back Pain at Work (Faculty of Occupational Medicine 2000).

Broadly the guidelines advise that:
- Red flags (serious medical conditions) are screened and managed
- The patient is reassured and given medication
- The patient is given clear up to date advice and responsibility to manage their problem - The Back Book (Roland et al 2002)
- Physiotherapy (manipulation) is effective in the first 6 weeks
- Patients who have not made a full functional recovery at 6 weeks should participate in a functional restoration programme

217

Functional restoration programmes or biopsychosocial rehabilitation is widely supported in current international research (Guzman et al 2001, Schonstein et al 2004) as the method most likely to achieve a functional recovery for people with chronic musculoskeletal problems. Functional restoration programmes achieve a higher proportion of patients returning to work reduced frequency of recurrences and reduced sickness absence (Lindstrom et al 1992, Mayer et al 1996, Bendix et al 1998, 1998a, Karjalainen et al 2004 2004a 2004b). Studies with longer term follow up report fewer days absence at 12 months (Mayer et al 1985) and 2 – 5 years (Bendix et al 1998, 1998a). Less self-reported disability was reported by Frost et al (1998) at 2 years follow up.

An evidence based management strategy for business and industry

Current practice in the NHS does not facilitate implementation of the guidelines in a way that assists business, industry or the individual. Proper management of these conditions by all stakeholders could significantly reduce the number of workers who develop long-term ill health and disability due to low back pain.

A three stage strategy is required comprising:

- **Primary prevention** - risk assessment and ergonomics in the workplace to identify potential causes of MSD and LBP, implement preventative measures and risk control where the problem can not be eliminated.

- **Secondary management** - case management by an occupational health professional supported by an occupational health physiotherapist, to provide timely and appropriate treatment and advice.

- **Tertiary treatment** - work focused rehabilitation (functional restoration) for workers having difficulty returning to work or resuming their full normal duties at 6 weeks.

Case study

The first company I started working with on an evidence based management strategy for musculoskeletal disorders was a water utilities company where the majority of workers had heavy manual jobs. The problems were:

1. The heavy and repetitive nature of the work may have contributed to the development of the problem and often it was not possible to modify the work (by ergonomics) to reduce the physical demands of the job.
2. Redeployment to lighter or lower risk work was often not possible as the workers were not skilled to undertake alternative work and frequently no suitable alternative work was available.

The programme was set up in partnership with the company's in-house occupational health and safety service. Commitment and communication throughout the organisation was essential to the success of the programme.

A case study of 'Kevin' will be used to illustrate the three-stage strategy and how a cohesive management approach can be effective in returning a worker with a heavy manual job back to work and fitness for life. Some details of the story have been changed to protect the identity of Kevin and his employer.

Kevin's Story

Kevin was a 39 year old utilities company worker. He was married with 2 boys ages 9 and 7. He enjoyed playing 5-a-side football once a week and football with his sons. He also liked walking and taking his sons swimming.

He had worked for the utility company for 10 years. His job required that he spent 30% of each day driving a small van visiting sewage treatment works to carry out routine maintenance. He spent 40% of his time walking. He had to stoop and bend to clean, sweep and dig channels for 30% of each day. Three or four times a day he had to climb ladders and lift manhole covers weighing up to 40kg.

Kevin's first back injury occurred in 1995 (aged 32) when he was lifting a manhole cover at work. He suffered acute, severe central lumbar pain. He saw his GP who prescribed pain killers and rest. He took one week off work.

His second incident of back pain occurred in 1996. The pain came on gradually after gardening. He saw his GP and an osteopath who helped relieve his symptoms. He took 2 weeks off work. His GP advised that the 5-a-side football was not good for his back. Kevin stopped football and decided that he should be extremely careful about all sport.

Kevin's third injury was in 1998. He hurt his back at work but managed to get an appointment with the osteopath quickly and took no time off. He continued to see the osteopath for 3 monthly checkups. The osteopath told him that this would prevent further recurrences.

In 2000, the pain recurred for no apparent reason. Osteopathy was of no benefit. He saw his GP who prescribed pain killers and advised rest. He said physiotherapy may also help and arranged an appointment at the local physiotherapy department. The physiotherapist prescribed exercises, but they hurt so Kevin stopped doing the exercises. He rated the physiotherapy treatment as of no real benefit. He had taken 6 weeks off work. On return to work he was suffering low back pain daily and was feeling very anxious about his back. He was struggling with heavier manual tasks such as lifting manhole covers. The company had a new OH service but he did not wish to be referred to see the Occupational Health Advisor (OHA) as he feared he may lose his job.

The fifth episode of pain came on gradually in March 2002 after an afternoon spent digging and sweeping channels. He reported this as a work accident. Kevin went straight to his GP. His GP decided that in view of his long-term recurrent problem he should not be at work and told Kevin that the job was obviously too heavy for him. Kevin was referred for an MRI scan and second opinion. The OHA contacted Kevin but was unable to intervene as Kevin wished to be managed by his GP. He was off work for 9 months until he saw the orthopaedic consultant who reviewed his scan. The scan showed a mild disc bulge at L4/5 and wear and tear changes. The consultant concluded that Kevin had wear and tear in his low back, surgery was not indicated and that there was nothing that he could do for Kevin.

Kevin was devastated and felt angry and let down. He could not work because he could not sit for very long and he could not bend or lift. He could not play football with his boys or walk the dog. His wife was fed up and they could not see a way forwards. Financial problems were going to occur. Kevin's salary had reduced to 50% after 6 months absence and would reduce to zero after 12 months absence.

Kevin decided that he would have to seek early retirement from the company on the ground of ill health and would have to make a claim for his original injury at work. He requested an appointment with the company's Occupational Health Advisor. The Occupational Health Advisor gave him a copy of The Back Book. She suggested that a functional restoration programme in line with evidence-based guidelines from Faculty of Occupational Medicine may help and referred Kevin to the Occupational Health Physician to ensure that a functional restoration programme would be appropriate management at this point. Kevin was very dubious. In 7 years of this problem no one had suggested this type of approach. His GP had suggested that his job was too heavy and the cause of his problem and now the company were suggesting a programme to get him back to his normal job.

Kevin's management would have been different if he had identified himself to the company and benefited from the 3-stage strategy that was introduced to manage musculoskeletal disorders.

Primary prevention

Back pain and musculoskeletal disorders arise in many work situations. The exact cause is often unclear. In a critical review of epidemiological evidence for work-related musculoskeletal disorders (Bernard 1997), The National Institute for Occupational Safety and Health (NIOSH) in the United States has identified activities, which may lead to, or aggravate, back pain. These include:

- Heavy physical work (strong evidence)
- Lifting and forceful movements (strong evidence)
- Bending and twisting (postures)
- Whole body vibration (strong evidence)
- Static work postures
- Combination of these factors

Devereux et al (2004) examined the role of work stress and psychological factors in the development of musculoskeletal disorders in The Stress and MSD Study. Physical work risk factors causing or contributing to low back pain are:

- Lifting 6-15 kilograms greater than 10 times per hour or lifting greater than 16kg at all and always/often working with the back in an awkward position.
- Pushing and pulling objects combined with tasks requiring lifting.

Devereux et al (2004) reported that workers highly exposed to psychosocial work risk factors and not physical work risk factors were 1.7 times more likely to report low-back complaints compared to workers with low exposure to both of these factors. Workers highly exposed to physical work risk factors and not to psychosocial work risk factors were approximately twice as likely to report low-back complaints compared to workers without high exposure to either physical or psychosocial work risk factors. The greatest likelihood of reporting low-back complaints was for workers highly exposed to both physical and psychosocial work risk factors. They were four times more likely to report problems compared to workers exposed to neither set of factors.

The evidence indicates that while physical risk factors in the workplace can cause or contribute to low back pain, psychosocial issues are of equal importance. Preventative programmes are a requirement in the UK under the Management of Health and Safety Regulations 1999. This and other associated legislation require employers to identify tasks or activities where there is a risk of injury or ill health. Employers must carry out formal risk assessments to identify the level of risk and to put into place control measures to reduce the risk. By law, all companies have a duty to:

- Identify hazards by risk assessment
- Remove potential for exposure by elimination or substitution
- Ergonomics for MSDs
- Control exposure by engineering & administrative systems
- Monitor controls – direct (audits of activity) & indirect (health & accident statistics)
- Train exposed employees and their supervisor
- Health surveillance (self, supervisory & occupational health – medical surveillance)

Primary Prevention:- Kevin

The Utilities Company employing Kevin was not acting in accordance with the law when he first injured his back in 1995 from lifting a manhole cover. A pre or post incident risk assessment would have identified that:

- *The tools and equipment Kevin used for digging and sweeping channels did not encourage him to work in good posture. Kevin could have been provided with long handled tools to improve working posture.*
- *Kevin's van had a poor seat with limited adjustment and no lumbar support. This was causing poor posture when sitting and driving. A van with adjustable seat and lumbar support could have been provided to improve sitting and driving posture.*
- *40kg manhole covers are too heavy to lift single-handed. Kevin could have been provided with a manhole lifter or requested to call assistance if a cover was too heavy. A manhole cover replacement programme would have meant that heavy covers or those in a poor state of repair and heavy to lift would have been replaced when identified as a manual handling problem.*
- *Kevin had not received any training in back care or manual handling that was relevant to his work tasks and activities.*

Had these measures been implemented, Kevin's risk of subsequent injury may have been less.

Secondary management

Once a person has gone off-work due to low back pain it has been shown that the longer they are off work the lower the likelihood of ever getting back to work. After 6 months absence an individual has a 50% chance of returning to work, after 12 months a less than 30% likelihood of returning to work and after two years this reduces to less than 10% (CSAG 1994). It is important that companies have in place a system to support injured and ill employees and to facilitate an early return to work. In large companies the Occupational Health team assist management to discharge their responsibility. In small or medium enterprises (SME's) the personnel department or line manager may undertake this role without support.

Important elements in facilitating a return to work are:

- The employer should keep in touch with the employee and reassure them that they are a valued member of the workforce.
- The employer should offer the opportunity for short term restricted or reduced duties to facilitate an early return to work.
- Many employers now offer treatment such as rapid access physiotherapy for musculoskeletal disorders.
- Some employers check fitness for work at pre employment and following illness and injury. This is often done by Occupational health.

Physiotherapy in the workplace has been shown to be effective in reducing the cost of absence in musculoskeletal injuries. Rennie (2000) reports that provision of on-site physiotherapy reduced sickness absent by 9%. Since 2000, the writer has run an Occupational Physiotherapy scheme for staff from a local NHS Trust, with annual absence costs due to musculoskeletal disorders in excess of £500K. Staff are referred by Occupational Health and receive a course of up to 6 physiotherapy treatment sessions commencing within 48 hours of referral. This scheme achieves a saving of £80 - £100k per annum for an average investment of £20K on treatment costs annually (National Audit Office 2003).

Manipulation and physical activity have been shown to be effective in reducing pain and speeding recovery within the first 6 weeks of a back problem (CSAG 1994, RCGP 1996).

Secondary Treatment:- Kevin

Kevin had treatment from an osteopath and from a physiotherapist between 1995 and 2000. A semi-structured interview with Kevin (Main & Spanswick 2000, Shorland 1998) revealed that the Osteopath used soft tissue techniques and manipulation as the main treatment.

The physiotherapist informed Kevin that the problem was likely to be a disc bulge and prescribed extension exercises. Kevin reported that this was effective in reducing the pain during the physiotherapy session but the pain returned after driving the car home. The advice from the physiotherapist seemed to conflict with the GP's advice to rest so Kevin did not continue the exercises at home. Kevin reported that physiotherapist's suggestion that the problem was due to a bulging disc was of concern and he felt that he should have been referred for further investigations and not just been given exercises.

In 2002 Kevin had a further severe episode of central low back pain. He went to see his GP and requested an MRI scan and a second opinion, as he was sure that there was something serious wrong in his back. His GP agreed and made the referrals.

Kevin was signed off work pending these investigations and joined a 6-month wait for MRI scan and a 9-month wait to see the orthopaedic surgeon.

The GP's decision in 2002 to refer for an MRI scan was contrary to the RCGP guidelines, as the investigations were not ordered to eliminate potential red flags. An assessment of psychosocial 'yellow flags' (patients beliefs and behaviours which may predict poor outcomes) should have been used as this may have identified that Kevin was at risk of developing chronic pain and disability. Kevin presented with:

- *A belief that his back pain was harmful and potentially serious*
- *Fear-avoidance behaviour and reduced activity levels (avoiding sports and work activities in the fear they may cause harm)*
- *Expectation that passive treatment would solve the problem rather than a belief that active participation will help (osteopathy, surgery and unwilling to try exercise)*

The real problem was that even if the yellow flags that were present had been identified, there was not a service available to the GP that could provide appropriate management for Kevin at this stage.

Had the GP been cognisant with FOM guidelines on management of back pain at work, he should have encouraged Kevin to continue ordinary activities as normally as possible despite pain and to remain at work. He should also have advised Kevin to request temporary restrictions to his job. The GP could have written to the companies OH department with this advice. This would have allowed the companies OH department to become involved in the management of Kevin at an earlier stage. Kevin would have had access to an occupational health physiotherapist and opportunity for restricted and reduced duties to help him remain at or return to work.

The action taken by the GP to put Kevin off work while he waited for a scan and second opinion gave him a less than 40% chance of returning to work, or put another way a 60% chance of losing his job and going onto incapacity benefit.

Tertiary Treatment

Deyo (1993) described the hypothetical course of a chronic low back disorder with acute onset, followed by episodic recurrence. The periods of remission become shorter until the patient has pain most of the time. It is at this point that long-term sickness absence occurs.

The Faculty of Occupational Medicine recommend that if medical treatment fails to produce recovery and return to work by 4-12 weeks, the emphasis should shift from symptomatic treatment to rehabilitation and self-management strategies. A rehabilitation programme for those with significant biopsychosocial factors is more likely to reduce pain and disability and achieve return to work (CSAG 1994, RCGP 1996, Carter & Birrell 2000, Watson 2001).

Effective rehabilitation is necessary in an overall strategy for back pain absence reduction. Cochrane systematic reviews by Guzman et al (2001) and Karjalainen et al (2004, 2004a & b) looked at the effectiveness of multidisciplinary bio-psycho-social rehabilitation. Guzman et al (2001) compared the approach with control treatments such as in or outpatient physiotherapy. The reviewers concluded that intensive multidisciplinary bio-psycho-social rehabilitation with a functional restoration approach improves pain and function. Less intensive interventions did not show improvements in clinically relevant outcomes.

Schonstein et al (2004) carried out a Cochrane review of work conditioning, work hardening and functional restoration for workers with low back and neck pain. The review identified that physical conditioning programs should include:

- a cognitive-behavioural approach
- intensive physical training (specific to the job or not) comprising aerobic capacity, muscle strength and endurance, and coordination;
- a work-related element

Programmes that are given and supervised by a physiotherapist or a multidisciplinary team seem to be effective in reducing the number of sick days for some workers with chronic back pain, when compared to usual care.

Our functional restoration programme was developed following a literature review and visits to functional restoration programmes in USA and Scandinavia.

The first step is that the patient attends for a detailed functional assessment. The purpose of the assessment is to obtain baseline measurements of the patient's attitudes and beliefs, physical condition and physical demand level capability against the requirements of their job.

The questionnaires and functional tests selected measure identified risk factors for low back pain and work capability. The questionnaire, physical and functional tests selected to monitor the patients progress through rehabilitation are published in peer-reviewed journals, have established reliability and validity and most have been shown to be sensitive to change.

The measures can be categorised as follows:
- **Biopsychosocial factors** are measured by structured interview (Shorland 1998, Main & Spanswick 2000) and the administration of four questionnaires. The Oswestry Disability Index (Fairbank et al 1980), The Acute Pain Screening Questionnaire (Kendall et al 1997) The Epic Spinal Function Sort (Matheson et al 1993) and 0 to 10 numeric pain scale.

225

- **Flexibility** of the trunk, shoulder girdle and hips are measured using dual inclinometry and electric goniometry following standardised protocols (Norkin & White 1985). The results are compared to the minimum documented normal value for the joint.

- **Trunk stability** muscles (transverse abdominals, quadratus lumborum and back extensors) are measured by timed endurance tests (McGill 1999) and results are compared to the minimum documented normal value for gender.

- **Manual handling capability** is measured by a range of tests, the results being compared to job requirements. The tests include static strength tests to the National Institute of Occupational Safety and Health protocol (Chaffin 1974, Chaffin et al 1974) covering carrying and lifting from the floor, mid shin, shoulder level and overhead.

- **Dynamic lifting capability** is measured in positions determined by the demands of the job such as floor to knuckle, knuckle to shoulder or waist to overhead (Snook et al 1983, Mayer et al 1998 1998a).

- **Aerobic fitness** is measured using the Chester step test (Sykes 1995). The result is one of 5 levels ranging from poor to above average by age and gender.

Figure 1 Key tests used for baseline functional measurement

Function	Measured by	Norms/ Job specific	Reference
Pain level	0-10 numeric pain rating scale	0 = no pain	
Risk of chronicity	Acute pain screening questionnaire	>105 = At risk	Kendall et al 1997
Perceived disability	Oswestry back pain disability questionnaire	0-20% mild, 21-40% moderate, 41-60% severe, 60% + bed bound	Fairbank et al 1980
Perceived work capability	EPIC Spinal function sort	Job specific, 135 light, 165 medium, 180 heavy	Matheson et al 1993

Function	Measured by	Norms/ Job specific	Reference
Spinal range of movement	Dual inclinometry	Norms	Mayer et al 1984 Porter & Wilkinson 1997 Adams et al 1999
Hip shoulder mobility	Goniometry	Norms	Norkin & White 1985
Trunk strength – static (stability)	Endurance exercises	Norms	McGill et al 1999
Lifting – static strength	NIOSH static strength tests	Job specific	Chaffin 1974 Chaffinn et al 1974
Lifting – dynamic	Maximal acceptable weight occasional and frequent lifting test	Job specific	Snook et al 1983 Mayer et al 1988, 1988a
Aerobic fitness	Chester step test	Related to age and gender	Sykes 1995

Functional restoration programme

A part time programme was designed in order that the patients could commence a graduated return to work alongside the programme. In addition the patient is expected to do 2 additional sessions of prescribed exercise each week. Residential places are available for more severe cases and patients who live a long distance away.

Patients join the rehab group on a rolling basis and attend for between 4 and 12 weeks. The group dynamics facilitate the rehabilitation process with new recruits able to learn of progress made by those nearing the end of their programme. This is an essential element of the psychological strategy of the programme.

A typical day comprises:

- Aerobic training.
- Individual exercise programme designed to address specific strength, flexibility and functional deficits.
- Individual review with physiotherapist to monitor progress towards goals
- Work conditioning activities such as lifting and handling tasks.
- Group cognitive behavioural therapy sessions addressing issues around pain management, stress, coping strategies, control (developed by a health psychologist).
- Sports activity such as swimming, walking etc.
- Work activities and job specific training.

The patients' progress is monitored through out the programme to ensure that they are making progress to achieve their goals, which are set by the patient and therapist at the start of the programme.

Changes that occur during the programme are measured by repeating baseline measurements taken at initial assessment on the last rehab session.

Tertiary Management Kevin

Kevin attended for a functional restoration assessment. The initial assessment indicated that his attitudes and beliefs about his problem were a risk factor for chronicity. The orthopaedic consultant had told Kevin there was nothing wrong except some wear and tear and nothing could be done for this. Kevin thought:

- *his back pain was harmful and potentially serious as his spine was wearing out.*
- *he should not resume his normal sports and activities as they may cause further wear and tear damage to his back*
- *that there was probably nothing to be done now to solve the problem or even to make the problem more bearable*

Kevin's physical examination indicated that he had poor posture with thoracic kyphosis and flattened lumbar spine. His lumbar movements were very stiff in all directions. His pelvis was immobile and his hips were stiff with tight hip flexor muscles and hamstrings. He had poor core stability. He had poor body mechanics and bending forwards movements were accomplished by flexing the thoracic and lumbar spine rather than the hips. This may have caused strain to the lumbar spine (Porter & Wilkinson 1997).

There was no sign of any serious medical condition or neurological involvement. Muscle power, jerks and sensation were normal in both limbs and SLR was negative.

Kevin's history and presentation indicated that the underlying problem could well have its origins in lumbar disc damage. Regardless of cause, it was clear that an important component of the ongoing problem was likely to be deconditioning caused by his fear avoidance beliefs and behaviour.

Kevin agreed to participate in a functional restoration programme and attended for 8 weeks alongside a graduated return to work programme. He set the following goals that he wished to achieve by the end of the programme:

Goal	To achieve the goal Kevin must be able to
To be able to return to work full-time and on normal duties.	• stand and walk for 3 hours a day • sit and drive for up to 3 hours a day • tolerate work in a forward flexed position for 2 hours a day in spells of 10 – 15 minutes • lift 45kg 3 to 4 times a day
To be able to put his socks on in the morning	• flex hips and pelvis so that he can reach his feet
To swim with his kids	• tolerate extension so that he can swim breaststroke as he is not a good swimmer

His manager was contacted by the OHA and the following workplace changes were undertaken to support Kevin's return to work:

- *Kevin worked with a colleague for 2 weeks to give him a chance to try work tasks in a safe environment where he could stop if having difficulty.*
- *A vehicle assessment was carried out by the OHA and Kevin was provided with a hired van with an adjustable seat as a short-term measure until a new vehicle could be ordered.*
- *Kevin was provided with long handled tools and long manhole cover keys.*
- *Kevin was told not to attempt to lift manhole covers single-handed and to call for help.*
- *A 'snapper' manhole lifter was obtained for him to try.*

Kevin's programme comprised:

- *45 minutes of aerobic exercise on bike, stepper, rower and cross trainer working at 65 - 70% maximum heart rate.*
- *Medical exercise programme comprising nine exercises to:*
  · improve lumbar, hip and thoracic mobility
  · improve core stability and trunk coordination

· *re-educate functional movements particularly squatting, and*
bending without overloading his lumbar spine.
· *strengthen legs.*
- *Lifting and handling education and training covering static lifts (for*
  when manhole covers are stuck), and dynamic lifts. This was
  progressed over the programme until he could lift 45kg with good
  technique and 30kg with good technique in a team lift.
- *Functional activities to educate him how to carry out forward*
  bending activities using his hips and legs and not overloading his
  spine, e.g. digging and sweeping. This built up over the programme
  until he could carryout these activities continuously for 15 to 20
  minutes without increasing his symptoms.
- *He participated in the group education and CBT sessions at each*
  attendance. These gave the therapist a chance to challenge Kevin's
  beliefs about his problem and help him come up with a more helpful
  alternative belief so that he could manage his problem and lead a
  normal and functional life.

Kevin's Outcome

Kevin's attitudes and beliefs about his back problem changed and he learned that
exercise and activity would help him recover and manage recurrence in the future.
This was shown by the reduction of his score on the acute pain screening
questionnaire from at risk to not at risk. His perceived disability reduced from
moderate to low on the oswestry disability questionnaire. Kevin's perceived work
capability increased from 'light-medium', which was not sufficient for his job, to
heavy, which was. While we didn't promise a reduction in pain, it is common for
pain to reduce and Kevin's reported pain reduced from very strong at the start of
the programme to mild at the end.

Questionnaire	Initial assessment	End of rehab	Target	Comment
Borg Pain Scale (0 -10+) Measures pain on worse and best days	5 - 7	0 - 2	1 – 3	Improved satisfactory
APSQ (Acute Pain Screening Questionnaire) Measures patients risk for long term disability	117	75	<90	Improved: satisfactory
Back ODI (Oswestry Disability Index) Measures patients disability due to back problem	38	6	<10%	Improved satisfactory

PACT (spinal function sort) measuring self efficacy and perceived work capability	145	198	180 – 190 Heavy	Improved: satisfactory

It was important to improve Kevin's range of movement, as this was a key feature of his deconditioned state. He was unable to bend forwards from the hips with his spine in neutral. To enable him to return to heavy manual work it was essential that we taught him to undertake tasks requiring forward flexion with out overloading his spine. The combination of specific and global exercise he undertook resulted in a significant improvement in his mobility over the 8 weeks of the programme. His posture improved and he became able to sit for longer in comfort and he learnt how to ease symptoms by changing position.

Spine	Initial	Discharge	Normal	Comment
Left lateral	12°	28°	25°+	Improved: Satisfactory
Right lateral	32°	33°	25°+	No change: normal
Flexion	31°	59°	60°+	Improved: Satisfactory
Extension	5°	25°	25°+	Improved: Satisfactory
Sacral hip flexion	35°	55°	45°+	Improved: Satisfactory
Straight leg raise left	64°	82°	80°+	Improved: Satisfactory
Straight leg raise right	66°	85°	80°+	Improved: Satisfactory
Thoracic kyphosis	45°	30°	20°	Improved – remains kyphotic

Flexibility of hips and shoulder girdle measured and compared to norms. Norkin and White (1985)	Initial	Discharge	Normal	Comment
Tight hip flexor muscle	10°/90°	0°/90°	0°/90°	Improved: Satisfactory
Reduced hip flexion	110° R 115° L	125°R 125°L	125°	Improved: satisfactory
Reduced shoulder girdle extension	4 cm	23 cm	23cm	Improved: satisfactory

Core stability and in particular early activation of transversus abdominis and miltifidus has been shown to be important in recovery from acute and sub acute low back pain (Hides et al 2001, Richardson et al 2002). Core stability was re-educated using a combination of specific exercises and functional medical exercise therapy. Timed hold tests devised by McGill are used to monitor improvements in core stability during the programme. While not ideal these are simple and quick to administer in a clinical setting.

Strength – measures trunk strength taken by timed static holds. McGill et al (1999)	Initial	Discharge	Normal	Comment
Reduced trunk extensor muscle strength tested by a timed hold	Unable to perform	140 secs	140 secs	Improved: Satisfactory
Reduced abdominal muscle strength tested by a timed hold	45 sec	140 secs	140 secs	Improved: satisfactory
Reduced trunk side flexor muscle strength tested by a timed hold	25 sec 25 sec	85 secs 90 secs	90 secs	Improved: satisfactory

Lifting and carrying capability was a key element of Kevin's job and much time was spent teaching him to risk assess lifting tasks, improving lifting technique and restoring his confidence in weight handling. Kevin's static and dynamic lifting capability improved to meet his job requirements. His results are shown on the chart below.

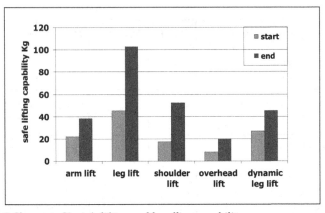

Figure 2 Change in Kevin's lifting and handling capability

Most *importantly Kevin was able to play football with his sons and walk the dog. Returning to work meant he was back on his full salary and his financial concerns were resolved.*

The cost of Kevin's back pain absence to the company was £350 in 2000 and £2,800 in 2001. In 2002 the absence cost was £10,500 plus £240 for physio, £700 for orthopaedic consultation and scan and £1,750 for the functional restoration programme (FRP) totalling £13,190.

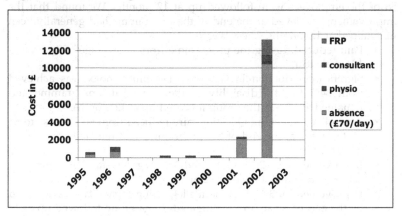

Figure 3 Cost of Kevin's Absence

If the functional restoration programme had commenced, as recommended by Faculty of Occupational Medicine guidelines on managing low back pain at work, after 6 weeks absence Kevin would have returned to work much sooner and the cost of the orthopaedic consultation and scan would have been saved.

Without the functional restoration programme, it is likely Kevin would never have returned to work. He would have pursued his request for ill health retirement and would have made a claim against the company for the accident at work. This would not have been a satisfactory out come for the company, for Kevin or his family.

Outcomes

A clinical audit was undertaken of outcomes of the first 85 employees with low back pain who were referred to our functional restoration programme. The employees had all had at least one course of physiotherapy for their back problem but had not recovered fully and at 6 weeks post injury remained off work or on restricted or reduced duties. They were all seen and assessed as suitable for the programme by a Consultant Occupational Health Physician.

233

Of the 85 employees who entered the rehabilitation programme: 83 completed and 81 returned to work on full duties; 2 returned to work on restricted duties; 2 dropped out and did not return to work. Absence due to musculoskeletal ill health declined by approximately 40% (from 1,170 days in the 24 months before rehab to 195 days in the 12 month post programme for the group).

58 of the employees were followed up at 12 months. We found that the improvements achieved at the end of the programme had generally been maintained at 12 months. These were:

- Pain reduced during the programme from an average of 4 on a 0 – 10+ scale to 1.5.
- Significant reduction in Oswestry Disability Index was achieved from 34% to 14% disability at the end of the programme and remained at 15% in the group followed up at 12 months.
- Acute Pain Screening Questionnaire reduced from 90 (at risk) to 63 (not at risk), at the end of the programme and remained at 63 at 12 months.
- Improvements of 20% in the NIOSH leg lift static strength was achieved and maintained at 12 months.
- Improvement of 30% in dynamic leg lifting capability was achieved by the end of rehab and maintained in the group followed up at 12 months.

At the end of the functional restoration programme 92% of participants reported that they were very satisfied with the programme and 8% reported being somewhat satisfied.

Summary

A three stage strategy for management of low back pain in an occupational health setting in line with evidence based guidelines appears to be both clinically effective in reducing symptoms and restoring function and cost effective. Early results indicate reduced claims against the company by mitigating the loss following a work accident and fewer ill health early retirements due to low back pain.

Employees with low back pain can develop the skills and confidence to return to work including heavy manual work. This reduces the chance of prolonged sickness absence and consequent loss of employment. It is better for the individual as loss of work results in low self-esteem, poorer physical health and mental health. It will also meet the government's agenda to reduce the numbers of people on incapacity benefit claims and the cost to the country of long-term disability.

Changing the way low back pain is managed in line with evidence-based guidelines appears to be of benefit to all. Physiotherapists are in a unique position to deliver an evidence-based service such as this in all settings.

References

Adams MA, Mannion AF, Dolan P 1999 Personal risk factors for first-time low back pain. Spine 24:2497-2505

Bendix AF, Bendix T, Haestrup C, Busch E 1998 A prospective, randomized 5-year follow-up study of functional restoration in chronic low back pain patients. European Spine Journal 7:111-119

Bendix AF, Bendix T, Labriola M, Boekgaard P 1998a Functional restoration for chronic low back pain: two-year follow-up of two randomized clinical trials. Spine 23:717-724

Bernard BP 1997 Musculoskeletal Disorders and Workplace Factors: A Critical Review of Epidemiologic Evidence for Work-Related Musculoskeletal Disorders of the Neck, Upper Extremity, and Low Back. Department of Health and Human Services, National Institute for Occupational Safety and Health, Cincinnati OH

Carter JT & Birrell LN (editors) March 2000 Occupational health guidelines for the management of LBP at work – principle recommendations Faculty of Occupational Medicine, London
http://www.facoccmed.ac.uk/content/BackPain.htm

Chaffin D B 1974 Human Strength Capability and Low Back Pain. Journal of Occupational Medicine 16:248-254

Chaffin, DB Caldwell, Dukes-Dobos et al 1974 A Proposed standard procedure for static muscle testing. American industrial hygiene association journal 35:201

CSAG 1994 Clinical Standards Advisory Group report on Back Pain HMSO, London

Devereux J, Rydstedt L, Kelly V et al 2004 The role of work stress and psychological factors in the development of musculoskeletal disorders. The stress and MSD study. Robens Centre for Health Ergonomics, University of Surrey HSE Research Report no 273

Deyo R 1993 Practice veriatios, treatment fads, rising disability. Do we need a new clinical research pradigm? Spine 18(15):2135 - 2162

Faculty of Occupational Medicine (2000) Occupational Health Guidelines on the management of low back pain. (www.facoccmed.ac.uk)

Fairbank J, Couper J, Davies J, O'Brien J 1980 The Oswestry Low Back Pain Disability Questionnaire. Physiotherapy 66(8):271-273

Frost H, Lamb SE, Klaber-Moffett JA, Fairbank JCT, Moser JS 1998 A fitness programme for patients with chronic low back pain: 2-year follow-up of a randomised controlled trial. Pain 75:273-280

Guzmán J, Esmail R, Karjalainen K et al 2001 Multidisciplinary Bio-Psycho-Social Rehabilitation for Chronic Low Back Pain (Cochrane Review). In: The Cochrane Library, Issue 1, John Wiley & Sons, Chichester

Hides J, Jull G, Richardson C 2001 Long term effects of specific stabilising exercises for first episodes of low back pain. Spine 26:E243-248

IUA/ABI Rehabilitation Working Party 2004   Psychology, Personal Injury and Rehabilitation. Sponsored By The International Underwriting Association Of London and The Association Of British Insurers

Karjalainen K, Malmivaara A, van Tulder M et al   2004 Multidisciplinary biopsychosocial rehabilitation for neck and shoulder pain among working age adults (Cochrane Review). In: The Cochrane Library, Issue 1. John Wiley & Sons, Chichester

Karjalainen K, Malmivaara A, van Tulder M, 2004a Multidisciplinary biopsychosocial rehabilitation for subacute low back pain among working age adults (Cochrane Review). In: The Cochrane Library, Issue 1, John Wiley & Sons, Chichester

Karjalainen K, Malmivaara A, van Tulder M, et al 2004b Biopsychosocial rehabilitation for upper limb repetitive strain injuries in working age adults (Cochrane Review). In: The Cochrane Library, Issue 1. John Wiley & Sons, Chichester

Kendall NAS, Linton SJ, Main CJ 1997 Guide to Assessing Psychosocial yellow flags in acute low back pain: Risk factors for long-term disability and work loss. Accident Rehabilitation & Compensation Insurance Corporation of New Zealand and the National Health Committee, Wellington, NZ (available online at: www:acc.org.nz)

Lindstrom I, Ohlund C, Eek C et al 1992 The Effects of Graded Activity on Patients with Subacute Low Back Pain: A randomised Prospective Clinical Study with an Operant-Conditioning Behavioural Approach. Physical Therapy 72(4) 279-293

Main C, Spanswick C 2000 Pain Management: an interdisciplinary approach. Churchill Livingstone, Edinburgh

Management of Health and Safety Regulations 1999 Health and Safety Executive HMSO

Matheson, LN, Matheson ML, Grant J 1993 Development of a measure of Perceived Functional Ability. Journal of Occupational Rehabilitation 3(1)15-30

Mayer TG, Kristoferson SG, Mooney V, Tencer AL 1984   Use of Noninvasive Techniques for Quantification of Spinal Range-of-Motion in Normal Subjects and Chronic Low-Back Dysfunction Patients, Spine 9(6)588-595

Mayer TG, Barnett J, Capra P et al 1985 Objective Assessment of Spine Function Following industrial Injury: A Prospective Study with Comparison Group and One-Year Follow –Up. Spine 10(6):482-493

Mayer TG, Barnes D, Kishino N et al 1988 Progressive Isoinertial Lifting Test I. Spine 13:993-997

Mayer TG, Barnes D, Kishino N et al 1988a Progressive Isoinertial Lifting Test 2. Spine 13:998-1002

Mayer TG, Garcy P, Gatchel RJT 1996 Recurrent or new injury outcomes after return to work in chronic disabling spinal disorders. Tertiary prevention efficacy of functional restoration treatment. Spine 21(8):952-959

McGill SM, Childs A, Liebenson C 1999 Endurance times for low back stabilization exercises: clinical targets for testing and training from a normal database. Arch Phys Med rehabil. 80(8):941-944

McKee-Ryan F, Song Z, Wanberg C, Kinicki A 2005 Psychological and physical wellbeing during unemployment: a meta analytic study. J Appl Psychol, 90(1):53-76

National Audit Office 2003 A Safer Place to Work: Improving the management of health and safety risks to staff in NHS trusts Report by the Comptroller and Auditor General HC 527 2002-2003 27 March 2003 ISBN: 0102921172 http://www.nao.org.uk/pn/02-03/0203527.htm

Nice K, Thornton P 2004 Job Retention and Rehabilitation Pilot: Employers' management of long-term sickness absence. Department for Work and Pensions Research Report No 227 HMSO

Norkin C, White D 1985 Measurement of Joint Motion – a guide to goniometry. FA Davis Company, Philadelphia

Porter JL, Wilkinson A 1997 Lumber-Hip Flexion Motion: A Comparative Study Between Asymptomatic and Chronic Low Back Pain in 18- to 36-year-old Men. Spine 22(13):1508-1514

RCGP 1999 Royal College of General Practitioners. Clinical Guidelines for the Management of Acute Low Back Pain. London, Royal College of General Practitioners (www.rcgp.org.uk)

Rennie F 2000 Getting Britain Back to Work, Report of three conferences on rehabilitation and job retention. TUC:36-39

Richardson C, Snijders C, Hides J et al 2002 The relation between transverses abdominis Muscles, Sacriiliac Joint mechanics and low back pain. Spine 27(4):399-405

Roland M, Waddell G, Klaber Moffett J et al 2002 The Back Book. The Stationary Office

Schonstein E, Kenny DT, Keating J, Koes BW 2004 Work conditioning, work hardening and functional restoration for workers with back and neck pain (Cochrane Review). In: The Cochrane Library Issue 1. John Wiley & Sons, Chichester

Securing Health Together – Occupational Health Strategy for England Scotland & Wales (download document)
http://www.ohstrategy.net/about_strategy/strategy_home.htm
http://www.ohstrategy.net/

Shorland S 1998 Patient assessment – case history. In: Gifford L (ed) Topical Issues in Pain 1. CNS Press, Falmouth 135-146

Snook SH, Ciriello VM, Hughes GJ 1983 Further studies of psychophysically determined maximum acceptable weights and Forces. Human Factors 35(1):175-186

Sykes K (1996) The Chester Step Test Manual Assist Pubs, Wrexham

Thacker M, Gifford L 2002 A review of physiotherapy management of Complex regional pain syndrome. In: Gifford L (Ed) Topical issues in pain 3. CNS press, Falmouth 119-141

Watson P 2001 Rehabilitation of unemployed patients with low back pain. Physiotherapy Pain Association News, 11:16

Web sites and pages referred to in this chapter:

www.hse.gov.uk
www.facoccmed.ac.uk
http://www.facoccmed.ac.uk/content/BackPain.htm
www.rcgp.org.uk
http://www.ohstrategy.net/about_strategy/strategy_home.htm
http://www.ohstrategy.net/

4

Cognitive behavioural

14

Psychosocial Approaches to Managing Pain: Current Status and Future Directions

FRANCIS KEEFE, CINDY SCIPIO AND LISACAITLIN PERRI

One of the most important changes occurring in pain practice and research over the past two decades has been the growing recognition of the importance of psychological and social factors in the pain experience (Keefe et al 2004). Pain clinicians working with patients having persistent pain, in particular, are increasingly interested in incorporating psychosocial treatment protocols into their pain management programs.

A variety of psychosocial approaches to pain management have been developed over the past 40 years. This chapter provides an overview of these interventions. The chapter is divided into six sections each covering a different type of psychosocial intervention. The interventions reviewed include multidisciplinary treatment-based psychosocial treatments, cognitive-behavioral treatment, partner-assisted cognitive-behavioral interventions, early interventions, emotional disclosure interventions, and meditation-based protocols. Within each section, we briefly describe the intervention, highlight the results of studies testing its efficacy, and provide a comment that addresses important issues and future directions.

Psychosocial Pain Management Interventions

Multidisciplinary Treatment-Based Psychosocial Treatments

The late 1960s and early 1970s witnessed the emergence of multidisciplinary treatment programs for chronic pain (Turk & Okifuji 2002). These programs were based on the notion that chronic pain is complex disorder that can best be understood and treated with input from pain specialists from medical, surgical, psychological, nursing, and rehabilitation disciplines. Psychosocial treatments figured prominently in many of these early programs. One of the earliest systematic applications of psychosocial intervention in the context of a multidisciplinary treatment program was Fordyce's (1976) operant behavioral program. This program had its roots in the operant learning perspective on pain which maintained that maladaptive pain behaviors could be acquired and maintained by positive reinforcement (e.g. pain-contingent delivery of positive rewards such as attention from a solicitous spouse or pain medication). Careful screening methods were used to select patients whose pain behavior appeared to be under the control of positive reinforcement, rather than primarily influenced by underlying tissue damage. Patients were admitted to an inpatient rehabilitation unit where they received multidisciplinary treatment. All patients received physical therapy interventions designed to increase their tolerance for activity and exercise. Pain medications were carefully controlled and patients were gradually weaned from medications using a "pain cocktail" that was delivered on a time-contingent rather than as needed (PRN) basis. A key feature of the inpatient unit was that staff members were trained to use their own attention and praise to reinforce adaptive, well behaviors (e.g. exercising) rather than to respond and reinforce pain behaviors. To generalize therapeutic gains, family members and significant others were also taught to use social reinforcement principles to reinforce patients' well behaviors following discharge from the program. Fordyce and his team published a number of reports documenting the efficacy of their multidisciplinary-based operant-behavioral treatment program (Fordyce 1976, Fordyce et al 1968, Fordyce et al 1973). What made their results so impressive was that the program was quite effective in increasing activity level and exercise tolerance and decreasing pain medication intake in patients with long-standing and treatment-resistant chronic pain.

From the 1970s to the 1990s there was rapid growth in multidisciplinary pain programs (Keefe et al in press). Although some of these programs were oriented around a particular intervention (e.g. nerve blocks, neurosurgical treatment) or a particular pain syndrome (e.g. headache), many were comprehensive in that they included a broad array of treatments and served a broad array of pain populations. Many of these programs were located on inpatient hospital units specially designed for pain management. Although the psychosocial component of some of the programs was modeled after Fordyce's operant-behavioral program, most used a broader array of cognitive-behavioral interventions designed to enhance patient's abilities to exert control over behavioral, cognitive-affective, and psychophysiological responses to pain. To enhance behavioral control over pain, patients in these programs typically were trained how to pace and gradually build up their activity level (activity pacing), how to identify and increase their level of pleasant activities (pleasant activity scheduling), and how to set specific and reasonable short- and long-term goals (goal setting). To enhance cognitive-affective control, patients were trained to recognize and alter overly negative pain-related thoughts (cognitive restructuring) and how to use imagery, distraction, and meditation methods to shift attention away from pain. Individual psychotherapy was also used in many programs to enhance patients' abilities to deal with issues such as rebuilding self-esteem, trauma, and grief. To enhance control over psychophysiological responses, patients in these programs were often trained in relaxation and biofeedback methods. Formats for delivering these psychosocial interventions varied from program to program, but most relied on a combination of daily group therapy sessions and individual therapy sessions. Many programs featured family involvement and follow-up sessions in the form of regular phone calls and/or regular return visits. Psychosocial intervention was typically delivered by psychologists, social workers, or psychiatric nurses having specialized training in pain management.

A large number of clinical reports published in the 1970s and 1980s described outcomes achieved in multidisciplinary-based psychosocial treatment programs (see Flor et al 1992). Overall, these studies showed that patients who complete such programs had quite substantial increases in activity level and decreases in opioid medication intake. Improvements in pain tended to be more modest, e.g. in the 30% range. Flor et al (1992) conducted a meta-analysis of multidisciplinary pain treatment programs, many of which featured psychosocial interventions. Over 300 articles reporting multidisciplinary treatment outcome data were screened and 65 articles included in the final meta-analysis. Data indicated that multidisciplinary treatment was superior to a variety of comparison conditions including no treatment, a waiting list, or single modality treatment (e.g. physical therapy alone). A particularly important finding was that the beneficial effects of multidisciplinary treatment were not limited to pain per se, but also apparent in a wide variety of other outcomes (e.g. improved mood, increased rates of return to work, and decreased health care utilization.). A limitation of the studies reviewed, however, was that many did not use random assignment to treatment and control/comparison conditions. As a result one must be cautious in drawing definitive conclusions from this meta-analysis.

Comment: Many of the psychosocial interventions currently being used in chronic pain management were first developed and refined in the context of multidisciplinary treatment programs. In particular, operant behavioral protocols and cognitive-behavioral treatment protocols had their roots in multidisciplinary treatment programs. Although multidisciplinary programs flourished in the period for the 1970s to 1990s, questions were raised about their costs. In the United States insurance coverage, particularly for inpatient-based multidisciplinary pain management programs has been cut back significantly. The lack of adequate reimbursement has led to closure of most specialized inpatient programs. Insurance coverage for comprehensive outpatient multidisciplinary treatment programs is also increasingly limited leading to a trend towards programs focused around a single intervention (e.g. nerve blocks, medication management, or spinal cord stimulation). These changes are unfortunate and unwarranted, particularly since there is evidence that multidisciplinary pain management is cost effective. Based on data from their meta-analysis, Flor et al (1992) estimated that, after completing multidisciplinary treatment, patients required one-third the number of surgeries and hospitalizations of patients treated by means of traditional medical and surgical approaches. Turk (2002) subsequently conducted a cost-effectiveness analysis that revealed that multidisciplinary treatment is 6 times more cost effective than surgery, 15 times more cost-effective than conservative care, and 25 times more cost-effective than spinal cord stimulation surgery.

Another key issue in evaluating multidisciplinary treatment programs is what represents the ideal mix of psychosocial versus other treatment components. Clearly, some multidisciplinary programs emphasize psychosocial intervention much more than others. Because multidisciplinary treatment programs typically combine psychosocial interventions with other interventions, outcome data from these programs do not enable one to definitively evaluate the efficacy of a specific psychosocial intervention. An important next phase in the development of psychosocial interventions was the use of randomized clinical trials to test the effectiveness of specific treatment protocols, e.g. cognitive-behavioral treatment.

Cognitive-Behavioral Treatment

The cognitive-behavioral model of pain that maintains that pain is a complex experience that can be influenced by thoughts, feelings, and behavior (Keefe et al 2005). A key tenet of cognitive-behavioral treatment (CBT) is that coping with persistent pain is a skill that can be acquired and mastered through systematic instruction, practice, and application. Training sessions are set up to facilitate learning and thus involve instruction in a coping skill, guided practice with the skill, therapist feedback, and home practice assignments. Patients are instructed in an array of coping strategies most often including progressive relaxation training, imagery, activity pacing, goal setting, methods for coping with overly negative pain-related thoughts, and problem solving. The training is conducted in a series of individual or group sessions. At the conclusion of treatment, patients are trained in strategies designed to help them maintain the strategies they have learned.

CBT is currently the most common for of psychosocial intervention used in managing persistent pain. There are several reasons for this. First, CBT teaches patients skills that enable them to manage pain on their own. Once these skills are learned, the patient can engage in self-management and is not dependent on a therapist or treatment provider. Second, CBT is quite flexible and can be easily modified for use with patients with different types of chronic pain (e.g. chronic low back pain, migraine headaches) and persistent disease-related pain conditions (e.g. cancer, arthritis). Finally, CBT is relatively inexpensive and represents a cost-effective approach to pain management.

The efficacy of CBT pain management protocols has been examined in numerous randomized clinical trials. A number of systematic reviews and meta-analyses have been published summarizing the findings of these studies. There is compelling evidence that CBT is effective in the management of both migraine and tension headache (Penzien et al 2004). CBT-based protocols have also been found to be effective in the treatment of chronic lower back pain and mixed chronic pain conditions (Morley et al 1999) and in the management of arthritis pain (Keefe et al 2002).

Comment: Clinicians interested in psychosocial interventions would benefit from learning more about CBT. CBT was one of the first psychosocial interventions to be used in pain management. It has also been found to be one of the more efficacious interventions. CBT is a flexible clinical approach that can be adapted to individual patients' needs and can be used in managing both chronic pain and disease-related pain conditions.

An important issue in the delivery of CBT is quality control. If CBT is to be effective, treatment must be structured in a way that promotes patients' sense of self-efficacy with regard to their pain coping skills. This means that sessions must be interactive, of sufficient length, and sufficient number to ensure that learned skills can be mastered. Time pressures and clinical demands may lead therapists to abbreviate CBT to the point that it no longer can be characterized as a skills-based approach. Highly abbreviated "CBT" protocols often consist of one or two sessions in which patients are simply presented with a great deal of information about pain coping methods, but given very few opportunities for guided skills practice, corrective feedback, or review of home practice efforts. As might be expected, these approaches to delivering CBT are not very effective.

Another issue in the delivery of CBT is the credentials of the persons delivering the treatment. In most of the controlled studies of CBT, the therapists have been clinical psychologists having extensive training and

245

supervised experience with behavioral and cognitive-behavioral therapies. There is a growing interest in CBT among allied health professionals (particularly physical therapists and nurses) who work with patients having persistent pain. At present, there is a great deal of variation in the amount of training and supervision of allied health professionals who are delivering CBT. The amount of training and supervision that a given therapist might receive can vary from a weekend workshop with no follow-up supervision to formal coursework combined with clinical practicum and weekly supervision. Clearly, standards for training and supervision need to be established for each discipline if allied health professionals are to be effective in using CBT in pain management.

Partner-Assisted Cognitive-Behavioral Intervention

Over the past decade, there has been increased interest in involving partners in cognitive-behavioral pain management. In partner-assisted pain management training, patients attend treatment sessions along with their partners and are taught both pain coping skills and couples skills for enhancing the acquisition and maintenance of learned skills. Involving a partner in pain management can be beneficial for a number of reasons. First, it can give the partner more familiarity with the skills the patient is learning to cope with the pain. Second, it can teach the partner methods (e.g. reinforcement methods, joint practice sessions) that they can use to promote the continued use of learned pain coping skills. Finally, it can give the patient and partner a common goal to work on.

We have conducted several studies of partner-assisted pain management protocols. We initially tested the efficacy of a spouse-assisted coping skills training intervention for osteoarthritis (OA) of the knee (Keefe et al 1996). Eighty-eight patients with OA and their spouses were randomized to spouse-assisted coping skills training, individual coping skills training, or arthritis education-spousal support control. The spouse-assisted intervention presented OA as a couples issue, and emphasized the role of the spouse in the patient's pain experience. The intervention included training in both pain coping skills and couple skills. The pain coping skills component focused on attention diversion, activity-based skills, and cognitive coping strategies. Couples skills training incorporated communication skills, behavioral rehearsal, mutual goal-setting, joint home and in vivo practice, and maintenance training. Data analyses indicated that, compared to patients in the arthritis education-spouse support condition, patients in the spouse-assisted coping skills training group experienced significant reductions in pain, psychological disability, and overt pain behavior and improvements in pain coping (i.e. increases in pain control and rational thinking, and coping attempts). These results suggest that spouse-assisted coping skills training has promise for helping patients manage the pain of OA. Furthermore, since patients in the arthritis education social support condition fail to show improvements, the results indicate that simply having a spouse present does not ensure better functioning if the patient and spouse are not taught pain coping and couples skills.

We recently tested the efficacy of partner-guided treatment for cancer pain occurring at end-of-life (Keefe et al 2005a). Seventy-eight hospice-eligible patients with pain due to advanced cancer and their partners were randomized to partner-guided pain management or usual care. The treatment protocol consisted of three 1-hour sessions during which dyads: 1) received information about cancer pain and its management, 2) were taught various pain coping strategies, and 3) partners were taught how to help the patients acquire and maintain coping skills. Results indicated that, after completing treatment, partners in the intervention group reported significantly higher levels of self-efficacy for helping patients control pain and other symptoms than partners in the usual care condition. In comparison to those in the usual care condition, partners in the intervention group also reported lower levels of caregiver strain.

Comment: The studies above suggest that partner-assisted approaches to pain management may be beneficial in both arthritis and cancer populations. Partner-assisted pain management can be important for several reasons. First, when a partner is taught pain coping skills, the patient can benefit more than if the partner is simply educated about the illness. Partners can be taught to help the patient maintain skills and to assist in setting future pain management goals. This point is important because it provides structure for a partner's involvement in the pain experience, whereas otherwise, a partner might not know how to assist the patient. Second, partners can benefit directly from participating in pain management. As was found in our cancer pain study, partners who were taught how to guide patients through pain coping skills reported a significant increase in their sense of self-efficacy in helping the patient manage pain and a reduction in caregiver strain. Third, the quality of relationship between the partner and the patient can benefit from the joint involvement in pain management. Along these lines, we found that arthritis patients undergoing spouse-assisted pain coping skills training reported significant improvements in marital satisfaction (Keefe et al 1996). These improvements may be due to the fact that the couple was actively working toward developing skills for reaching the common goal of pain reduction, and felt closer together because of it. Fourth, partner-assisted treatments can be easily incorporated into current pain management settings. Many patients have family members or friends who are interested in and willing to play an active role in treatment and can be incorporated with minimal effort.

Although there are many benefits to partner-assisted pain management interventions, they do have some potential limitations. First, partner-assisted pain management is based on the assumption that the person having pain and their partner have an ongoing and reasonably satisfied relationship. This approach may not be appropriate for couples with dysfunctional relationships. Such couples may need a course of couples or marital therapy before being candidates for partner-assisted training. Second, some people prefer to cope in an individual fashion instead of in a communal manner, i.e. with their partner. These people might be reluctant to fully involve another person in their pain management program. When working with such individuals it is often helpful to hold a sharing conference to outline treatment goals with both patient and their partner and then conduct the actual treatment with the patient alone. Third, partners might have feelings and beliefs about the patient's pain experience that impede successful collaboration. These include blaming the patient for his/her pain, feeling resentful for the patient's limitations, and feeling hopeless about the potential for improvement. By directly addressing these thoughts and related feelings early in treatment, one can enhance the effects of partner-assisted treatment approaches.

Early Psychosocial Intervention

One of the most important, recent trends in psychosocial pain management has been a growing emphasis on early intervention. The basic notion that underpins this approach is that, if one can identify and treat maladaptive pain coping patterns early, one can prevent much of the psychological and physical disability associated with persistent pain. Several studies have examined the efficacy of early psychosocial intervention protocols. Linton & Ryberg (2001), for example, conducted a study investigating the effects of a cognitive-behavioral group intervention for reducing pain-related disability in people experiencing episodic neck and back pain. Participants in this study were considered to be at risk for developing chronic pain in that they experienced significant pain ($\geq 7/10$ on pain scale), had 4 or more pain episodes over the previous year, and had missed at least 30 days of work over the previous year. The early intervention protocol consisted of six group sessions of training in pain coping skills including problem-solving, applied relaxation, scheduling activities, cognitive appraisal, warning signals, communication, and flare-up control. Data analyses revealed that, six months after completing treatment, participants who had received the early intervention protocol had one-third the incidence of long-term sick leave compared to the control group. The early intervention group also had significantly more pain-free days and significantly lower levels of fear avoidant behaviors than the control group. These findings suggest that systematically intervening early with group training in pain coping skills can help prevent long-term pain-related disability in persons with episodic pain.

A recent study by van den Hout et al (2003) tested the efficacy of early intervention protocol that emphasized training in problem solving methods. Participants for this study were identified on the basis of having a recent work absence due to lower back pain and met several criteria suggesting they were at risk for chronic pain (i.e. had lower back pain for greater than 6 weeks, were on sick leave less than 20 weeks, and had less than 120 days sick leave for back pain over the previous year). An interesting aspect of the problem solving intervention used in this study was that it was integrated into ongoing physical therapy sessions. The intervention included instruction in five steps of problem solving: 1) problem orientation, 2) problem definition, 3) generation of alternatives, 4) decision-making, and 5) implementation and evaluation. Results showed that, six months after completing treatment, participants who received the problem solving protocol had significantly fewer sick days than those in education control condition. Furthermore, those who received training in problem solving were significantly more likely to achieve 100% return-to-work status than those in the education control group. An impressive aspect of this study was that all data on sick absenteeism and return to work were obtained from actual work records rather than self-report data. These results are important because they indicate that training in behavioral problem solving strategies can have a significant and long-term positive impact on sick leave and return to work.

Comment: Taken together, the findings of the studies reviewed suggest that relatively brief psychosocial interventions can prevent pain-related problems such as fear of pain and work absenteeism due to pain. Early intervention is potentially quite cost-effective, particularly if as in the van den Hout (2003) study, it is incorporated into ongoing physical therapy treatments. To our knowledge, formal cost-effectiveness studies of such early interventions have not been carried out. This is obviously an important direction for future research.

Another important aspect of the studies profiled is that the researchers were able to identify individuals during an early stage in the development of persistent pain. Eligible study participants showed indications of becoming disabled, but were still early in the course of developing persistent pain and pain-related disability. One of the most important directions for future early intervention research is developing the best strategies for early identification of patients who are at-risk and determining the optimal time point for early intervention.

Emotional Disclosure

Persistent pain is quite emotionally stressful. Major stressors include the pain itself, inability to fulfill home or work responsibilities, and uncertainty about the future. These stressors can induce an array of strong emotions including anger, frustration, depression, anxiety, and guilt. Patients vary in their willingness and ability to express these distressing emotions.

Converging lines of evidence suggest that people who inhibit emotional expression are more likely to experience long-term negative psychological and physiological consequences (Pennebaker 1995). Pennebaker designed a protocol that encourages individuals to openly discuss their thoughts and feelings. In this four-day protocol, individuals are encouraged to write (or talk into a tape recorder) for thirty minutes each day about difficult, traumatic events they have not discussed with others. Emotional disclosure interventions, in general, encourage people to "volitionally recall the event, access and experience the emotions stemming from it, explore how the event has changed their beliefs, and then integrate these new perspectives into their developing sense of self" (Greenberg & Stone 1992). To date, most of the research on emotional disclosure interventions has been conducted in healthy pain-free populations. A large number of studies have documented the psychological and physiological benefits of emotional disclosure in healthy populations (Pennebaker 2000).

Emotional disclosure interventions might be particularly beneficial for persons suffering from persistent pain. Through writing or talking about stressful pain-related experiences, patients may alter how they emotionally and cognitively process these experiences, and, as a result have less psychological distress. A further benefit of emotional disclosure is that it may improve how patients and their loved ones communicate about pain and its consequences for their relationships. Finally, emotional disclosure may enhance the ability of a person with persistent pain to confront and manage future highly emotional and stressful experiences.

Several recent studies have tested the efficacy of emotional disclosure interventions in persons having persistent pain. Norman et al (2004) tested the effects of written emotional disclosure in a study of 48 patients suffering from chronic pelvic pain. In this study, patients were randomly assigned to either an emotional disclosure condition that involved three days of writing about the stressful consequences of their pain, or a control condition that involved three days of writing about positive events. Data analyses revealed that, when compared patients in the control condition, patients who received the emotional disclosure intervention had a significant reduction in pain. Interestingly, participants who were the most emotionally upset by their pain (i.e. who reported the highest level of negative affect and pain catastrophizing prior to treatment) benefited the most from the emotional disclosure intervention.

Kelley et al (1997) conducted a study of the effects of emotional disclosure in patients having pain due to rheumatoid arthritis. In this study, 72 rheumatoid arthritis patients were assigned to four days of either spoken emotional disclosure or a control group. Data analyses showed that immediately after disclosure, patients who received the emotional disclosure experienced a significant increase in negative affect. At three months follow-up, however, the emotional disclosure group experienced a significant reduction in pain and improvement in physical functioning. Interestingly, participants whose negative affect increased the most during

250

emotional disclosure reported a greater decrease in joint pain at the three-month follow-up. These findings suggest that emotional disclosure may have long term benefits for rheumatoid arthritis patients and that those patients who work the hardest during disclosure sessions (i.e. who experience the largest increases in negative emotion when they engage in disclosure) are likely to have the best long-term outcomes.

Comments: Although emotional disclosure interventions have been tested in relatively few studies, the initial results are promising. These findings, if confirmed in a larger number of studies, have interesting clinical implications. For example, clinical observations suggest that many patients who suffer from persistent pain are emotionally inhibited. This style might cause some patients to ignore the influence of their emotions on their health and on their own attempts to manage their health (e.g., by exercising, monitoring activity levels). Such patients may particularly benefit from an emotional disclosure intervention. This raises the interesting possibility that patients who are emotionally inhibited may well benefit from more from an exercise regimen if they first receive an emotional disclosure intervention.

Several issues need to be explored before emotional disclosure interventions are widely incorporated into clinical practice. First, we need to learn more about which patients benefit versus fail to benefit from emotional disclosure. The study by Norman et al (2004) suggests that patients who are emotionally upset by pain may benefit from emotional disclosure. However, patients who are in the acute phase of dealing with a psychiatric disorder (e.g. recovering from trauma) are unlikely to benefit from this intervention. In fact, patients who are acutely emotionally distressed are typically excluded from research studies of emotional disclosure. Second, little is known about the physiological benefits of emotional disclosure in patients suffering from persistent pain. In healthy populations there is evidence that emotional disclosure can improve immune function (Pennebaker 2000). This raises the possibility that emotional disclosure might be particularly beneficial in patients whose pain is related to an autoimmune disorder (e.g. rheumatoid arthritis). Finally, more needs to be learned about the effects of emotional disclosure that occurs in an interpersonal context. All of the studies reviewed above have tested the effects of private emotional disclosure, i.e. disclosing either in written or spoken form while being alone in a quiet room. A great deal of emotional disclosure clinically, however, occurs in the context of a patient and practicing clinician. Clinical observations suggest that such disclosure is often helpful, but research data on the effects of such interpersonal disclosure is lacking.

Mindfulness Meditation

Although meditation has been used for centuries, it has only recently been systematically studied as a psychosocial approach to pain management. Kabat-Zinn (1982) pioneered the development of a mindfulness meditation protocol which combines traditional meditation practices with pain education and coping skills training. Kabat-Zinn (1982) theorized that the mindfulness meditation could be particularly helpful in pain management because it fosters the development of a disassociated view of sensory experiences that helps patients distinguish between sensory aspects and affective-emotional aspects of pain. The protocol described by Kabat-Zinn (1982) involves eight to ten weekly group sessions with one day serving as a retreat. The central goal is to promote the development of mindfulness, defined as an awareness of thoughts and feelings, as well as recognition of thoughts and feelings as mental events, not aspects of the self or reflections of reality. Other goals of this protocol include the reduction of patients' negative thinking patterns and the incorporation of mindfulness into patients' daily lives. These goals can be achieved through education about mindfulness, in-session and at-home practice of mindfulness meditation, and audiocassettes that contain guided meditation sessions. Beginning about twenty years ago, Kabat-Zinn and his colleagues conducted several studies to understand the role of mindfulness meditation in the treatment of patients experiencing persistent pain. In a set of three uncontrolled studies, Kabat-Zinn et al (1985) demonstrated patient improvement on a variety of psychological and physical outcome measures through the use of a mindfulness-based stress reduction program. Results showed decreases in mood disturbance and emotional distress both directly after treatment as well as maintained levels at follow-up. Many participants also experienced a significant decrease in pain intensity and pain-related disability, although pain intensity returned to pre-treatment levels for some participants. Kabat-Zinn et al (1987) reported on the results of a mindfulness meditation program with 225 persistent pain patients. Outcome data indicated that the protocol was associated with "great improvement" in pain for 30-55% of the participants, and at least "moderate improvement" in pain for 60-72% of the 225 participants. Significant improvements were maintained from post-treatment through follow-up in the following outcomes: emotional distress, severity of psychiatric symptoms and pain-related disability; however, follow-up results showed that pain levels had returned to pre-treatment levels.

Until recently, however, no randomized, controlled trials had been performed to test the efficacy of mindfulness meditation program for pain management (Bishop 2002). Speca et al (2000) conducted a randomized, controlled study to test the effects of mindfulness-based stress reduction with patients having cancer pain. In this study, 90 cancer patients were randomly assigned either to mindfulness meditation-based stress reduction or to a waitlist control condition. Data analyses revealed that, at the completion of treatment, patients who received mindfulness-based stress reduction had improvements in mood, anxiety, depression, anger, stress, confusion and energy. Interestingly, there was a strong link between participation in treatment and treatment outcome. Participants who improved the most (i.e., better mood, decreased stress) attended more of the sessions and also completed more of the homework practices.

Comments: Mindfulness meditation is a psychosocial intervention that one would assume could have a role in pain management. At present, however, there are few controlled studies examining the effects of this intervention in persons having persistent pain. Mindfulness meditation could be quite useful clinically, particularly by increasing patients' awareness of how thoughts, feelings, behaviors, and daily stressors affect pain. The practice of mindfulness meditation could also help patients suffering from pain shift their focus from pain to improving other facets of their lives. Mindfulness meditation, in fact, might have particular benefits from improving patients' relationships with loved ones. Along these lines, Carson et al (2004) recently described a novel mindfulness-based relationship enhancement intervention that was used in pain-free, non-distressed couples. The intervention involved training couples in both formal and informal meditation and yoga-based practices and involved structured exercises in which they were encouraged to practice together on a daily basis. Data analyses showed that, after completing the intervention, the couples achieved significantly higher levels of satisfaction with their partners and themselves, as well as lower levels of psychological distress. These benefits were maintained through the three-month follow-up. This novel mindfulness meditation intervention could be extended to couples in which one member has chronic pain and might produce beneficial outcomes for patients and their partners.

One factor limiting the use of mindfulness meditation training is that patients vary in their readiness to use this technique. Some patients find the idea of meditation appealing, while others are much less interested. Along these lines, it should be noted that attrition rates in some studies of mindfulness meditation have been high. These problems may reflect overly negative attitudes and beliefs about meditation that are popular in our current culture (e.g. "Meditation is just a fad", "Meditation means mind control"). To better address these concerns, more emphasis needs to be placed on incorporating educational and cognitive-behavioral interventions (e.g. motivational interviewing) into mindfulness meditation protocols. Such a strategy very likely could enhance the appeal and potential efficacy of mindfulness meditation in the management of persistent pain.

Conclusions

Over the past 40 years, psychosocial interventions have become recognized as an important option in the array of strategies for managing chronic pain. Evidence for the efficacy of these strategies is accumulating. Newer studies are exploring the benefits of early intervention and partner-assisted interventions. Novel interventions such as emotional disclosure and mindfulness meditation also are being developed and refined. In the coming years, psychosocial interventions are likely to be used by a wider array of practitioners with a wider array of patient populations. These developments are important clinically and hold the promise of reducing pain and suffering experienced by many chronic pain patients.

Acknowledgements

Preparation of this chapter was supported by several grants from the National Instsitutes of Health (AR50245; NS46422-01, CA91947, AR047218, MH63429, AR46305) and in part, by funds provided by the Arthritis Foundation and the Fetzer Institute.

References

Bishop SR 2002 What do we really know about mindfulness-based stress reduction? Psychosomatic Medicine 64:71-84

Carson JW, Carson KM, Gil KM, Baucom DH 2004 Mindfulness-based relationship enhancement. Behavior Therapy 35:474-494

Flor H, Fydrich T, Turk DC 1992 Efficacy of multidisciplinary treatment centers: A meta-analytic review. Pain 49:221-230

Fordyce WE 1976 Behavioral methods for chronic pain and illness. CV Mosby. St Louis

Fordyce WE, Fowler RS, Delateur B 1968 An application of behavior modification technique to a problem of chronic pain. Behaviour Research & Therapy 6:105-107

Fordyce WE, Fowler RS, Lehmann JF, DeLateur B, Sand PL, Trieschmann RB 1973 Operant conditioning in the treatment of chronic pain. Archives of Physical Medicine and Rehabilitation 54:399-406

Greenberg MA, Stone AA 1992 Emotional disclosure about traumas and its relation to health: Effects of previous disclosure and trauma severity. Journal of Personality and Social Psychology 63:75-84

Kabat-Zinn J 1982 An outpatient program in behavioral medicine for chronic pain patients based on the practice of mindfulness meditation: theoretical considerations and preliminary results. General Hospital Psychiatry 4:33-47

Kabat-Zinn J, Lipworth L, Burney R 1985 The clinical use of mindfulness meditation for the self-regulation of chronic pain. Journal of Behavioral Medicine 8:162-190

Kabat-Zinn J, Lipworth L, Burney R, Sellers W 1987 Four-year follow-up of a meditation-based program for the self-regulation of chronic pain: treatment outcomes and compliance. Clinical Journal of Pain 2:159-173

Keefe FJ, Caldwell DS, Baucom D, Salley A, Robinson E, Timmons K, Beaupre P, Weisberg J, Helms M 1996 Spouse-assisted coping skills training in the management of osteoarthritis knee pain. Arthritis Care and Research 9:279-291

Keefe FJ, Smith SJ, Buffington ALH, Gibson J, Studts J, Caldwell DS 2002 Recent advances and future directions in the biopsychosocial assessment and treatment of arthritis. Journal of Consulting and Clinical Psychology 70:640-655

Keefe FJ, Rumble ME, Scipio CD, Giardano L, Perri LM 2004 Psychological aspects of persistent pain: Current state of the science. Journal of Pain 5:195-211

Keefe FJ, Abernathy M, Campbell L 2005 Psychological approaches to understanding and treating disease-related pain. Annual Review of Psychology 56:601-630

Keefe F J, Ahles TA, Sutton L, Dalton J, Baucom D, Pope MS, Knowles V, McKinstry E, Furstenberg C, Syrjala K, Waters SJ, McKee D, McBride C, Rumble M, Scipio C 2005a Partner-guided cancer pain management at end of life: a preliminary study. Journal of Pain and Symptom Management 29:263-272

Keefe FJ, Dixon KE, Pryor R (in press) Psychological Contributions to Understanding and Treatment of Pain. In: Merskey H (Ed.) The Paths of Pain . Elsevier: New York

Kelley JE, Lumley MA, Liesen JCC 1997 Health effects of emotional disclosure in rheumatoid arthritis patients. Health Psychology 16:331-340

Linton SJ, Ryberg M 2001 A cognitive-behavioral group intervention as prevention for persistent neck and back pain in a non-patient population: a randomized controlled trial. Pain 90:83-90

Morley S, Eccleston C, Williams A 1999 Systematic review and meta-analysis of randomized controlled trials of cognitive behaviour therapy and behaviour therapy for chronic pain in adults, excluding headache. Pain 80:1-13.

Norman SA, Lumley MA, Dooley JA, Diamond MP 2004 For whom does it work? Moderators of the effects of written emotional disclosure in a randomized trial among women with chronic pelvic pain. Psychosomatic Medicine 66:174-183

Pennebaker JW (Ed) 1995 Emotion, disclosure and health. American Psychological Association, Washington DC

Pennebaker JW 2000 Telling stories: the health benefits of narrative. Literature & Medicine 19:3-18

Penzien DB, Rains JC, Lipchik GL, Creer TL 2004 Behavioral interventions for tension-type headache: overview of current therapies and recommendation for a self-management model for chronic headache. Current Pain & Headache Reports 8:489-499

Speca M, Carlson LE, Goodey E, Angen M 2000 A randomized, wait-list controlled clinical trial: The effect of a mindfulness meditation-based stress reduction program on mood and symptoms of stress in cancer outpatients. Psychosomatic Medicine 62:613-622

Turk DC 2002 Clinical effectiveness and cost-effectiveness of treatments for patients with chronic pain. Clinical Journal of Pain 18:355-365

Turk DC, Okifuji A 2002 Psychological factors in chronic pain: Evolution and revolution. Journal of Consulting and Clinical Psychology 70:678-690

van den Hout JH, Vlaeyen JW, Heuts PH, Zijlema JH, Wijnen J A 2003 Secondary prevention of work-related disability in nonspecific low back pain: Does problem-solving therapy help? A randomized clinical trial. The Clinical Journal of Pain 19:87-96

15

Post Traumatic Stress Disorder: A Cognitive Behavioural Perspective

SHARON WILDAY

Post traumatic stress disorder (PTSD) is an anxiety disorder that is triggered by the experience of extreme trauma and is distinguished by symptoms of re-experiencing, avoidance and hyper arousal. Approximately 5% of men and 10% of women will suffer from it at some point in their lifetime (NICE 2005). Over the past two decades it has received increasing attention from academic and clinical research areas, which has led to the growing awareness of both its prevalence and impact upon society.

Cognitive behavioural therapy (CBT) encompasses a range of therapeutic techniques that aim to reduce people's distressing emotions by changing their thoughts, beliefs and/or behaviour. It is the current treatment of choice for PTSD (Roth & Fonagy 1996, NICE 2005).

The subject of PTSD brings into sharp focus the range of profound consequences that can arise from the experience of a traumatic event. The symptoms highlight the dynamic interplay between the physical and psychological domains, which until comparatively recent times have been separated from one another within the context of health models, and professions. The cognitive behavioural (CB) model opens up these boundaries and provides a useful perspective from which to view the disorder including an understanding of the range of potential symptoms as well as the processes for change.

This chapter will consider PTSD through its development, starting with the traumatic event itself followed by information about how we process situations, looking especially at the impact of trauma. Normal symptoms that can develop will be considered along with the mechanisms by which they can develop into disordered responses. Finally the current CB interventions for PTSD will be explained along with their evidence base and mechanisms of change.

What is a Traumatic Event?

The risk of exposure to trauma has been part of the human condition since we evolved as a species with a majority of people experiencing at least one traumatic event (Kessler et al 1995). According to the 4th edition of the diagnostic and statistical manual of mental disorders (DSM IV) of the American Psychiatric Association (1994) a situation would be called traumatic if a person had experienced or been witness to an event that involved actual or threatened death or serious injury. There might also have been a threat to this persons or other people's physical integrity, so that they feared physical harm would come to them. This threat could have been so overwhelming that the person would have experienced intense fear, helplessness or horror at least some of the time during the event. The intensity of the traumatic experience is related to both the type of trauma as well as the individual's perception of the trauma.

With respect to the impact of the type of trauma, a study by Kessler and his colleagues (1995) found high PTSD rates associated with rape, combat exposure, childhood neglect and physical abuse, sexual molestation and for women only, physical attack and being threatened with a weapon, kidnapped or held hostage. Accidents, witnessing death or injury, and natural disasters were associated with lower PTSD rates.

However, in addition to the type of trauma another significant factor in whether or not an event is considered traumatic is the individual's perception. Lazarus (1966) explains that a situation will be appraised as threatening in response to a primary appraisal of the situation, and a secondary appraisal of our perceived ability to cope with it. When there is a shortfall between these two appraisals we perceive the situation as threatening.

Thus the exposure to a specific event may lead to the appraisal of threat to one and not for another. Friedman (1990) highlights how such observations have prompted the recognition that trauma, like pain, is not an external process separate from subjective influence. Like pain the experience of trauma is filtered through cognitive and emotional processes before it can be considered an extreme threat.

As such it is the difference in individual appraisal processes that can explain some of the variances observed between peoples vulnerability to developing clinical symptoms following exposure to trauma (Foa et al 1999, Ehlers & Clarke, 2000). This is perhaps indicative of why a CB approach to the disorder is so valuable, being grounded as it is in the philosophy that we are influenced not by events but by the meaning of those events (Epictetus, first century AD: cited in Trower et al 2004).

How Do We Process Traumatic Events?

Traumatic events can alter the way in which we process and store information. This change in processing is one of the key reasons for the problems that can arise. To understand what happens when we experience trauma it is helpful to first look at our processing of normal events.

Processing of Normal Events

CB theory proposes that as we make our way through life we develop core beliefs about self, others, the world and the future via various learning experiences. These beliefs then help to form rules for living that enable us to get by in life with the beliefs that we hold. For most of the time these beliefs are unconsciously governing and directing our cognitive, behavioural, biological and emotional appraisals and responses in the daily circumstances in which we find ourselves. We feel, think and behave based on the beliefs that we hold and the rules that we live by. Our unique set of life experiences lead us to perceive our world in a unique way and this is one of the basic principles of CB theory (Beck 1976, Beck et al 1979, Salkovskis 1996, Wells 1997).

For example if you have a core belief that 'people are generally trustworthy' then a rule for living might be 'relax and enjoy meeting new people'. Someone who had the opposite core belief 'people are generally untrustworthy' might have a very different rule for living, 'don't relax around others until you know you can trust them'. It is clear to see how these two people with opposing beliefs would enter situations differently. At a party for example where there are lots of new people the trusting person is likely to appraise the situation as within their ability to cope, and the untrusting person is likely to appraise it in a more threatening way. Consequently the trusting person would likely feel relaxed, be actively meeting others and perceiving others actions in a mostly positive way; the untrusting person would probably be tense and be avoiding contact, spending time on assessing who was trustworthy and avoiding others. Their core beliefs and rules for living would ultimately influence their perceptions within the situation and their behavioural, emotional and biological responses.

259

These responses then influence one another in a reciprocal way (Beck 1976, Beck et al 1979, Persons et al 2001). In the example above this can be seen as the untrusting person's ability to cope and get through the party by the avoidance of others, reinforcing their beliefs that others are untrustworthy and that they did well to avoid them. This behaviour tends to prevent them from gaining alternative evidence that people can be trustworthy. However even if trustworthiness of others is found the experience is likely to be disregarded as incongruent with their current beliefs.

This process can be further understood by Piaget's theory of human adaptation and cognitive development (see Gruber & Voneche 1995 for a summary of his work) which suggests that we attempt to make sense of our life experiences and adapt to our environments via the two cognitive processes of assimilation and accommodation. It proposes that when we experience new information about ourselves, others, the world and/or the future that is different from our current understanding, we experience dissonance (a form of distress), at which point we have the choice to assimilate or accommodate the new information.

Assimilation is the process by which we adapt our experiences to fit with our existing body of information (core beliefs), and accommodation is where we attempt to alter our current beliefs to fit with the new information. Mostly we assimilate. It is usually only in extreme and/or highly emotive circumstances (such as traumatic experiences) when we struggle to assimilate, that we consider challenging what we already know and accommodate our own beliefs to fit the new information. As such, mostly our unique perspectives go unchallenged.

We tend to view the world in our own way and use our current template with which to organise new experiences and information so that it fits our established view.

Processing of Traumatic Events

Traumatic experiences are believed to affect the way in which we process information and consequently lay down memory (Foa & Kozak 1986, NICE 2005). This is due to the impact of the extreme emotional and biological changes that are triggered when we face an event that is so different from our normal life events and coping skills.

We have a highly sensitive mechanism that is designed to protect us from danger and help us to survive when we are faced with life threatening traumatic events. This mechanism is called our 'fight or flight response'. It is triggered by our appraisal of threat and is switched into action in a fraction of a second. Its main aim is to provide us with the energy that we will need to either fight or flight from the danger. It is this process along with the extreme nature of the event that can interfere with our ability to process information during the trauma.

This difficulty in information processing causes the traumatic event to be laid down in fear-based memory. Consequently the experience is not fully processed or correctly stored. This leads to frequent re-experiencing of the memories as if they are happening now rather than as a past event (NICE 2005, Foa & Kozak 1986, Brewin et al 1996, McNally 2003). Mc Farlane (1988) suggests that it is the intrusive reliving of the trauma rather than the trauma itself that is responsible for the complex changes indicative of PTSD.

The experience of high levels of peri-traumatic dissociation (the separation of mental processes during the trauma experience) is also likely to further disrupt processing and increase the frequency of later intrusions (Shalev et al 1996, Spiegel & Cardena 1991).

How Do We Respond to Trauma?

There is a range of normal responses that can occur following trauma. It is believed that our perceptions and responses to these symptoms are paramount in the eventual outcome of the trauma. Either the symptoms reduce and the individual naturally recovers or alternatively the natural processes of recovery are hindered and the symptoms worsen leading to a disordered response.

Normal Response

Foa et al (2005) suggest that it is common to experience a range of unusual symptoms following exposure to a traumatic event. The intensity with which the symptoms are experienced will vary between individuals. A high percentage of people will feel improved within three months but for some this process is slower and a small proportion will need help to recover.

Emotional Symptoms

Anxiety is a natural response to a dangerous situation. However, following a traumatic event we often experience anxiety long after the trauma has ended. This can be as a consequence of the increased re-experiencing of the trauma or can be indicative of a continuing perception of a reduced capacity to cope; both of which can lead to the triggering of the fight/flight arousal. Anger and irritability are common emotions following trauma and they can occur as a consequence of an increased arousal response. Alternatively the emotion can be related to our beliefs about the trauma as unfair or unjust.

Grief and Depression following trauma are often related to a sense of loss. This may be associated with actual loss (depending on the trauma) or a perception of loss related to the changes in how we now see the world, ourselves and or others.

Cognitive Symptoms

The reliving of the traumatic event is common and is activated by the need to fully process and correctly store the event in memory. Re-experiencing can be in the form of unwanted thoughts, vivid flash backs and nightmares.

Change in our beliefs about self, others, the world and the future can develop following trauma. The event is so far removed from our beliefs that we find it difficult to fit it into our current understanding, which can be very distressing. New information that would assist in giving perspective to our beliefs is often absent because of the increased avoidance (see behavioural symptoms)

Biological Symptoms

Increased arousal is related to the fight or flight response and can lead to a number of physical symptoms ranging from being easily startled, having difficulty concentrating and sleeping, as well as generally feeling on edge. Following a trauma we can often believe that we are still in danger and our body responds by keeping us in this state of readiness and arousal as if we were on 'red alert'. This is further exacerbated by the range of triggers for the memory of the trauma that have been learned via the processes of classical conditioning. Through these processes objects, situations and sensory perceptions present at the time of the trauma may have become conditioned to the trauma (Keane et al 1985). These conditioned events will then come to elicit the fight/flight response.

Prolonged arousal can lead to increased irritability and is further compounded by poor sleep.

Behavioural Symptoms

Avoidance is a common coping strategy for trauma related distress. Most commonly we avoid anything that reminds us of the trauma; such as the actual situation in which the trauma occurred, talking or thinking about what happened, blocking out intrusive recollections and drinking or taking drugs to blot out the memories.

Social avoidance and relationship problems are also a common reaction to trauma. Problems commonly arise because of increased irritability with others. It is also often difficult for people who have not experienced trauma to understand the symptoms that can be experienced.

Disordered Response

The recognised disorders following a trauma are acute stress disorder (ASD) and PTSD. Both will be defined and the processes by which they develop will follow.

Acute Stress Disorder (ASD)

ASD is a psychiatric diagnosis that was introduced into the DSM-IV in 1994 to describe stress reactions that occur between 2 days and 4 weeks following a trauma. The current diagnostic criteria for ASD are similar to those for PTSD; the difference is in the former having a greater emphasis on extreme avoidance and dissociation. The diagnosis can only be given within the first month after a traumatic event but has been found to be highly predictive of subsequent diagnosis of PTSD. Criteria for ASD involves A) exposure to a stressor with a response of fear or helplessness; where the individual goes onto experience symptoms including B) at least three of five symptoms of dissociation C) at least one re experiencing symptom D) marked avoidance and E) marked arousal. (American Psychiatric Association 1994).

Because ASD is a relatively new diagnosis, research on the disorder is in the early stages. Early studies suggest that the prevalence of ASD following a traumatic experience is 6% to 33%. This variance is believed to be dependant on the type of trauma (Gibson 2005).

Post Traumatic Stress Disorder (PTSD)

It was not formally recognised as a disorder until 1980 when it appeared for the first time in the DSM III (American Psychiatric Association 1980). Since then it has further been refined and today is defined as a disorder which involves A) exposure to a life threatening experience, with intense subjective distress upon exposure, and where by the individual goes on to experience symptoms inclusive of B) re experiencing the trauma, C) persistent avoidance or numbing, as well as D) persistent symptoms of increased arousal (American Psychiatric Association1994).

A diagnosis of PTSD would be relevant only after a month. Approximately 30% of individuals exposed to extreme trauma develop short-term PTSD, and approximately 10% will develop chronic symptoms (duration of 3 months or more). The risk of developing PTSD after a traumatic event is 8.1% for men, and 20.4% for women (Kessler et al 1995).

Associated symptoms that can occur alongside PTSD but do not need to be present for the diagnosis include; issues such as guilt, depression, suicidal ideation, substance use, and other anxiety disorders. Other possible complications of PTSD include somatisation, chronic pain, and poor health (Schnurr & Green 2004). Ouimette and his colleagues (2004) have also cited the greater incidence of medical conditions in individuals diagnosed with PTSD.

How Does A Disordered Response Develop?

As with most emotional disorders the CB formulation suggests that it is the responses that an individual makes to their condition that can determine the duration and severity of the problem. This is no different for trauma (Foa et al 1999, Ehlers & Clark 2000). Disordered responses can be seen as an increase in the normal symptoms of trauma, or a prolonging of their presence. This is a consequence of the avoidance of behaviour that would naturally assist with the necessary processing of the trauma memory (Ehlers & Clark, 2000). Symptoms are extremely distressing and confusing (Ehlers & Steil 1995) and the individual often develops avoidant coping techniques to manage them.

Avoidance includes effortful suppression of trauma memories and emotions, dissociation, social withdrawal, substance abuse and physical avoidance of the trauma reminders (Ehlers & Clarke, 2000). This leads to the reduction of the distress, which is associated with them (e.g. following an assault in a bank, the avoidance of banks prevents the onset of distress and potential reminders of the trauma). This avoidance behaviour is negatively reinforced (i.e. likely to be repeated because of its success in preventing distress).

However, these avoidance behaviours are frequently counterproductive (Wells 1997; Salkovskis 1991 and Ehlers and Clarke 2000) in that they:

- Prevent the emotional processing of the memory thus leaving it fragmented and easily triggered.

- Reduce our immediate distress leading us to believe they are helpful coping mechanisms, which encourages their continued use.

- Prevent experiences of the conditioned events and therefore inhibit learning that would give a more realistic perception of them and assist in natural cognitive restructuring.

- Enhance the continued preoccupation with the appraisals of danger thus maintaining symptoms.

As such despite providing short term relief from distress avoidance ultimately prevents the processing of the fragmented trauma memory and maintains symptoms of re-experiencing, increased arousal and the maintenance of potentially faulty beliefs about self, the world and others. The consequences of which are development of the disordered responses of ASD and PTSD.

Interventions For Trauma

Evidence Base for CBT Interventions:

Interventions for trauma can be offered in the acute aftermath of traumatic events (e.g. psychological debriefing), as well as post diagnosis of either ASD or PSTD. Further details can be obtained from the National Collaborating Center for Mental Health (NICE 2005).

Psychological debriefing is an early intervention that was originally developed for rescue workers but has been widely applied in the acute aftermath of potentially traumatic events. It is commonly offered in a group format to all individuals soon after a traumatic event. However a review of the literature on debriefing (Litz et al 2002) concluded that there is little evidence to support its continued use with acutely traumatised individuals.

CBT interventions are offered usually on a one to one basis once an individual has been diagnosed with either ASD or PTSD. The evidence suggests that where CBT is offered between 1-6 months post trauma it is effective in reducing the severity of PTSD and anxiety as well as increasing quality of life at 9-13 months follow up (NICE 2005). It is more effective at preventing the development of chronic PTSD than wait list, supportive counseling, relaxation or self help literature. 8-12 sessions of CBT are recommended for those who present with PTSD within the first 3 months following the incident and this can be reduced to 5 sessions if treatment is started within the fist month (NICE 2005).

Components of CBT Intervention:

The CBT treatment components that are used in the treatment of PTSD are psycho education, exposure, cognitive restructuring and anxiety management (Harvey et al 2003).

Psycho Education

Providing a plausible explanation for the intrusive re-experiencing of trauma memory can help to correct dysfunctional appraisals that are believed to contribute to the development and/or maintenance of PTSD (Ehlers at al 1998, Ehlers & Steil 1995, Dunmore et al 2001)

This involves the provision of information about the common symptoms during the initial treatment session. This session highlights the symptoms of the post trauma response and discusses the way in which the core symptoms will be treated during the course of therapy. The aim is to normalise the trauma reaction, to help the patient develop a formulation of their symptoms, and to assist in establishing a rationale for treatment. This aspect of the intervention can offer considerable reassurance. It can enable an individual to perceive their symptoms differently and can impact positively on their associated coping responses to them. This in turn reduces the intensity and severity of problems overall.

Exposure Therapy

Exposure therapy has been used with great success for many years to treat a variety of disorders including phobias, panic, and obsessive-compulsive disorder. In the last 15-20 years exposure has been applied and adapted for treatment of PTSD. It has more empirical evidence for its efficacy than any other treatment for trauma, is cited as the quickest acting treatment for PTSD and is a preferred treatment across trauma populations (Foa & Meadows 1997; Astin & Rothbaum 2000, Grey at al 2002).

Exposure entails the client reliving the trauma experience by describing it aloud in as much detail as possible to encourage habituation. The therapist assists the client in the provision of the narrative of their trauma. Typically these reliving sessions will last at least 90 minutes to enable time to describe the trauma, discuss the experience afterwards and have time to become calmer before leaving the session (Grey at al 2002).

This process activates the reliving of the trauma and enables the individual to process the traumatic memory allowing the modification of the fear memory (Astin & Rothbaum 2000). This process will have been actively avoided by the individual and is likely to increase the client's distress and fear during the exercise. It is important that the therapist actively assist with the process of encouraging the client to stay with the distress as much as possible as the exposure to the experience will enable the memories to be adequately processed leading to the longer term reduction in distress. Each time the client exposes to the trauma the intensity of the experience reduces and becomes more of a memory than the re-experiencing of the trauma. This becomes apparent to the client and the process becomes easier as they realise the benefit of it (Astin & Rotherbaum 2000).

Cognitive Restructuring

Cognitive restructuring is a cognitive technique involving the identification of negative automatic thoughts that may serve to maintain and worsen symptoms of distress. The thoughts are representative of deeper cognitive structures (core beliefs), which may have come into question since the trauma. It encourages patients to evaluate the evidence for their negative thoughts as well as assisting in the evaluation of their beliefs about the trauma, the world and the future (Marks et al 1998).

Research has highlighted the role of a range of negative core beliefs that are commonly associated with trauma patients and include beliefs around: personal safety/vulnerability, dangerousness of the world, lessened trust in others, loss of confidence in the fairness/benevolence of the world, self blame and guilt, low self efficacy or perceived self competence, negative future outcome expectancies, low self esteem/worth and the loss of spiritual beliefs (Follette et al 1998). The impact of such negative core beliefs can lead to distress and consequential avoidance of the situations that could ultimately provide alternative evidence to diminish the strength of the beliefs (Ehlers & Clark, 2000).

Traditionally it is believed that most cognitive change takes place at times of high affect (Beck 1995). Imagery based restructuring of meaning is therefore also believed to be more effective at these times as much of the trauma memory is stored in this way (Ehlers & Clarke 2000). Cognitive restructuring can be considered both during the reliving sessions or the discussion time afterwards.

It is likely that intervention would also involve behavioural experiments. This would include the development of a list of situations currently being avoided in increasing levels of perceived distress. The client would expose to the situation of least perceived distress and stay until they experienced their levels of distress reducing (i.e. as a consequence of habituation). This process would ultimately provide evidence that would dis-confirm faulty beliefs and reduce the conditioned fear response. Exposure can be real or imaginary.

Anxiety Management

Anxiety management training aims to provide individuals with coping skills to assist in the mastery over their fear. Specific approaches often include aspects of psycho education, relaxation skills, thought stopping, and self-talk. However it should be noted that the use of thought stopping has been challenged (Rassin et al 2000) because there is evidence that attempting to stop or suppress thoughts relating to a trauma may actually fuel these thoughts (Harvey & Bryant, 1998).

Conclusion

PTSD occurs following exposure to a trauma and most people will experience at least one such event in their lifetime. Whether or not people develop PTSD depends on their subjective perception of the experience as well as the objective facts.

The majority of literature relating to trauma focuses on the consequential disorders of ASD and PTSD. However the occurrence of distressing symptoms in the immediate aftermath of a traumatic event is common and does not constitute a disordered response (Foa et al 2005). The symptoms are unusual compared to those of everyday life and are extremely unpleasant. It is easy to focus on the abnormal nature of their occurrence; however the author believes that they are mostly natural experiences indicative of the body's healing processes. As such they need to be understood and normalised.

We have many such adaptive responses to adverse conditions (e.g. stress, depression, pain). Our stress response is triggered in threatening conditions and provides us with the necessary energy to deal with danger. Depression is a natural mechanism for slowing us down for a short time to enable us to deal with loss. Acute pain can inform us of potential damage and a need to be cautious. These systems are only designed to be active for a short duration. The mechanism by which they become enduring and mal-adaptive is often related to our perceptions and associated coping. The role of avoidance of distress for those experiencing anxiety, for example, becomes an integral component of their reduced self-efficacy and increasing focus on threat (Salkovskis 1991, Wells 1997). The impact of inactivity and social isolation in those with depression serves to maintain their negative appraisals of self (Beck et al 1979, Teasdale & Bernard 1993). Fear avoidance behaviour activated by our ongoing beliefs of pain meaning damage leads to a heightened awareness of pain sensations and maintains our belief in disability (Vlaeyen & Linton 2000). All of these perceptions and coping behaviours serve to perpetuate the responses, which they were attempting to reduce.

Trauma is no different. It becomes a diagnostic condition when we actively prevent the completion of processes that would extinguish it. CBT provides the psycho-education to assist the normalisation of symptoms and provides insight into the function of the treatment interventions. It includes exposure sessions that enable the processing of trauma memories and provides instruction and encouragement through the techniques of cognitive restructuring. It can help in the early stages post trauma (less than 3 months) and is also seen to be an effective intervention regardless of the time delay following the event (NICE 2005).

There are always exceptions to rules and there may well be cases that do not fit with this formulation, however in the majority of situations the development, severity and duration of conditions such as PTSD would be reduced via the introduction of early intervention, education and general normalisation of the experience.

References

American Psychiatric Association (1980) Diagnostic and Statistical Manual of Mental Disorders (3rd edition) Washington DC: American `psychiatric Association

American Psychiatric Association 1994 Diagnostic and statistical manual of mental disorders (4th ed). Washington DC: Author

Astin MC, Rothbaum BO 2000 Exposure therapy for the treatment of posttraumatic stress disorder. National center for post traumatic stress disorder clinical quarterly 9(4):1052-7168.

Beck A T 1976 Cognitive therapy and emotional disorders. Penguin Books, London

Beck AT, Rush AJ, Shaw BF, Emery G 1979 Cognitive therapy of depression. The Guilford Press: New York

Beck JS 1995 Cognitive Therapy: Basics and Beyond. The Guildford Press, New York

Brewin CR, Dalgleish T, Joseph S 1996 A dual representation theory of posttraumatic stress disorder. Psychological Review 103:670–686

Dunmore E, Clark DM, Ehlers A 2001 A prospective investigation of the role of cognitive factors in persistent posttraumatic stress disorder (PTSD) after physical or sexual assault. Behaviour Research and Therapy 39:1063-1984

Ehlers, A Steil R 1995 Maintenance of intrusive memories in posttraumatic stress disorder: A cognitive approach. Behavioural and Cognitive Psychotherapy 23:217-249

Ehlers A, Clark DM 2000 A cognitive model of posttraumatic stress disorder. Behaviour Research and Therapy 38:319-345

Ehlers A, Mayou RA, Bryant B 1998 Psychological predictors of chronic posttraumatic stress disorder after motor vehicle accidents. Journal of Abnormal Psychology 107:508-519

Foa EB, Kozac MJ 1986 Emotional processing in fear: exposure to corrective information. Psychological Bulletin 99:20-35

Foa EB, Meadows E 1997 Psychosocial treatments for post traumatic stress disorder: A critical review. Annual Review of Psychology 48:449-480

Foa EB, Steketee G, Rothbaum BO 1989 Behavioral/cognitive conceptualisations of post-traumatic stress disorder. Behavior Therapy 20:155-176

Foa EB, Ehlers A, Clark DM 1999 The Post-traumatic cognitions inventory (PTCI): development and validation. Psychological Assessment11:303–314

Foa EB, Hembree EA, Riggs D, Rauch S, Franklin M 2005 Common reactions to trauma. A national center for PTSD fact sheet www.ncptsd.org

Follette VM, Ruzek JI, Abueg FR 1998 Cognitive-behavioral therapies for trauma. Guilford Press, London

Friedman MJ 1990 Interrelationships between biological mechanisms and pharmacotherapy of posttraumatic stress disorder. In: Wolf ME, Mosnaim AD (eds) Post traumatic stress disorder, aetiology, phenomenology and treatment. American Psychological Association Washington DC

Gibson LE 2005 Acute stress disorder: A brief description. A national center for PTSD fact sheet www.ncptsd.org

Grey N, Young K, Holmes E 2002 Cognitive restructuring within reliving: A treatment for peritraumatic emotional hotspots in post traumatic stress disorder. Behavioural and Cognitive psychotherapy 30(1):37-56

Gruber HE, Voneche JJ (eds) 1995 The essential Piaget: An interpretative reference and guide. Jason Aronson, Northvale NJ

Harvey AG, Bryant RA 1998 The effect of attempted thought suppression in acute stress disorder. Behaviour Research and Therapy 36:583-590

Harvey AG, Bryant RA, Tarrier BN 2003 Cognitive behaviour therapy for posttraumatic stress disorder. Clinical Psychology Review 23:501-522

Keane TM, Zimering RT, Caddell JM 1985 A behavioural formulation of posttraumatic stress disorder in combat veterans. Behaviour Therapist 8:9-12

Kessler RC, Sonnega A, Bromet E 1995 Post traumatic stress disorder in the National Comorbidity Survey. Archives of General Psychiatry 52:1048-1060

Lazarus RS 1966 Psychological stress and the coping process. McGraw-Hill: New York

Litz BT, Gray MJ, Bryant RA 2002 Early intervention for trauma: Current status and future directions. Clinical Psychology – Science and Practice 9:112-134

Marks I, Lovell K, Noshirvani H 1998 Treatment of posttraumatic stress disorder by exposure and/or cognitive restructuring: a controlled study. Archives of General Psychiatry 55:317-325

McFarlane AC 1988 The phenomenology of post traumatic stress disorders following a natural disaster. The journal of mental and nervous disorders 176:22-29

McNally R J 2003 Remembering Trauma. Harvard University Press, Cambridge MA

NICE, National Institute of Clinical Excellence 2005 Post Traumatic Stress Disorder (PTSD): The management of PTSD in adults and children in primary and secondary care. Clinical Guideline 26, NICE, London

Ouimette P, Cronkite R, Henson BR 2004 Post traumatic stress disorder and health status among female and male medical patients. Journal of Traumatic Stress 17:1-9

Persons JB, Davidson J, Tomkins MA 2001 Essential components of cognitive behavioural therapy for depression. American psychological association: Washington DC

Rassin E, Merckelbach H, Muris P 2000 Paradoxical and less paradoxical effects of thought suppression: A critical review. Clinical Psychology Review 20:973-995

Roth A, Fonagy P 1996 What works for whom?: A critical review of the psychotherapy research. Guilford Press, London

Salkovskis PM 1991 The importance of behaviour therapy in the maintenance of anxiety and panic: A cognitive account. Behavioural Psychotherapy 19:16-19

Salkovskis PM 1996 Frontiers of Cognitive Therapy. The Guilford Press, New York

Schnurr PP, Green BL (eds) 2004 Trauma and health: physical consequences of exposure to extreme stress. American Psychological Association, Washington DC

Shalev AT, Peri T, Canetti L, Schreiber S 1996 Predictors of PTSD in injured trauma survivors: a prospective study. American Journal of Psychiatry 153:219-225

Spiegel D, Cardena E 1991 Disintegrated experience: The dissociative disorders revisited. Journal of Abnormal Psychology. 100(3):366-378

Teasdale JD, Barnard PJ 1993 Cognition, Affect and Change: Re-modelling Depressive Thought. Erlbaum, Hove

Trower P, Casey A, Dryden W 2004 Cognitive Behavioural Counselling in Action. Sage, London (page 1)

Vlaeyen JWS, Linton SJ 2000 Fear avoidance and its consequences in chronic musculoskeletal pain: a state of the art. Pain 85:317-322

Wells A 1997 Cognitive therapy of anxiety disorder. Wiley and sons, Chichester

16

Learning to Facilitate Change in Cognition and Behaviour

MARK A. JONES AND IAN EDWARDS

Patients' thoughts and feelings have been shown to be positively associated with greater disability and risk of chronicity necessitating therapists not only understand these relationships but also develop skills of assessment, reasoning and management directed to these aspects of patients' pain and disability experiences. While the biopsychosocial model has encouraged a better appreciation of the psychological alongside the biomedical, there may still be too superficial an approach by some therapists' assessment and management (e.g. application of cognitive-behavioural strategies) of this dimension of patients' presentations. Superficial judgements of patients' expressed cognitions without adequate exploration of the basis for those thoughts, or their unique evaluations of their experience, and over focus on behavioural strategies to alter patient cognitions and behaviours are not uncommon. Similarly the sociological influences (either as precipitating factors or consequences) on patients' pain and disability experiences are not always adequately explored or addressed. Schema theory may provide further insight of the extent that patient's cognitions can be affected which we believe may be useful to assist therapists' more thorough assessment of psychosocial factors creating a fuller appreciation of patients' pain and disability experiences and avenues to effect change.

This chapter aims to discuss changes in patient cognition and behaviour within a biopsychosocial framework of health. How might such a discussion influence strategies such as the cognitive-behavioural approach? We propose that changes in cognition and behaviour are best achieved through a particular adult learning process (Transformative learning) which embraces the different understandings of health that are implicit within the biopsychosocial framework. Narrative reasoning is put forward as the preferred clinical reasoning strategy for understanding the person behind the problem and communicative management is suggested as the means by which the cognitive dimension of cognitive-behavioural therapy can facilitate deep, transformative patient learning.

Patients' Thoughts and Feelings Contribute to their Disabilities and Prospects for Recovery/Improvement and Risk of Chronicity:

Patients' thoughts and beliefs (i.e. their cognitions) have been found to interact with reports of pain intensity, attempts to adjust or cope (Jensen et al 1991, 1994, 2003) mood and pain-related disability (Keefe 1991, Turk & Rudy 1992, Williams &, Wilson et al 1993, Jensen et al 1994). Patients' preoccupation with negative thoughts and self-statements about their circumstances and future prospects, or what has been labelled "catastrophising" (Pincus 2004) is also identified as a risk factor for pain-related fear (Vlaeyen & Linton 2000) and long-term disability (Pincus et al 2002). Greater worry about pain has been associated with greater hypervigilance, or somatic attention, with potential for amplification of somatosensory input and subsequent validation of patients' beliefs and fears (Eccleston 1995, Eccleston et al 1997, Crombez et al 1998, 1998a). Somatic vigilance may also be related to catastrophic cognitions which in turn may be related to the "meaning" individuals attribute to their pain as reflected in their attitudes and beliefs about pain (Moseley 2004).

Interpretation of pain as being indicative of more damage appears to be at the core of many chronic pain patients' beliefs with general acceptance that perspectives such as this are positively associated with increased avoidance and greater disability (Phillips 1987, Vlaeyen et al 1995, Waddell 1998, Vlaeyen & Linton 2000). The meaning patients ascribe to their pain (e.g. pain equals damage) is believed to be strengthened by their subsequent avoidance behaviours. When activities are attempted they are commonly overdone, further reinforcing the association of activity with aggravation of symptoms. Combined with this, complete avoidance of activities, or failure to attempt them in reduced, less aggravating dosages, results in patients' beliefs never being disconfirmed (Sharp 2001). Patients' self-efficacy or perception and general confidence of their ability to cope with their circumstances and make a change is considered significant to the success of treatment with those patients showing low self-efficacy tending toward beliefs that their own efforts will not be successful and hence are less likely to use constructive coping strategies (Williams & Keefe 1991, Turk & Rudy 1992, Pincus et al 2002, Strong & Unruh 2002, Pincus 2004).

A clear trend in physiotherapy practice directed toward health promotion, minimisation of chronicity and management of chronicity is education aimed to address patients' health behaviours, thoughts and feelings judged either to put them at risk of progressing from an acute to a chronic condition or as contributing to the maintenance of their chronicity (e.g. Spanswick & Parker 2000, Main & Watson 2002, Muncey 2002, Unruh & Harman 2002, Butler & Mosley 2003,). In a systematic review investigating the prognostic strength of psychosocial factors influencing chronicity, Linton (2000, p1153) concluded that "psychosocial variables are clearly linked to the transition from acute to chronic pain disability", and that "psychosocial factors may be used as predictors of the risk of developing long-term pain and disability." Unfortunately the methodological quality of the research into psychosocial risk factors for chronicity varies considerably (Linton 2000, Pengel et al 2003) and is mostly limited to the quantitative paradigm where patients' perspectives (e.g. beliefs, thoughts, feelings) regarding their pain experience is arguably only superficially assessed (Hunt 1997, Dijkers 1999, Buetow & Kenealy 2000, Mallinson 2002). Nevertheless there is growing acceptance that patients' thoughts, feelings and health behaviours can functionally become maladaptive in that they become barriers to their recovery.

Cognitive-behavioural Approach:

The cognitive-behavioural approach situated in the biopsychosocial model is increasingly put forward as the preferred approach for the management of chronic pain and disability (e.g. Morley et al 1999, Strong & Unruh 2002). The evolution of this approach is described elsewhere (Gamsa 1994, 1994a) but in general it is based on the theory that patients' thoughts, feelings and behaviours are inter-related in their pain experience. Based on individual patient assessment cognitive-behavioural management then draws on a combination of explanation/education directed at facilitating restructuring of unhelpful or maladaptive thoughts and associated feelings, and operant behavioural techniques to strengthen patients' constructive thoughts, self-efficacy and active coping behaviours while discouraging the reverse. Some of the management strategies commonly recommended in the cognitive-behavioural management of chronic pain include the following:

- Explanation/education (based on thorough biopsychosocial assessment) directed toward assisting patients to understand their condition and management recommended.
- Specific strategies to help patients recognise their own cognition (thoughts, beliefs, fears, etc.) and unpleasant emotions along with any antecedents (i.e. cues) to unhelpful thoughts, self-statements, coping behaviours, emotions, with the aim of addressing/ challenging these through provision of alternatives in order to facilitate patients' recognition, understanding and control.

275

- Collaborative specific goal-setting toward meaningful achievements (see chapters 2 and 13 this volume].
- Instruction in specific coping strategies (e.g. pacing, graded exposure, relaxation, set-back and flare-up planning, etc.).
- Pacing of aggravating activities (in place of common overactivity/ underactivity cycle many patients experience) by making them time or quota-dependent instead of symptom-dependent.
- Graded exposure of feared stimulus (e.g. activity, situation, environment, etc.) with the intent of systematically desensitising the learned fear.
- Selective reinforcement (i.e. operant learning), generally in the form of encouragement/praise but also via self-reinforcement, of desired health behaviours, coping behaviours, self-statements.
- Selective in-attention (based on behavioural technique of extinguishing unwanted behaviour) to unhelpful pain/coping behaviours, self-statements (e.g. catastrophising).

Barriers to Adopting a Biopsychosocial Approach

There is also now very helpful physiotherapy literature providing suggestions on assessment and management strategies specifically targeting patients' unhelpful thoughts, feelings and behaviours (e.g. Harding & Williams 1995, Wittink et al 1997, Harding 1998, 1998a, Kendall & Watson 2000, Main & Watson 2002, Muncey 2002, Strong & Unruh 2002). However, it is our experience that many therapists have yet to take up these strategies in practice, likely due to a variety of factors. Some therapists' personal and professional perspectives of health, pain and disability are clearly more biomedically, as opposed to biopsychosocially based, leading to either a lack of attention to these dimensions of patients' presentations (e.g. view that 'psychological' aspects of patients' problems are separate from physical and it is not the physiotherapist's role to manage 'psychological' issues) or to an overly superficial, and hence less effective, assessment, reasoning and management of psychosocial barriers. This may also be associated with a view that psychosocial factors only become relevant when working with patients in chronic pain and disability and hence are not relevant to the more acute patient presentations. While physiotherapists may claim to be biopsychosocially oriented in their assessment, reasoning and management, on closer inspection this may prove to be mere lip service where their conception of "biopsychosocial" remains dualistic with the patient's presentation viewed as a combination of biomedical and psychosocial problems rather than seeing biopsychosocial as a genuine integration of mind and body where each influences the other (Engel 1978, Leventhal 1993, Duncan 2000, Borrell-Carrió 2004, Pincus 2004,), or where appreciation and focus is given to psychological factors without appropriate recognition and attention to the social circumstances that have contributed to shaping those cognitions and remain as barriers to change (Osborn & Smith 1998, Sim & Smith 2004).

The intent of the biopsychosocial model as it was originally proposed (Engel 1977) was:

"...to provide a framework within which can be conceptualized and related as natural systems all the levels of organization pertinent to health and disease, from subatomic particles through molecules, cells, tissues, organs, organ systems, the person, the family, the community, the culture, and ultimately the biosphere."

"Predicated on the systems approach, the biopsychosocial model dispenses with the scientifically archaic principles of dualism and reductionism and replaces the simple cause-and-effect explanations of linear causality with reciprocal causal models." (Engel 1978, p175)

We need therefore, as physiotherapy clinicians, to consider our patients carefully within each component and also in the interaction between each of the components in the biopsychosocial model. Additional factors that may contribute to whether therapists genuinely practice within a biopsychosocial framework and take up cognitive-behavioural strategy suggestions now available in the literature include:

- Lack of cognitive-behavioural education. While traditional physiotherapy education provides good grounding in biomedically based assessment, reasoning and management of physical impairment, explicit instruction in pain science and biopsychosocially related assessment, reasoning and management is less common and less developed;
- Lack of experience and hence confidence in assessing and making judgements regarding patients' thoughts, feelings and pain behaviours;
- Lack of experience in implementing, monitoring and progressing cognitive-behavioural strategies;
- Lack of a reasoning framework within which to place this dimension of their thinking and practice.

The superficial way in which cognitive-behavioural assessment and management is interpreted and practiced by some therapists may also relate to a tendency for it to be used 'on', as opposed to 'with', a patient, possibly in a manner similar to how some therapists approach their assessment and management of physical impairment. That is, if a therapist is already biomedically biased and uses a therapist-centred (as opposed to patient-centred, Ersser & Atkins 2000) approach, where the patient is an inactive object of assessment, and diagnostic and management decisions are made by the therapist with the patient being a passive recipient of advice and therapeutic procedures, it is likely that any attempt by such therapist to integrate cognitive-behavioural assessment and management will be done superficially in the same mechanistic way. In fact, in a critical review of cognitive-behavioural theory and practice, Sharp (2001a) argues that the cognitive dimension of cognitive-behavioural therapy for chronic pain reported in the literature is inadequate and that behavioural management inappropriately dominates the cognitive-behavioural interventions.

Sharp (2001a) also cites Turk's (1996) concerns regarding the 'pain behaviour' construct noting pain behaviours are commonly assumed to be maladaptive when in reality any judgement regarding pain behaviours requires interpretation to establish their 'raison d'être'. This would not be disputed by those explaining the use of cognitive-behavioural therapy in the management of chronic pain but clearly there is a risk for such superficial and potentially unethical judgements to be made if the behavioural component outweighs the cognitive. It is not uncommon to find recommendations for operant behavioural management strategies to selectively ignore maladaptive coping behaviours and self-statements while reinforcing patients' adaptive responses without explanation as to how judgements regarding adaptive versus maladaptive should be made. It is as though there is an assumption that maladaptive thoughts, statements and behaviours can be defined out of context and some sort of universal truth exists that defines for everyone what is normal versus abnormal. For example, praying is classically given as an example of a passive coping behaviour that should be challenged and ideally replaced with something more active. However, judgements such as this simply cannot be made out of context. While praying for one person may well be a passive coping behaviour linked to their excessively negative perspective, for another praying functions as an active coping mechanism with links to positive thoughts providing for them a source of strength and conviction to fight on. We certainly take issue with the positivist position that judgements about normality regarding superficial assessments of patients' beliefs, emotions and behaviours can be made without deeper understanding of the person (including personal perceptions and social influences) and the basis for their perspectives. Kleinman et al (1992) highlight the challenge this creates to the epistemological premise that underpins traditional biomedical theory and research '...namely that there is objective knowledge, knowledge apart from subjective experience.' (page 6). While it may not be the intent of those promoting cognitive-behavioural therapy it is very common to see these sorts of superficial judgements being made in practice.

Need for Physiotherapy Curriculum to Embrace the Biopsychosocial Model

Clearly there is a need for Physiotherapy schools not already doing so to provide explicit instruction and opportunity for students to practice assessment, reasoning and management of psychosocial factors. Importantly, this must occur in a manner that discourages dualistic separation of mind and body as can easily be inadvertently communicated to students when theory and practice directed to physical impairment is not clearly linked to theory and practice of psychosocial impairment. For example, it has been our experience that guest lecturers providing separate theory related to chronic pain and cognitive-behavioural assessment and management is ineffective on its own in promoting students' holistic understanding of mind-body relationships. Not surprisingly, presentation of theory alone also is ineffective in promoting application of theory in practice. Students need to be given practical supervised experience in applying this theory to practice, something all school and program coordinators will recognise as challenging as its success is directly related to the knowledge and experience of the clinical supervisors charged with facilitating application of this knowledge and skill in practice. Elsewhere we have suggested that presentation of contemporary models of health and disability, such as the latest World Health Organisation model (WHO 2001), the 'Mature Organism' model (Gifford 1998) and the Main et al (2000) disability model, is one strategy to facilitate a more holistic understanding of health and disability that recognises integration of physical, environmental and psychological factors in all patients' health and disability (Jones et al 2002). This, combined with dedicated instruction in pain science, biopsychosocial and cognitive-behavioural theory, mental representation and learning/cognitive restructuring theory, reinforced with supervised clinical experience seems essential if practice paradigms of future therapists are to change. As the relevance of this theory is clearly not limited to 'musculoskeletal' problems or patients with pain, it is important the models adopted and the theory presented are related to all states of health (e.g. 'musculoskeletal', 'neurological' and 'cardiorespiratory' problems from paediatrics to old age) and integrated across the entire physiotherapy curriculum. For this, the World Health Organisation model provides an excellent introductory model, as it is appropriately generic to all states of health. Essentially what is needed is a deeper understanding of the person behind the problem, including the basis for any beliefs, self-statements and coping behaviours initially identified. We recognise this is precisely what is suggested by previous authors discussing application of cognitive-behavioural therapy in physiotherapy management of chronic pain but as this does not always occur we would like to suggest additional measures to link with the traditional descriptions of cognitive-behavioural therapy that may assist in promoting this fuller, more critical understanding and more holistic approach.

279

Dimensions of the Pain Experience

In discussing the multidimensional construct pain Sim and Smith (2004) present the following diagram (Figure 1) to depict the various dimensions of the pain experience.

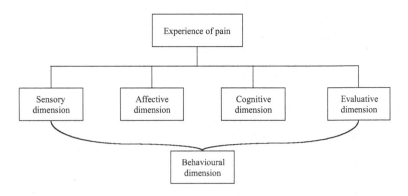

Figure 1.   The dimensions of the pain experience.
From Physiotherapy a psychosocial approach, French S and Sim J (eds.), Sim J and Smith MV, The Sociology of Pain, p 119, Copyright (2004), Reprinted with permission from Elsevier.

While the sensory, affective, cognitive and behavioural dimensions of pain are well described in contemporary pain literature, it is our view that the evaluative dimension Sim and Smith (2004) describe is typically subsumed within the cognitive dimension and as such may not be adequately attended to by practicing therapists. Sim and Smith (2004) make the distinction that the cognitive dimension relates to patients' more generic pain (or health) beliefs while the evaluative dimension relates to the way in which pain is experienced and interpreted in the context of the individual's specific circumstances. This account of patients' evaluative dimension of pain is consistent with the phenomenological perspective that considers patients' physical presentations, cognitions, emotions and behaviours relating to pain and disability can only be understood, and hence evaluated, with respect to their particular pain/disability experiences (e.g. Steen & Haugli 2000). We readily acknowledge this evaluative dimension is well recognised and discussed under the heading of cognitive factors (e.g. Main & Booker 2000) but believe that signposting the importance of considering health and pain beliefs from the perspective of patients' specific circumstances (e.g. what they think and why) as this theoretical division of cognitive and evaluative encourages, may assist in better communicating the importance of this depth of understanding of patients' perspectives to practice. As Duncan (2000) highlights, understanding chronic pain necessitates understanding the familial, cultural and socio-political circumstances of the person in pain. This enlarged understanding, both deeper and broader, that considers biomedical, psychological and sociological perspectives, should enable therapists and patients to identify factors that may be contributing to their pain or disability experience while also influencing their ability to participate in therapeutic efforts directed toward restructuring of unhelpful thoughts and feelings and reactivation in life activities.

Schema Enmeshment Model of Pain

Another construct we find promising for encouraging therapists to seek a fuller understanding of patients' pain experiences so that patients' thoughts are not oversimplified as simply internal behaviours that can be managed through operant behavioural strategies is the notion of pain, illness and self schema and how they are influenced by a person's pain/disability experience. Pincus and Morley (2001) review the literature on selective information processing bias in chronic pain patients, and based on conflicting research findings related to attention, interpretation and memory bias, propose a 'schema enmeshment' model of pain. Of particular interest to us is their conceptualisation of the schemas people construct related to pain, illness and the self which we believe may assist therapists' understanding of the depth of influence pain can have, the role of learning in pain experiences and schema shifts and the importance of assisting patients to explore their own, often unconscious schemas or perspectives in order to successfully promote transformation to more constructive ones.

The experience of pain is integrally associated with personal perceptions and social influences such that patients' pain perceptions, experiences and coping combine into a pain experience lived as a whole (Kleinman et al 1992, Sim & Smith 2004). As such the various elements can never truly be isolated. However, greater understanding of the components of the pain experience and their interrelationships provides further insight into the depth that management strategies, such as the cognitive restructuring element of cognitive-behavioural therapy, need to be applied. Research in medical anthropology, medical sociology and cognitive psychology has all contributed to the understanding of illness representations or schemas (Bishop 1991, Skelton & Croyle 1991, Turk & Rudy 1992, Pincus & Morley 2001, Sim & Smith 2004). In what has been described as a 'groundbreaking article' (Skelton & Croyle 1991, pg 2), Leventhal et al (1980) put forward the notion that patients' mental representations of health threats determine how they respond to those threats. Illness schemata are defined as individuals' 'implicit theories of illness' that they use in order to interpret and respond to health threats. These illness (or pain) representations are like imprints, or patterns of interconnected features, learned through social and personal experiences. Skelton and Croyle (1991, pg 4) report on illness cognition research supporting lay illness schema being comprised of the following elements:

1. concrete *symptoms* and a *label* (e.g. a common cold vs. pneumonia) that facilitate identification of the health problem, beliefs about
2. the immediate and long-term *consequences* of the problem and
3. its *temporal course*, and attributions concerning
4. the *cause* of the problem and
5. the means by which a *cure* may be affected.

In addition, research has also identified a number of dimensions that people use in evaluating these elements including such things as seriousness, social desirability, personal responsibility, controllability and changeability (Bishop 1991). Therefore it is not only the person's existing beliefs and assumptions that make up their mental representation and contribute to determining their coping but also their appraisal of the threat their problem/pain or the situation poses. Salkovskis' (1996) illustration of the factors that make up this internal 'threat analysis', discussed in the context of anxiety, offers further insight into some of the issues that may similarly contribute to patients' interpretation of threat with respect to pain (Figure 2).

$$\text{Anxiety} = \frac{\text{Perceived probability of threat x Perceived cost/Awfulness of danger}}{\text{Perceived ability to cope with danger + Perceived "rescue factors"}}$$

Figure 2: Factors that comprise the cognitive component of anxiety (Salkovskis 1996 p 51).

Schema evolve over time and the repeated simultaneous activation of aspects from different schema is thought to be a mechanism of learning that results in a blurring of representations such that elements from one schema become incorporated in another. This 'enmeshment' of schema is believed to be one explanation for why events leading to activation of one schema with relatively benign consequences can develop into a schema eliciting more significant effects (Pincus & Morley 2001). Recognising overlap exists, Pincus and Morley (2001) portray the pain schema as being comprised of the immediate sensory-intensity, spatial and temporal features of pain along with the initial affective responses and self-protective behaviours that ensue. Illness schema include the elements identified by Skelton and Croyle (1991) above along with further evaluative dimensions relating to disability, quality of life and emotional expectations. Self schema is a complex multifaceted construct that relates to who you are with reference to who you used to be (prior to your perceived change in self) and who you would like to be in the future. It includes an evaluative dimension that contributes to an individual's sense of self-worth. Pain has the ability to disrupt aspects of the self such that repeated failures to function 'normally' and the negative emotions that result, can lead to changes in a person's self-image (Steen & Haugli 2000).

Pincus and Morley (2001) put forward examples of possible interrelationships that can exist between a person's pain, illness and self schemas (Figure 3). Figure 3A is used to portray the relationship in a healthy person where there is only partial overlap. The extent of overlap in acute pain is reported to depend on the context and the authors provide the example of pain occurring with needle puncture during blood donation having no significance to general physical well-being and little relevance to the sense of self other than perhaps strengthening the person's sense of altruism. In contrast, the same needle puncture pain occurring with a blood test for a potentially fatal disease would clearly activate both pain and illness schemas but also contemplation of the self and what the future may hold. Figure 3B is suggested as an enmeshment that might be found with a chronic pain patient who is adaptively coping with their condition and their 'self' is largely unchanged and their self-worth retained. Figure 3C portrays a situation where the pain and self schemas are enmeshed without change to the illness schema. Here they offer the example of the athlete whose pain following a traumatic injury has impacted on their self-identity but without any significant activation of illness scenarios. Lastly, in Figure 3D all three schemas are enmeshed as might occur in the chronic pain patient who is not coping and where the threats associated with their pain/illness experience have led to serious changes in their concept of who they are and their self-worth.

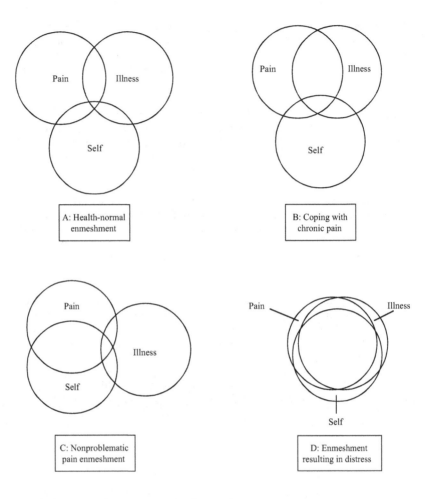

Figure 3:   Variations in the overlap of pain, illness, and self-schemas. From, Psychological Bulletin, Vol 127(5), Pincus T and Morley S, Cognitive-processing bias in chronic pain: a review and integration, p 608, Copyright © 2001 by the American Psychological Association. Reprinted with permission.

Continuums of Stress and Distress

Pincus and Morley (2001) go on to discuss the continuum from affective distress to depression and their theory that these states, characterised by cognitive processing biases ranging from a focus on negative aspects of health, in the case of the distressed chronic pain patient, to a focus on negative aspects of the self (manifest as low self-worth), in the case of clinical depression. Pincus (2004) expands on this with the notion of two continuums, one for stress and another for distress. At the lowest levels of the stress continuum are people manifesting with selective attention to sensory information and fear-avoidance of movement perceived as dangerous and likely to increase their pain and injury. Many of these will either adjust to this themselves over time or respond well to education, behavioural interventions and gradual exposure to activity (i.e. to desensitise their fear). Further along the stress continuum the fear of pain is generalised to health and the person begins to manifest symptoms of stress including catastrophising cognitions, somatisation and some physical symptoms of stress such as panic attacks, dizziness and shortness of breath. Pain is no longer simply perceived as likely to cause further injury, instead pain perception is generalised as a broader threat to overall health and well-being. Attention bias at this end of the continuum is now towards health-related information and this is where Pincus (2004) suggest more extensive cognitive-behavioural interventions are recommended.

The distress continuum ranges from loss and frustration associated with restrictions in "participation" due to pain, made worse when the pain cannot be explained, and responsive to education, social support and maintenance of activity, to higher levels of distress where the person's representation of pain and illness becomes integrated with their self-schema. Here past concepts of the self are compared with future predictions of the self leading to greater distress, loss and emotions of helplessness and hopelessness. Cognitive-behavioural management is recommended to encourage increase in activities not associated with pain in order to "restructure" the self-schema. Pincus (2004) puts depression at the highest level of the distress continuum where feelings of hopelessness and helplessness are further generalised and intermixed with other emotions such as guilt and despair. Acceptance and management of normal life in the presence of pain and/or disability is put forward as the key to reducing distress.

We present this schema and stress/distress continuum theory supported by cognitive biasing research, not to suggest new discrete psychological categorisations are needed. Rather, we put this literature and these concepts forward as we feel they assist in highlighting the range of pain, illness, self, and likely other (e.g. see Schwoebel et al 2001 on "pain and the body schema") potential influences of pain, disability and associated social consequences that patients may present. Patients are clearly not homogenous in their psychosocial presentations. We feel this literature may facilitate this recognition and as such should discourage therapists from making superficial judgments about patients' cognitions, emotions and pain behaviours.

Salkovskis (1996) discusses the excessively negative interpretations of stimuli, events, or situations with respect to maintaining negative thinking and anxiety proposing three principal factors contribute to perpetuating threat cognitions, selective attention, physiological change and changes in behaviour (Figure 4).

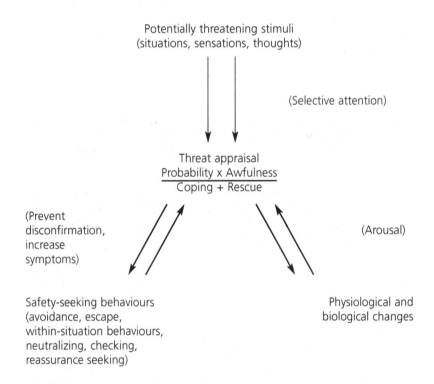

Figure 4: Factors contributing to the maintenance of threat cognitions. From Frontiers of Cognitive Therapy, Salkovskis P (ed.), The cognitive approach to anxiety: threat beliefs, safety-seeking behaviour, and the special case of health anxiety and obsessions, p 53, Copyright (1996), reprinted with permission from The Guilford Press.

Of particular interest to us in this discussion is the avoidance, or safety-seeking behaviours that are now a well recognised feature of chronic pain. One effect of avoidance responses, which Salkovskis (1996) emphasises is a normal, not a pathological, response (the perception of danger being the problem or misinterpretation), is that they can prevent the person from discovering or learning that their fears are not substantiated. While graded exposure is a valid strategy to enable the person to experience success, Salkovskis (1996) stresses the importance of combining this with challenges to the patient's negative appraisal. Support for this in the context of chronic low back pain is evident in research where experimentally modifying chronic low back pack pain patients' pain cognitions has been shown to produce significant change in traditional measures of physical impairment (i.e. forward bending, straight leg raise, Moseley 2004), (EMG Flexion Relaxation Response, Watson et al 1997) and where exposure in vivo, producing disconfirmations of expected consequences of physical activity, has been shown to decrease pain-related fear, pain catastrophizing, pain disability and pain vigilance while increasing physical activity levels (Vlaeyen et al 2002).

Evidence of the Chronic Pain Experience

A large body of literature exists relating to the pain experience and pain, illness and self-representations or schema in patients with chronic illness and pain (e.g. Skelton & Croyle 1991, Good et al 1992, Pincus & Morley 2001, Sim & Smith 2004). We encourage readers to follow these lines of research which hold promise for improving our understanding of how patients' cognitions can be restructured through their pain experiences and consequently the extent of enquiry needed to truly understand patients' pain experiences and associated cognitions.

For example, in a qualitative study investigating the personal experience and psychological processes involved in maintaining pain, distress and disability in subjects presenting with benign chronic low back pain, Osborn and Smith (1998) used an interpretative phenomenological analysis to identify four themes common to the participants: 1) searching for an explanation; 2) comparing this self with other selves; 3) not being believed; and 4) withdrawing from others. The notion that patients will search for an explanation for their symptoms is consistent with schema theory discussed above and the frustrations regarding inadequate explanation from the medical system these subjects reported is well recognised as an iatrogenic contributing factor to maintained disability (e.g. Main et al 2000, Main & Watson 2002). Evidence for influence to a person's self-image or schema is also available in the second theme as participants were consistently found to compare themselves to others and to their memory of their past selves while also projecting who they were likely to be in the future (Osborn & Smith 1998, p72):

"Through their selective use of social and personal comparison participants highlighted the impact of their pain on their self-regard and the equivocal nature of their attempts to cope with its imposition. Pain denied them the chance to be who they once were and preferred still to be. Their contemporary self-regard contrasted with a nostalgic recall of their past and those around them, and their comparisons served almost inevitably as an index of their sense of threat and loss. Attempts to buttress self-esteem by comparison with those more unfortunate often proved counterproductive and served only to remind participants of their own gloomy prognosis."

The impact of chronic pain and disability on a person's concept of 'self' is also recognised by other authors. Pincus (2004, p107) describes suffering and distress as common features of the chronic pain experience when pain has had a significant impact on the person's life and suggests the main features of this sort of suffering are "...a sense of hopelessness, helplessness, lack of control and direct threat to integrity of the self." Sim and Smith (2004) note that this loss of a former self is a common finding in people suffering with chronic disability and pain and describe the circumstances that leave these people with a fundamental choice of trying to maintain their former self in spite of the pain; to suspend the former self in the hope that it can be regained once the pain is gone; or to come to terms with a new painful self.

The third theme identified by Osborn and Smith (1998) of not being believed created for them a continual need to justify their pain and the incongruity of being mobile or appearing healthy created a sense that they should appear ill in order to conform to the expectations of others. The participants' tendency to withdraw from others was the final theme. The researchers' related this to participants' fear of misunderstanding and rejection highlighting the various and complex forms in which fear-avoidance may take (Phillips 1987). In other words, fear-avoidance may have a social basis and not just a biomedical one.

We draw attention to the findings from this study, consistent with other research and social theory relating to pain (e.g. Borkan et al 1995, Sim & Smith 2004) because we feel they support the importance of acquiring a more critical understanding of patients' pain experiences that should include their illness and 'self' perspectives or schema. Superficial snapshots of patients' cognitions and perceptions gleaned through questionnaires alone or from patient statements made in an initial assessment, clearly are insufficient to understand their pain, illness and self cognitions or schemas. While many physiotherapists may not have the time or skills to assess patient cognitions to this extent in current paradigms of physiotherapy practice, we believe a greater appreciation of the complexity of patients' cognitions will discourage superficial cognitive assessment and management and strengthen the case for this material to make its way into basic physiotherapy education. While physiotherapy paradigms of practice may never fully embrace this domain of understanding and practice as being their responsibility, appreciating these cognitive interactions seems important if therapists are going to provide their physical management and education, with at the very least, care for how their interventions may impact on the various dimensions of patients' cognitions and associated schema.

Application of the biopsychosocial model to clinical practice is facilitated through understanding contemporary models of health and disability and through understanding and skilfully directing the focus of your thinking, or clinical reasoning, to the biomedical, psychological and sociological dimensions of patients' problems (Jones et al 2002).

The Evolution of Clinical Reasoning Theory and Understanding in Physiotherapy

The initial formulation of clinical reasoning in physiotherapy was diagnostically focussed and likened the clinical reasoning process of physiotherapy clinicians to that of physicians (Payton 1985, Thomas-Edding 1987). In this understanding hypotheses related to diagnostic features concerning a case would be first generated and then tested (generally in an empirical manner) until they were either negated or confirmed leaving a best or strongest hypothesis (Elstein et al 1978). The notion that hypotheses could be formulated in a number of different aspects of clinical practice and not just diagnosis was put forward by Jones (1992) with his framework of hypothesis categories. These have continued to evolve and now incorporate elements of the current World Health Organisation's (2001) International Classification of Functioning, Disability and Health with concepts such as activity and participation restrictions and capabilities (Jones & Rivett 2004). A further change in emphasis in the understanding of clinical reasoning in physiotherapy concerned its interactive and collaborative elements as expressed in Figure 5 (Edwards & Jones 1995).

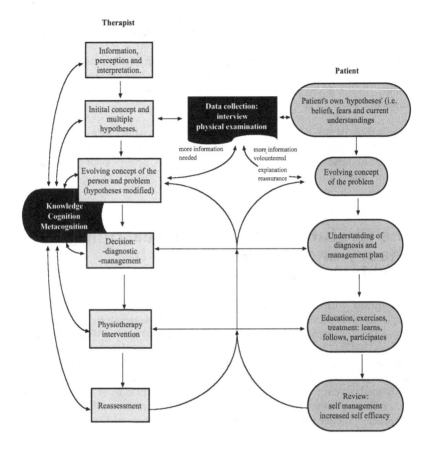

Figure 5:   Collaborative decision making (Edwards & Jones 1995)

In this model the notion of parallel processes of reasoning between therapist and patient were introduced. The model illustrated an understanding of reasoning where the therapist reasoned using a hypothesis oriented process towards diagnostic and management decisions. At the same time the therapist was attentive to the patient's thoughts and interpretations regarding his or her understanding of diagnosis and management decisions. More recently a model of clinical reasoning known as 'Dialectical reasoning' (Edwards et al 2004) proposes that therapists' reasoning occurs through various particular strategies and within different paradigms. A dialectic in this context is a debate intended to reconcile a contradiction (in this case between fundamentally different processes or paradigms of reasoning) without attempting to establish either view as intrinsically truer than the other. Such paradigms are discussed further in Edwards et al

(2004a) and can be considered analogous to the different assumptions underlying different research paradigms. Clinical reasoning strategies encompass a range of diverse reasoning and foci of action in clinical practice (see Table 1). These are considered under the headings of 'diagnosis' and 'management' where 'diagnosis' is broadly defined as an inquiry that incorporates the different reasoning paradigms represented by hypothetico-deductive and narrative reasoning. Hypothetico-deductive reasoning uses a scientific or experimental research method where hypotheses are generated and then tested in an empirical manner in relation to diagnosis (and management procedures). In this method findings are held to be objective and empirically 'testable' and thus hold true for larger populations under specified conditions. In contrast narrative reasoning is based on similar assumptions to a qualitative research method where there is broad agreement that knowledge is constructed and that truth and meaning are contextually bound. The particular perspective and experience of a patient expressed in a narrative or story like manner is, therefore, valued as being true for this person at this time and not necessarily generalizable to others. Narrative reasoning sets out to understand the particularity of such a perspective and experience (White & Epston 1990, O'Dowd 2000, Edwards et al 2004a).

- **Diagnostic reasoning:** the formation of a diagnosis related to physical disability and impairment with consideration of associated pain mechanisms, tissue pathology and the broad scope of potential contributing factors.
- **Narrative reasoning:** the comprehension and understanding of patients' illness experiences, 'stories', contexts, beliefs and cultures.
- **Procedural reasoning:** the determination and implementation of treatment procedures.
- **Interactive reasoning:** the purposeful establishment and ongoing management of therapist-patient rapport.
- **Collaborative reasoning:** the nurturing of a consensual approach towards the interpretation of examination findings, the setting of goals and priorities and the implementation and progression of treatment.
- **Reasoning about teaching:** the activity of individualized and context sensitive teaching.
- **Predictive reasoning:** the active envisioning of future scenarios with patients including the exploration of their choices and the implications of those choices.
- **Ethical reasoning:** the apprehension of ethical and practical dilemmas that impinge on both the conduct of treatment and its desired goals, and the resultant action towards their resolution.

Table 1. Clinical Reasoning Strategies (Edwards 2000)

Under management are listed the reasoning strategies of procedure, interaction, collaboration, teaching, prediction and ethics. Edwards et al (2004) argue that clinical reasoning occurs as an interplay of reasoning paradigms (represented by hypothetico-deductive and narrative reasoning) within each of the identified reasoning strategies. Furthermore these reasoning paradigms both make use of and result in different learning processes, for both therapist and patient. These are *instrumental learning* – learning to control and manipulate the environment or other people, as in task oriented problem solving (hypothetico-deductive manner) to improve performance – and *communicative learning* – learning (in a narrative manner) what others mean when they communicate with you, a deeper form of learning which often involves feelings, intentions, values, and moral issues (Mezirow 2000 p8). When used effectively together these two learning processes lead to a *transformatory* learning which is based on an ability to examine existing understandings and beliefs, how they have been formed and whether they continue to be adequate and reliable for a new or current situation (Mezirow 2000).

The Relationship between Reasoning and Learning

In this discussion of clinical reasoning we argue that processes of reasoning and learning cannot be separated either in life or in clinical practice. We reason and make decisions based on our existing knowledge frameworks or, in other words, on what we already know. Similarly, we either generate new understandings (i.e. knowledge) or confirm existing understandings via the integrity of our reasoning processes. And this is a strong reason for considering the integrity of our clinical reasoning in practice so that we learn well from our decision making in diverse areas of practice whether it be diagnosis making, management issues or even the ethical conduct of practice.

Figure 5, cited earlier, (Edwards & Jones 1995), illustrates how there are essentially two sets of reasoning processes in any given physiotherapy clinical encounter: the therapist's and the patient's. It is the physiotherapist's responsibility to seek to achieve some kind of coherence between these two processes, initially at least, with the aim of formulating a 'diagnosis', as used in the wider sense of the term described above. However, in the interests of effective management we would also propose that there needs to be more than just this coherence of reasoning between therapist and patient. That is, there has to be more than just an accurate communication of what each other is thinking even though this is an indispensable first step. We also propose that a subsequent transference of knowledge and learning take place between the two parties in a range of decision making areas and that this need not always or necessarily be a one way transference in the direction of therapist to patient (Edwards et al 2004a). Just as Evidence based practice requires physiotherapists to challenge the assumptions underlying particular management choices or strategies, so too, particular patients and their situations may challenge a therapist to re-examine the assumptions underlying their decision making in a range of areas from treatment selection to ethical decision making. We also believe, consistent with cognitive restructuring principles of cognitive-behavioural therapy, that therapists can play a vital role in assisting patients to understand and challenge the assumptions underlying their own reasoning with its implications for subsequent decisions and/or actions regarding their health. As stated earlier such decision-making may have significant effects on the course and nature of patients' pain experience, their physical impairments and on their daily participation in physical and social activities (e.g. Borkan et al 1991, Duke et al 2002, Moseley 2003).

Clinical reasoning is therefore not only concerned with how physiotherapy clinicians interpret a broad range of data in the conduct of practice and then learn from their reasoning, through the 'outcomes' or consequences of their decision making. Clinical reasoning is also concerned with fostering a process of adult learning with patients that involves both *instrumental* and *communicative* forms of learning. Unhelpful schema enmeshment is proposed to be a product of learning related to patients' pain and disability experiences (Pincus & Morley 2001) and we suggest narrative reasoning leading to communicative management and learning is the logical approach by which patients' may successfully alter unhelpful cognitions or schemas. Framing therapy in adult learning terms, therefore, involves another kind of skill building with patients than just teaching exercise or behavioural strategies. It involves patients learning how to critically reflect on their situations. In this sense 'critical' does not mean reflecting more profoundly but reflecting with a critical examination of the assumptions underlying a presently held set of values and conclusions (Brookfield 2000).

Such a concept of clinical reasoning (including its emphasis on the learning which takes place in clinical practice on the part of both therapists and patients) requires particular communication skills. If we consider the nature of communication within a reasoning and learning context we need to ask the following questions:

- What are the conditions under which true communication can occur?
- How can we assess for the presence, distortion or absence of such conditions and the resultant effects on our communication with (and the learning ability of) patients?
- How can we assist patients to adopt new perspectives or interpretations of previous or present experiences / frames of reference towards Transformatory learning?

In our experience physiotherapists are generally good communicators and recognise the importance of patient therapist communication. However, this does not mean that they would not benefit from reviewing their understanding of the dynamics of communication. The importance of communication in clinical or professional practice, although anecdotally valued by experienced clinicians has received further corroboration as an indispensable feature of expertise (Goleman 1998, Jensen et al 1999, Resnik & Jensen 2003, Edwards et al 2004). However, our purpose here is to briefly highlight why it is important to consider the conditions under which people communicate and, therefore, learn.

A fundamental issue impacting on what Habermas (1984) terms "ideal communication" has to do with power and rank and therefore, whose 'voice' is privileged in any encounter. This differential in perspective between people of different power and rank is a common source of conflict (Mindell 1995). Such conflict may be expressed explicitly (as anger) or implicitly (as passivity). In either case they have to do with a perceived or real loss of autonomy or power (Osborne & Smith 1998, O'Dowd 2000). For example, patients' apparent passivity toward self-management or taking self-responsibility commonly will be judged as a lack of motivation or passive coping. And yet, such behaviours or attitudes may well have their seeds in the actual nature of the patient - therapist relationship and be an expression of the fundamental differences in perspective and power between the patient and therapist (Mindell 1995, O'Dowd 2000). An imbalance of power is a prime cause of chronic relationship problems and the unconscious use of power can lead to significant difficulties in the functioning of a relationship. Unconscious use of rank marginalizes the 'problem' of the other person. When the 'problem' is not part of one's experience, and when one's power and/ or rank is used unconsciously, there is no room to understand difficulties that the other person is having (Mindell 1995).

The issue of failed treatment (Main et al 2000) is perhaps the greatest source of distress in patients with chronic pain. With chronic pain patients several such failed treatments could also often be thought of as several failed patient – practitioner relationships at least in terms of communication (Turk & Okifuji 1998, O'Dowd 2000). In this light, one can view the treatment encounter as not only requiring that the patient's unhelpful beliefs and behaviours be addressed but also that fundamental problems of communication which arise as a result of the difference in perspective, rank and power between therapist and patient be considered. While we recognise the inherent nature of differences in power and perspective (between the professional health practitioner and patients), we argue that at least recognising these differences and their influences allows for these to be taken into account in order to foster a more positive process of communication.

We would propose, therefore, that early on the therapist needs to do some preparatory work before "point(ing) out to patients the likely effects of persistent negative thinking and begin(ning) to help them make some changes" (Main & Watson 2002, p180). Prior to, or at least in parallel with this we would advocate, therapists evaluating and then creating the conditions for more equal participation of the patient in therapy. Earlier we read how chronic pain sufferers experience a loss of self and identity (Osborne & Smith 1998). From a narrative perspective this may also be expressed as a loss of an authentic 'voice' and this is concurrent and consistent with the expression of "thin" and "stereotyped" kinds of patient narratives and behaviours compared to "rich" and preferred narratives and behaviours (White & Epston 1990, O'Dowd 2000). The therapist has a responsibility to help create the conditions for truer communication and, therefore, learning through assisting the patient to participate fully in the relationship between patient and therapist and also the therapy process.

Mezirow (2000 p15) cites other conditions necessary for what he terms 'reflective discourse' or the ability to exchange views in the context of communication. These include values like freedom, equality, tolerance, social justice and rationality. As health professionals we would generally take the first set of values as givens in our practices. However, O'Dowd (2000) states, and the discussion on parallel processes of reasoning between patients and therapists above also reminds us, that health practitioners and patients are likely to be thinking and acting in very different spheres. The clinical reasoning strategy of collaboration may not be as straightforward as we imagine (Edwards et al 2004a). To the general values above Mezirow (2000) adds that being hungry, homeless, desperate, threatened, sick or frightened has a significant influence on the ability to effectively participate in discourse and, therefore, the capacity to critically reflect on experiences. One could certainly add pain, and especially chronic pain, to that list.

One implication of the factors affecting communication and learning as discussed above is that physiotherapists may need to carefully assess patients' capacities to learn under a wide set of criteria. The notions of instrumental and communicative learning can be very useful here. For example, some of the excellent behavioural strategies may fall under the process of instrumental learning where patients are taught particular ways of responding and coping with pain; ways which might be useful in common with many other patients in a similar situation. The evaluation of such learning is amenable to an empirical evaluation in terms of performance or non-performance of particular tasks. On other occasions communicative learning may be primary where discerning the particular meaning which a patient attributes to their pain experience (in the wider sense) may be paramount. The communicative learning approach will emphasize the uniqueness of this particular patient's circumstances. Such an understanding may re-order entirely the order or choice of existing strategies or even obviate particular strategies in favour of others. An example of this is discussed below. This kind of learning would be evaluated in a consensual agreement of new perspectives or what White and Epston (1990) call 'preferred narratives'. We argue that both instrumental and communicative approaches to promoting learning will always be necessary.

How to frame problems for instrumental and communicative learning

What follows is an exercise that we teach to final year physiotherapy students and physiotherapists participating in clinical reasoning workshops for clinical educators. The aim of the exercise is to demonstrate that the way in which we frame a particular problem dictates the kind of reasoning or logic through which we further inquire, make decisions and then take subsequent actions concerning the problem. We should stress that this exercise is only one of many examples of patient and therapist learning in practice. They are asked to consider this common scenario:

> As part of a management strategy a patient is taught some home exercises, following discussion and with their consent. When the patient returns the following week and the physiotherapist, as part of the reassessment, asks the patient how he or she found the exercises the reply is given that he or she didn't do them or, at least, didn't carry them out to anywhere near the extent they were prescribed and taught.

The participants are asked in small groups to hypothesize some of the reasons for the patient not doing or continuing the exercises as prescribed. These are some actual responses that commonly arise:

- They were too painful
- The patient forgot – to do them or how to do them
- There was a perceived lack of time expressed by the patient
- The comment above may be an excuse because the patient didn't really want to do them
- There were too many exercises or they were wrongly prescribed and were therefore too hard and caused pain
- Or, they were correctly prescribed but the patient experienced a 'normal' increase in discomfort and was afraid
- The patient lacks motivation or is lazy
- The patient was afraid that the exercises would make their pain worse
- The patient wants a passive approach to treatment

Framing the problem for further inquiry

Although the hypotheses above are the responses of the final year students and workshop participants, it is our experience that they are not so different to the responses of many therapists. Such responses may be based on what the patient has said or they may be based on the therapist's past experiences (e.g. a kind of pattern recognition) or a mixture of the two. In any case we teach that these responses represent hypotheses requiring some kind of further inquiry. In this sense they parallel research processes: what do we know about this particular phenomenon and how can we validate it? When we talk about different research processes (e.g. quantitative and qualitative research) we are also talking about different logics or reasoning processes. If we translate these concepts to clinical practice then the terms *instrumental learning* and *communicative learning* (for both therapist and patient) become particularly useful.

As previously mentioned *Instrumental learning/ reasoning* represents a task oriented problem solving. This is the type of learning used when one wants to manipulate or control the environment or people in order to improve performance (Mezirow 2000). Like the quantitative research paradigm it is interested in cause and effect and therefore seeks to describe processes or interventions that, under specified conditions, hold true in a generalizable sense for wider situations or populations.

If we take the first hypothesis that the exercises were too painful let's begin by framing the problem instrumentally. As we do this we may also pick up some of the other points or hypotheses (e.g. the exercises were too hard or there were too many of them). In framing the problem instrumentally we are using a logic or reasoning which says that this point can be examined in an empirical manner. For example, the following situations are quite possible:

- The exercise(s) were appropriate but performed with a poor technique by the patient thus leading to not only the exercises being less effective but also causing excessive pain. In this case the validity or not of this hypothesis is empirically determined by assessing the technique and correcting it.
- The exercises were done with correct technique but the patient did too many of them leading to pain. The patient may have done too many because of an over enthusiasm on his or her part or because there were too many prescribed. In either case the number of sets or repetitions can be adjusted.
- The exercises were carried out with the patient endeavouring to follow the correct technique and number but they caused pain anyway. In this case it may be that the exercise was instructed at too advanced or difficult a level and so the attempted performance of them led to increased symptoms.

297

In each example above the therapist is able to examine and validate the underlying assumptions not only by empirically testing them but by doing so in relation to accepted standards or suggested measures. In other words, the therapist is not pulling a number 'out of the hat' in relation to choice, frequency or intensity of exercise but is basing it on either research evidence or a rule of thumb which has been determined by some forum of physiotherapists (e.g. journal, special interest group, outcome measure) and which is applied to many other patients with similar presentations.

Inquiry regarding the hypothesis "the exercises were too painful" may therefore take place through an instrumental form of learning on the part of both patient and therapist.

Communicative learning/ reasoning stands in contrast to instrumental learning in that it involves learning what others mean when they communicate with you (Mezirow 2000). As discussed above this means that such things as feelings, intentions, values and even morals may be involved. The same response by different patients regarding why they didn't do their exercises can have a different basis and be associated with quite different feelings. Instead of cause and effect we are dealing with interpretation. Since a person's interpretation is based on an incredibly diverse set of criteria such as their situation in life, their past experiences and a variety of beliefs, patient meaning or interpretation arising from this kind of learning cannot be generalized but is unique for this person at this time. If we therefore frame the statement "The exercises were too painful" in communicative reasoning and learning terms, we use an entirely different learning or reasoning process of logic. The therapist is only able to examine the assumptions underlying this statement in a narrative sense. That is, by understanding the particular 'story' and subsequent interpretations of experience by our patient. Goleman (1998) reminds us that our interpretations of another's behaviour can be fraught with unreliability. Someone yawns at a meeting when we are making a presentation. We interpret this based perhaps on our own past experience as disinterest or boredom and this quite naturally 'colours' our attitude towards that person. However, the yawn may have an entirely different basis. Perhaps the person was up most of the night nursing a sick child. Similarly, a patient may be afraid of or have a negative view of an exercise for many reasons. They may have someone in or close to the family who had a very negative or damaging experience of doctors, physiotherapists and exercises following a similar (or perceived similar) problem.

Earlier it was emphasized that instrumental and communicative learning go hand in hand. For example, a patient's ability to be taught and then perform an exercise using an effective technique, although an example of instrumental learning, is significantly influenced by their interpretation of the exercise or by the imputed meaning which they give to that exercise or similar movements. In this instance, communicative learning assumes an important role. It needs to be re-stated that unless the climate for communication has been carefully considered such interpretations may not necessarily come to light (or at least not until much later). However, it is also clear from the hypotheses above that physiotherapists also need to understand the assumptions or validity of their assumptions regarding patient behaviours. We do not deny the reality of the constructs of either laziness or being unmotivated. At some time in our lives all of us may be guilty of such behaviours. However, we agree with Steen and Haugli (2000) that often there are good and rational reasons for someone exhibiting a particular behaviour. These reasons are not necessarily generalizable from one person to another. And yet, if we use the incorrect learning or process of logic in these situations of communicative learning then we as therapists can end up having hypotheses that aren't validated. Working hypotheses such as the patient is lazy or unmotivated aren't amenable to empirical testing or instrumental learning. The only way to validate a hypothesis in a communicative learning is through consensual validation where others have communicated to you what they mean by certain language or actions. This does not mean that we accept what others say without any form of critical appraisal. It does mean that any reasoning process that has integrity would require that the therapist validate with the patient a working hypothesis that the patient is lazy or unmotivated. When we use an instrumental logic to understand patient behaviour there is the danger of labelling or 'diagnosing' the behaviour in terms of generalizable 'norms'. As a result terms such as 'lazy', 'unmotivated', 'abnormal illness behaviour', 'functional overlay', 'secondary gain', and 'malingerer' are judgements that are rarely validated. They are also judgements that severely damage the therapist – patient relationship, the climate for communication and therefore, the conditions for genuine learning on both the therapist's and patient's part.

We have said that patients like all people have reasons for what they do. These reasons may often be tacit or 'unreflected on' and so the task of 'transformatory learning' is to assist patients to examine the underlying assumptions for decisions, actions and behaviours in response to (and in possibly perpetuating) their pain, impairments and levels of participation in various situations of their lives. This examination of assumptions includes the patient assessing alternative assumptions or propositions for their particular lives and their particular situations. They may not hold true for everybody. However, it must be concluded that everyone has the right to choose to learn and transform their thinking or to not do so. In the end we are assisting the development of a learning skill and not just replacing views/ ideas or behaviours which are 'wrong' or inadequate per se. These skills are needed to resume participation (Duke et al 2002) and to resume identity in community. This also has implications for how management 'success' is judged – while the patient may still have pain and disabilities, when successful, they will acquire new or modified perspectives that assist their acceptance and coping with their new 'self'. This in turn hopefully leads to resumption of life participation.

299

So what? / Suggested narrative reasoning and communicative management strategies emerging from above theory/discussions:

What follows is a series of suggested issues to explore with the patient, centred on trying to understand patients' pain and disability experiences through narrative reasoning with the aim of encouraging a fuller understanding of patients to better inform our communicative management. While the focus of the issues suggested may not be new to those experienced in cognitive-behavioural assessment, we feel that an exploration of them with consideration of the schema enmeshment theory put forward by Pincus and Morley (2001) may assist therapists to avoid the error of over-generalizing the interpretations of patients' cognitions, emotions and behaviours. Clearly the issues need to be raised at the appropriate time with questions carefully worded and clarification of meaning as required. Often overt questions about a particular issue are not even required, as patients will commonly spontaneously volunteer valuable information reflecting their pain, self and illness schemas and how these have been affected by their unique pain or disability experiences. Central to these strategies is interpretation of patient meaning.

For the communicative learning to be adequately implemented the therapist and the patient must first unpack the patient's cognitions and feelings in order to understand their basis and the circumstances in which they occur. While this is a clear aim of cognitive-behavioural therapy, we feel the scope in which this is approached may be strengthened if therapists have a better understanding of the elements of patients' mental representations (e.g. pain, self, illness schemas discussed above) that contribute to their cognitions and feelings, and the various ways in which these schemas may or may not be affected as suggested by Pincus and Morley (2001). Pain schemas are perhaps most familiar to practicing therapists but the concept and variations (i.e. patterns) of illness and self-schemas are from our experience less familiar. Understanding these enable the therapist to listen to patients' comments with perhaps a broader perspective. Thus, trends in the things they say about their pain, their general health and other health complaints, their self with respect to how they believe others view them and how they view themselves, may all be better recognised as actual plots in the story of their pain or disability experience. In addition, this broader perspective of what underpins cognitions and feelings can assist therapists to specifically screen for clues to these different schemas while also appreciating the social circumstances that may be at work in creating or maintaining them. The narrative reasoning and communicative management we are recommending relate well to existing taxonomies of psychosocial screening put forward by others (e.g. Watson & Kendall 2000):

A – Attitudes and Beliefs about the pain

B – Behaviours

C – Economic and Compensation issues

D – Diagnosis and treatment issues

E – Emotion

F – Family

W – Work

The story of the patient's pain and disability experience and clues to how their pain, illness and self-schemas have been affected will emerge through exploration of all of these A-W issues. This focus of inquiry and thinking, referred to above as Narrative Reasoning, is different from the biomedically-based physical impairment/pathology oriented thinking, as absolute criteria for interpreting what are adaptive versus maladaptive cognitions, emotions and behaviours, do not exist. Rather, these judgements can only be made in the context of each patient's cognitions and emotions with careful consideration of their associated social circumstances. Within the exploration of the patient's understanding and/or feelings about their pain, disability, compensation situation, diagnosis, recommended treatment, family and work influences, additional issues to attend to include the following:

- **Pain and illness perceptions** – Skelton and Croyle (1991) report that lay schemas typically include the symptoms, a label of some kind, the immediate and long term consequences, the temporal course for the condition, beliefs about its cause, and means by which it will be cured. While therapists should explore all these, they should also be alert to other dimensions of the illness or pain schemas that people have been shown to use in evaluating these elements. This includes the patient's perceptions of seriousness, social desirability, personal responsibility, controllability and changeability. While picking up on the common belief that pain equals harm is important, to limit your search and understanding of a patient's schemas to this one manifestation, as sometimes occurs, is inadequate and equivalent to summarising a paraplegics disability experience with the biomedical diagnosis that they are an L1-L2 spinal cord patient. Obtaining the fuller story of their understanding, thoughts, beliefs and feelings also provides greater options when considering where communicative management may start when later challenging and assisting the patient to reflect on and confront what may be misconceptions in beliefs.

301

- **How informed is the patient about their pain/condition and the appropriate strategies for managing and coping with it?** – Uncertainty is a common experience with chronic pain and has been shown to correlate with distress, helplessness and levels of reported pain intensity (e.g. Jensen et al 1991). In the absence of clear explanations patients with chronic illness will resort to their own "common-sense" explanations (Leventhal & Diefenbach, 1991).

- **How does the patient's pain/disability effect them?** – While this will often provide useful insight into activity and participation restrictions/capabilities, interpretations from this line of questioning should also consider the patient's perception of their "self", that is who they have become with reference to who they were and how they see themselves in the future. As discussed, Pincus (2004) proposed the concept of stress and distress continuums linked to cognitive processing bias where the stress continuum ranges from over-attention of sensory information and fear-avoidance to more generalised over-attention of overall health with catastrophising cognitions and more overt symptoms of stress. The distress continuum spans from natural and still harmless feelings of frustration to higher levels of distress (e.g. depression) that affect the "self". This consideration of continuums of patients' focus of attention and negative thoughts about their health and/or their self with greater consideration of their threat appraisal and safety-seeking behaviours should encourage therapists to more critically consider where patients are along these sorts of continuums thereby minimising the error of over generalising from more superficial assessments. Better understanding of the patient's cognitions and feelings, by both therapist and patient, should in turn assist attempts to promote cognitive-restructuring or transformative learning.

- **How is the patient perceived by others and how does this effect how they feel about themself?** – Pain behaviour is often explained as a form of attention seeking. While this clearly does occur, it could be simply related to the desire (conscious or otherwise) for attention, or instead, it may relate more to society's expectation of what a person with chronic pain should behave like. If engaging in activities of daily living without overt expressions of pain and disability is perceived by others to be inconsistent and hence suggestive of symptom exaggeration it should not be surprising that some learn to display "appropriate" pain behaviours, not necessarily to seek attention, but just to avoid not being believed. Others may do just the opposite and disguise their disability and despair because they have come to learn that they are often poorly accepted by society. Making judgments about patients' pain or safety seeking behaviours can only be done through exploration of these issues.

- **How does the patient compare themself with others (explored not just with respect to what the patient can and cannot do, but also with regard to their pleasures, their self-worth, and their perception of their contributions)?** – Chronic pain patients may highlight their comparisons with others positively where self-esteem is strengthened (e.g. I could be worse off, I could be stuck in a wheelchair) or negatively where their comparison with someone worse off only serves to reinforce their own sense of despair and threat of rejection. Clearly there is no universal truth with regard to how a chronic pain person will or will not perceive themselves but exploration of this issue should assist your understanding of their self-schema.

- **Does the patient think others believe them and how do they say or imply this makes them feel?** – Commonly chronic pain patients will feel they need to justify their pain as real and not just in their head, sometimes even leading to pain behaviours expected of someone with a "real" problem (Osborne & Smith 1998). Perceptions of whether others believe them can then impact on the chronic pain sufferer's self-schema creating perceived threats of being misjudged or rejected by others (spouses, family and workmates).

- **Does the patient ever find themself avoiding activities or withdrawing from others because of their pain/disability?** – Understanding this and the reasons that underpin it seems important to inform management strategies such as graded exposure and pacing so that appropriate discussions regarding these perspectives can take place to complement and maximise these more behaviourally based techniques. It also highlights that chronic pain patients' cognitions, feelings and pain behaviours are not simply of their own doing, and hence their responsibility alone to recognise and change. There are countless examples of where society does not place equal value on those with disability (e.g. Rotholz 2002, Sim & Smith 2004). Also, many with chronic pain live in social and economic circumstances that disempower them from making changes or moving on. Successful prevention and management of chronic pain is not just about changing patient's cognitions and behaviours, but also about changing society's views, understanding and acceptance of disability (from government policy to lay understanding of health, pain and disability).

Summary

So what are the clinical implications from the key issues discussed through this chapter? Issues discussed have included: schema enmeshment and clinical reasoning and in particular here, narrative reasoning and communicative management to promote transformative learning. As discussed at the start, the physiotherapy, chronic pain and pain science literature already provide us with good theory and evidence establishing the importance of psychosocial assessment and management. Pain is now recognised as not simply a biophysical event; instead it exists in a biomedical, psychological and sociocultural context.

Despite the excellent literature that is now available, in our opinion, there continues to be a problem with some therapists grouping all chronic pain patients with apparent psychosocial contributing factors into a single homogenous group as though their cognitions, feelings and behaviours all have a similar basis that will be responsive to some generic application of cognitive-behavioural principles. When this occurs the obvious risk is that management becomes a recipe like protocol with cognitive-behavioural strategies being employed superficially, instead of with the patient and tailored to their individual cognitive, affective and behavioural presentation. Surely this is no less an error than uncritically finding a painful low back joint and simply mobilising it because it reproduces the patient's pain?

Schema and health representation theory provide some insight into how people structure their understanding of health, disability and pain. The importance of the meaning patients attribute to their problems, in terms of their health related behaviours (constructive and non-constructive), emotions, coping and views of the future, is well-recognised in the chronic pain literature. People do not simply react to stimuli (pain sensations, physical impairments, disabilities or social interactions) with a straightforward, 'behavioural', hard wired response. The constructivist philosophy of learning and knowledge acquisition maintains that people make sense of life (in this case their problem, their pain, their medical and social interactions) by constructing meaning of their experience. Schema and representation theory holds that this occurs through a process of relating (consciously and unconsciously) their interpretation of events to pre-existing schemata that have been culturally and socially acquired through past experiences (personal or observed). Responses (thoughts, emotions, behaviours) to stimuli can then be seen as elements of coping based on the person's evaluation or appraisal as shaped by the enmeshment of their pain, illness, self and possibly other schema. Learning theory similarly accounts for how people change (e.g. acquire new knowledge, alter points of view, and modify behaviour).

Consideration of learning from the learning theorist/research perspective provides a look, from a different angle, at how our patients acquire their beliefs, their perspectives, that we believe contribute to understanding the depth of what comprises patients' pain experience cognitions and feelings while further substantiating the importance of emphasising the 'cognitive' aspect of a cognitive-behavioural approach.

Management of unhelpful cognitions, feelings and behaviours identified through narrative reasoning typically occurs through explanation/education, or what we have called communicative learning and management, directed to assisting patients to recognise unhelpful thought and feeling structures (or schemas) that may have become barriers to their recovery. This also represents the "cognitive" aspect of cognitive-behavioural therapy. It is important this is approached from a transformative, deep learning framework that aims to promote genuine change in patient perspectives, and not simply through a behavioural approach of selectively attending and not-attending to desired or undesired behaviours (spoken or actions). While behavioural strategies are clearly important, on their own they are less likely to result in altered perspectives, instead only shaping "appropriate" behaviours in the therapist's presence without generalisation to the rest of life's circumstances. This is not dissimilar to the ignoring or punishment of a child's unwanted behaviour without further exploration of what underpins it and explanation of why it is inappropriate resulting in the child's superficial learning not to do that in front of you rather than genuinely understanding and changing this behaviour.

References

Bishop GD 1991 Understanding the understanding of illness: lay disease representations. In: Skelton JA, Croyle RT (eds) Mental Representation in Health and Illness. Springer-Verlag, New York 32 – 59

Borkan JM, Quirk M, Sullivan M 1991 Finding meaning after the fall: Injury narratives from elderly hip fracture patients. Social Science and Medicine 33:947–957

Borkan J, Reis S, Hermoni D, Biderman A 1995 Talking about the pain: a patient-centred study of low back pain in primary care. Social Science and Medicine 40:977-988

Borrell-Carrió F, Suchman AL, Epstein RM 2004 The biopsychosocial model 25 years later: Principles, practice, and scientific inquiry. Annals of Family Medicine, www.annfammed.org 2(6):576-582

Brookfield S 2000 Clinical reasoning and generic thinking skills. In: Higgs J, Jones M (eds) Clinical Reasoning in the Health Professions (2nd edn). Butterworth-Heinemann, Edinburgh 62–77

Buetow S, Kenealy T 2000 Evidence-based medicine: the need for a new definition. Journal of Evaluation in Clinical Practice. 6:85-92

Butler D, Moseley L 2003 Explain Pain. Noigroup Publications, Adelaide

Crombez G, Eccleston C, Baeyens F, Eelen P 1998 When somatic information treatens, catastrophic thinking enhances attentional interference. Pain 75: 187-198

Crombez G, Eccleston C, Baeyens F, Eelen P 1998a Attentional disruption is enhanced by the threat of pain. Behaviour Research and Therapy. 36:195-204

Dijkers M 1999 Measuring quality of life. American Journal of Physical Medicine and Rehabilitation 78:286-300

Duke J, Leventhal H, Brownlee S, Leventhal EA 2002 Giving up and replacing activities in response to illness. Journal of Gerontology 57B:P367–P376

Duncan G 2000 Mind-body dualism and the biopsychosocial model of pain: what did Descartes really say? Journal of Medicine and Philosophy. 25:485-513

Eccleston C 1995 Chronic pain and distraction: an experimental investigation into the role of sustained and shifting attention in the processing of chronic persistent pain. Behaviour Research and Therapy 33:391-405

Eccleston C, Crombez G, Aldrich S, Stannard C 1997 Attention and somatic awareness in chronic pain. Pain 72:209-215

Edwards IC 2000 Clinical reasoning in three different fields of physiotherapy - a qualitative case study approach. Vols. I and II. Unpublished thesis submitted in partial fulfilment of the Doctor of Philosophy in Health Sciences. University of South Australia, Adelaide, Australia. The Australian Digitized Theses Program. 2001. Available at: http://www.library.unisa.edu.au/adt-root/public/adt-SUSA-20030603-090552/index.html

Edwards IC, Jones MA 1995 Collaborative reasoning. Unpublished paper submitted in partial fulfilment of the Graduate Diploma in Orthopaedics. University of South Australia, Adelaide, Australia

Edwards I, Jones MA, Carr J, Braunack-Mayer A, Jensen GM 2004 Clinical reasoning strategies in physical therapy, Physical Therapy 84:312–335

Edwards I, Jones MA, Higgs J, Trede F, Jensen GM 2004a What is collaborative reasoning? Advances in Physiotherapy 6:70–83

Elstein AS, Shulman LS and Sprafka SA 1978 Medical Problem Solving. An Analysis of Clinical Reasoning. Harvard University Press, Cambridge MA

Engel G 1977 The need for a new medical model: a challenge for biomedicine. Science 196:129-136

Engel G 1978 The biopsychosocial model and the education of health professionals. Annals New York Academy of Sciences 310:535–544

Ersser SJ, Atkins S 2000 Clinical reasoning and patient-centred care. In: Higgs J, Jones M (eds) Clinical Reasoning in the Health Professions (2nd edn). Butterworth-Heinemann, Edinburgh 68–77

Gamsa A 1994 The role of psychological factors in chronic pain. I A half century of study. Pain 57: 5 – 15

Gamsa A 1994a The role of psychological factors in chronic pain. II A critical appraisal. Pain 57: 17 – 29

Gifford LS 1998 The mature organism model. In: Gifford L (ed) Topical Issues in Pain 1. Whiplash - Science and Management, Fear-Avoidance Beliefs and Behaviour. CNS Press, Falmouth 45–56

Goleman D 1998 Working with emotional intelligence. Bloomsbury, London

Good MJD, Brodwin PE, Good BJ, Kleinman A (eds) 1992 Pain as Human Experience: An Anthropological Perspective. University of California Press, Berkeley

Habermas J 1984 Theory of communicative action. Vol 1 Beacon Press, Boston

Harding V 1998 Application of the cognitive-behavioural approach. In: Pitt-Brooke J, Reid H, Lockwood J et al (eds) Rehabilitation of Movement: Theoretical bases of clinical practice. WB Saunders, London 539 – 583

Harding V 1998a Cognitive-behavioural approach to fear and avoidance. In: Gifford L (ed) Topical Issues in Pain 1. Whiplash-Science and Management, Fear-Avoidance Beliefs and Behaviour. CNS Press, Falmouth 173–191

Harding V, Williams AC de C 1995 Extending physiotherapy skills using a psychological approach: Cognitive behavioural management of chronic pain. Physiotherapy 81:681–688

Hunt SM 1997 The problem of quality of life. Quality of Life Research 6:205–212

Jensen MP, Turner JA, Romano JM, Karoly P 1991 Coping with pain: a critical review of the literature. Pain 47:249–283

Jensen MP, Turner JA, Romano JM 1994 Relationship of pain-specific beliefs to chronic pain adjustment. Pain 57:301–309

Jensen GM, Gwyer J, Hack LM, Shepard KF 1999 Expertise in physical therapy practice. Boston: Butterworth-Heineman

Jensen MP, Nielson WR, Turner JA, Romano JM, Hill ML 2003 Readiness to self-manage pain is associated with coping and with psychological and physical functioning among patients with chronic pain. Pain 104:529–537

Jones MA 1992 Clinical reasoning in manual therapy. Physical Therapy 72:875–884

Jones MA, Edwards I, Gifford L 2002 Conceptual models for implementing biopsychosocial theory in clinical practice. Manual Therapy 7:2–9

Jones MA, Rivett D (eds) 2004 Clinical Reasoning for Manual Therapists. Butterworth Heinemann, Oxford

Kendall N, Watson P 2000 Identifying psychosocial yellow flags and modifying management. In: Gifford L (ed) Topical Issues of Pain 2. Biopsychosocial assessment and management. Relationships and pain. CNS Press, Falmouth 131–139

Kleinman A, Brodwin PE, Good BJ, Good MJD 1992 Pain as human experience, an introduction. In: Good MJD, Brodwin PE, Good BJ, Kleinman A (eds) Pain as Human Experience: An Anthropological Perspective. University of California Press, Berkeley 1–28

Leventhal H 1993 The pain system: a multilevel model for the study of motivation and emotion. Motivation and Emotion 17:139–146

Leventhal H, Meyer D, Nerenz D 1980 The common sense representation of illness danger. In: Rachman S (ed) Contributions to Medical Pscychology, Vol 2. Pergamon Press, New York

Leventhal H, Diefenbach M 1991 The active side of illness cognition. In: Skelton JA, Croyle RT (eds) Mental Representation in Health and Illness. Springer-Verlag, New York 247–272

Linton SJ 2000 A review of psychological risk factors in back and neck pain. Spine 25:1148–1156

Main CJ, Booker CK 2000 The nature of psychological factors. In: Main CJ, Spanswick CC (eds) Pain Management: An Interdisciplinary Approach. Churchill Livingstone, Edinburgh 19–42

Main CJ, Spanswick CC, Watson P 2000 The nature of disability. In: Main CJ, Spanswick CC (eds) Pain Management: An Interdisciplinary Approach. Churchill Livingstone, Edinburgh 89–106

Main C, Watson P 2002 The distressed and angry low back pain patient. In: Gifford L (ed) Topical Issues in Pain 3. Sympathetic nervous system and pain. Pain management. Clinical effectiveness. CNS Press, Falmouth 175–192

Mallinson S 2002 Listening to respondents: a qualitative assessment of the Short-Form 36 Health Status Questionnaire. Social Science & Medicine 54:11–21

Mezirow J 2000 Learning to think like an adult. Core concepts of transformation theory. In: Mezirow J (ed) Learning as Transformation. Critical Perspectives on a Theory in Progress. Jossey-Bass, San Francisco 3–33

Mindell A 1995 Sitting in the fire: large group transformation using conflict and diversity. Lao Tse Press: Portland, Oregon

Morley S, Eccleston C, Williams A 1999 Systematic review and meta-analysis of randomized controlled trials of cognitive behaviour therapy and behaviour therapy for chronic pain in adults, excluding headache. Pain 80:1–13

Moseley GL 2003 A pain neuromatrix approach to patients with chronic pain. Manual Therapy 8:1–11

Moseley GL 2004 Evidence for a direct relationship between cognitive and physical change during an education intervention in people with chronic low back pain. European Journal of Pain 8:39–45

Muncey H 2002 Explaining pain to patients. In: Gifford LS (ed) Topical Issues in Pain 4. Placebo and nocebo, Pain management, Muscles and pain. CNS Press, Falmouth 157–166

O'Dowd H 2000 Pain 'stories'. In: Gifford L (ed) Topical Issues in Pain 2. Biopsychosocial assessment and management. Relationships and pain. CNS Press, Falmouth 155–163

Osborn M, Smith JA 1998 The personal experience of chronic benign lower back pain: An interpretative phenomenological analysis. British Journal of Health Psychology 3:65–83

Payton OD 1985 Clinical reasoning process in physical therapy. Physical Therapy 65:924–928

Pengel LHM, Herbert RD, Maher CG, Refshauge KM 2003 Acute low back pain: systematic review of its prognosis. British Medical Journal 327:1–5

Phillips HC 1987 Avoidance behaviour and its role in sustaining chronic pain. Behaviour Research and Therapy 25:273–279

Pincus T 2004 The psychology of pain. In: French S, Sim J (eds) Physiotherapy a Psychosocial Approach. Elsevier, Edinburgh 95–115

Pincus T, Morley S 2001 Cognitive-processing bias in chronic pain: a review and integration. Psychological Bulletin 127:599–617

Pincus T, Vlaeyen JWS, Kendall NAS 2002 Cognitive-behavioral therapy and psychosocial factors in low back pain. Spine 27:E133–E138

Resnik L, Jensen G 2003 Using clinical outcomes to explore the theory of expert practice in physical therapy, Physical Therapy 83:1090–1106

Rotholz JM 2002 Chronic Fatigue Syndrome, Christianity, & Culture. The Harworth Medical Press, New York

Salkovskis P 1996 The cognitive approach to anxiety: threat beliefs, safety-seeking behaviour, and the special case of health anxiety and obsessions. In: Salkovskis P (ed) Frontiers of Cognitive Therapy. The Guilford Press, London 48–74

Schwoebel J, Friedman R, Duda N, Branch Coslett H 2001 Pain and Body Schema: evidence for peripheral effects on mental representations of movement. Brain 124(10):2098–2104

Sharp TJ 2001 The "safety seeking behaviours" construct and its application to chronic pain. Behavioural and Cognitive Psychotherapy 29:241–244

Sharp TJ 2001a Chronic pain: a reformulation of the cognitive-behavioural model. Behaviour Research and Therapy 39:787–800

Sim J, Smith MV 2004 The sociology of pain. In: French S, Sim J (eds) Physiotherapy a Psychosocial Approach. Elsevier, Edinburgh 117–139

Skelton JA, Croyle RT 1991 Mental representation, health, and illness: an introduction. In: Skelton JA, Croyle RT (eds) Mental Representation in Health and Illness. Springer-Verlag, New York 1–9

Spanswick CC, Parker H 2000 Clinical content of interdisciplinary pain management programmes. In: Main CJ, Spanswick CC (eds) Pain Management: An Interdisciplinary Approach. Churchill Livingstone, Edinburgh 255–265

Steen E, Haugli L 2000 Generalised chronic musculoskeletal pain as a rational reaction to a life situation? Theoretical Medicine 21:581–599

Strong J, Unruh AM 2002 Psychologically based pain management strategies. In: Strong J, Unruh AM, Wright A, Baxter GD (eds) Pain. A Textbook for Therapists. Churchill Livingstone,Edinburgh 169–185

Thomas-Edding D 1987 Clinical problem solving in physical therapy and its implications for curriculum development. In Proceedings of the Tenth International Congress of the World Confederation for Physical Therapy, World Confederation for Physical Therapy, May 17-22, Sydney, Australia, pp 100–104

Turk DC 1996 Cognitive factors in chronic pain and disability. In: Gatchel R, Turk D (eds) Psychological Approaches to Pain Management – A Practitioner's Handbook. The Guilford Press, New York

Turk DC, Rudy TE 1992 Cognitive factors and persistent pain: a glimpse into pandora's box. Cognitive Therapy and Research 16:99–122

Turk DC, Okifuji A 1998 Directions in prescriptive chronic pain management based on diagnostic characteristics of the patient. American Pain Society Bulletin Sept/ Oct:5-11

Unruh AM, Harman K 2002 Generic principles of practice. In: Strong J, Unruh AM, Wright A, Baxter GD (eds) Pain. A Textbook for Therapists. Churchill Livingstone,Edinburgh 151–167

Vlaeyen JWS, Kole-Snijders AMJ, Boeren RGB, van Eck H 1995 Fear of movement/(re)injury in chronic low back pain and its relation to behavioural performance. Pain 62:363–372

Vlaeyen JWS, Linton SJ 2000 Fear-avoidance and its consequences in chronic musculoskeletal pain: a state of the art. Pain 85:317–332

Vlaeyen JWS, de Jong J, Geilen M, Heuts PHTG, van Breukelen G 2002 The treatment of fear of movement/(re)injury in chronic low back pain: further evidence on the effectiveness of exposure in vivo. The Clinical Journal of Pain 18:251–261

Wadell G 1998 The Back Pain Revolution. Churchill Livingstone, Edinburgh

Watson PJ, Booker CK, Main CJ, Chen ACN 1997 Surface electromyography in the identification of chronic low back pain patients: The development of a flexion relaxation ratio. Clinical Biomechanics 12(3):165-171

Watson P, Kendall N 2000 Assessing psychosocial yellow flags. In: Gifford L (ed) Topical Issues in Pain 2. Biopsychosocial assessment and management. Relationships and pain. CNS Press, Falmouth 111–129

White M, Epston D 1990 Narrative means to therapeutic ends. WW Norton and Company, New York

Williams DA, Keefe FJ 1991 Pain beliefs and the use of cognitive-behavioral coping strategies. Pain 46:185–190

Wilson P, Henry J, Nicholas M 1993 Cognitive methods in the management of chronic pain and tinnitus. Australian Psychologist 28:172–180

Wittink H, Michel TH, Cohen LJ, Fishman SM 1997 Physical therapy treatment. In: Wittink H, Michel TH (eds) Chronic Pain Management for Physical Therapists. Butterworth-Heinemann, Boston 119–56

World Health Organization 2001 ICF Checklist Version 2.1a, clinician form for international classification of functioning, disability and health. [Online] Available http://www.who.int/classification/icf/checklist/icf-checklist.pdf,April 15, 2002

17

Pain Management: Integrating Physiotherapy and Clinical Psychology Practice

RICHARD JOHNSON AND LORRAINE MOORES

Introduction

The importance of psychosocial factors in the development and maintenance of chronic pain disability has become widely recognised (Kendal et al 1997, Linton 2000, Watson 2000). This increasing awareness has led to a gradual progression from the provision of specific treatments focused on pain reduction, toward active rehabilitative approaches based on a biopsychosocial model (Klaber Moffet & Frost 2000, Roland et al 1996, Underwood et al 2004, Waddell et al 2001). Treatment from a biopsychosocial perspective focuses on providing the patient with techniques to help them gain control over the effects of pain on their life through modification of the sensory, cognitive, affective and behavioural aspects of the pain experience. Interdisciplinary Pain Management Programmes are particularly suited to such an approach and over recent years there has been an increase in the number of such programmes in the United Kingdom. To date, there are approximately eighty Pain Management Programmes registered on the British Pain Society's Pain Management Programme Directory (www.britishpainsociety.org/ February 2005).

Critical reviews of this treatment approach conclude there is strong, if not overwhelming evidence for the efficacy of cognitive-behavioural rehabilitation programmes in the restoration of function, improved mood and reduction of disability in adults with chronic pain. The interested reader is directed to the reviews and meta-analyses carried out by Flor et al (1992), Morley et al (1999), Rossy et al (1999). This treatment approach is delivered by an interdisciplinary team, as the range of clinical knowledge and skills required is not encompassed within any single profession.

The Pain Society's[1] (1997) document, 'Desirable Criteria For Pain Management Programmes' (currently under review) identifies the minimum clinical staff required to run a Pain Management Programme as a medical doctor, clinical psychologist and physiotherapist. The interdisciplinary team possesses generic skills common to all team members and specific skills of individual professions.

As mentioned, the evidence for the efficacy of Pain Management Programmes is strong, and there are resources available to assist clinical teams in gaining the skills to carry out this form of intervention (e.g. Main & Spanswick 2000). However, for a number of reasons (such as available resources or patient suitability), not all patients are offered a Pain Management Programme. A significant amount of interdisciplinary teamwork may therefore take place outside a Pain Management Programme context. Good teamwork does not happen automatically; it is important that clinicians involved in such work are guided by a clear understanding of the contributions of their colleagues from other disciplines, and of the ways in which they can effectively work together. This chapter aims to illustrate a model of how physiotherapists and clinical psychologists can effectively work together in a pain management setting to ensure that both physical and psychological aspects of the patients' pain problem are addressed. Once high quality teamwork is established then we think that this can lead to better clinical outcomes and optimal efficiency. It can also lead to a stimulating and rewarding environment in which to work.

[1] Known as The british pain Society since August 2004

A model of the interface between physiotherapy and clinical psychology work in chronic pain management

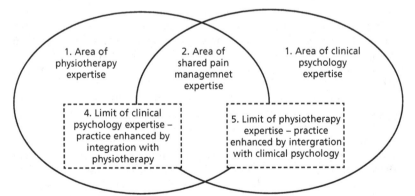

Figure 1 illustrates a model of the interface between physiotherapy and clinical psychology skills in chronic pain management.

Area 1 indicates the specific strengths and expertise that the physiotherapist brings to pain management, for example, musculoskeletal assessment of patients, knowledge of exercise and physical rehabilitation including education about fitness and deconditioning. Area 3 represents the specific strengths and expertise possessed by the clinical psychologist, for example, the assessment of primary mental health problems, treatment of comorbid problems such as post-traumatic stress disorder, and specific psychological therapy to address barriers to the implementation of pain management strategies. Area 2 represents the overlapping pain management knowledge and skills of the physiotherapist and clinical psychologist. Knowledge of pain physiology, pacing skills and goal setting are examples of the generic pain management expertise possessed by both disciplines. The boundaries labelled 4 and 5 denote the areas where the each clinician has the opportunity to draw upon the specific skills and strengths of the other discipline to enhance clinical treatment. The interaction of the disciplines at these boundaries in delivering integrated treatment may be seen as a hallmark of interdisciplinary (as opposed to multidisciplinary) care (Melvin, 1980; cited in Main & Spanswick 2000). Handling these boundaries successfully is one of the major challenges of interdisciplinary work; arguably these boundaries represent the most rewarding and interesting aspect of teamwork. In the next section we will illustrate this process by reference to case examples from our clinical practice.

Case examples to illustrate the interface between physiotherapy and clinical psychology

Handing over clinical management to a colleague

The first two case examples illustrate scenarios where one clinician has assessed a patient and recognises a specific issue that falls within their colleague's expertise and outside their own.

Case 1: physiotherapist recognises the need for clinical psychology assessment

A 26-year old female was being assessed by a physiotherapist to determine their suitability for inclusion on an interdisciplinary Pain Management Programme. As the patient described the onset of her pain, she outlined the road traffic accident she had been involved in two years previously in which she sustained serious injury. During this discussion the patient became tearful and distressed, explaining that her close friend had been killed in the accident.

She described intrusive memories of the accident, especially at night, and frequent thoughts of the friends she had lost. The physiotherapist listened empathically and acknowledged the impact of the traumatic event. She recognised the possibility of post-traumatic stress disorder and unresolved grief, and considered that these issues required more in depth assessment to establish whether specific psychological intervention was needed. The physiotherapist outlined the rehabilitative approach and gave a careful explanation of the importance of clinical psychology assessment. She stressed that pain management rehabilitation may be intensive and that distress relating to the accident may have a detrimental affect on the patient's ability to gain optimum benefit from any physiotherapy input. The patient was given time to consider this, and consented to being assessed by a clinical psychologist. Clinical psychology sessions were commenced, with a long term plan for joint physiotherapy and clinical psychology review to establish rehabilitation options once post traumatic stress disorder and grief issues had been fully addressed.

In this example, the physiotherapist was aware of the potential impact of post-traumatic stress disorder and grief issues on the patient's ability to rehabilitate, and was able to help the patient understand this impact. A key skill was to make the prospect of psychological assessment of these issues acceptable to her. The patient reported that this was the first time in two years she had felt able to discuss her feelings about the accident, and readily agreed to an appointment with the psychologist.

Case 2: clinical psychologist recognises the need for physiotherapy assessment

A 28-year old female was being reviewed by a clinical psychologist four months after her attendance on a Pain Management Programme. During the review the patient complained of a six week history of new symptoms. These included a new area of pain in the left leg with numbness and pins and needles in the leg and foot. The clinical psychologist was aware that this may indicate new pathology requiring further assessment. He asked the physiotherapist to join him to discuss these symptoms with the patient. The physiotherapist established that the symptoms fitted a specific pattern and were accompanied by altered bladder function. The physiotherapist felt that this pattern of new symptoms merited re-referral to the medical pain consultant. The consultant agreed, and the patient's symptoms were investigated by magnetic resonance imaging.

In this example, the clinical psychologist had been concerned that the patient may be distracted from her self-management skills by the presence of new symptoms. The physiotherapist's involvement at this stage ensured that the new symptoms were appropriately investigated, but allowed a continued focus on self management skills. If working alone, then it would have been more difficult for the clinical psychologist to resist a return to an entirely medical approach given the need to investigate the new symptoms.

Sharing clinical management

The following two examples illustrate how having a colleague available supports each discipline's own practice at the limit of their expertise. Supporting each others' practice in this way optimises the patient's treatment.

Case 3: physiotherapist draws upon clinical psychology to enhance the patient's management

The physiotherapist was working with a 45-year old man with the aim of helping him to increase his level of function to a point where inclusion on to a Pain Management Programme would be possible. The physiotherapist was aware that the patient had marked low mood associated with their chronic pain problem. As the sessions continued, it became clear that the patient's depression was posing a barrier to functional improvement. The physiotherapist discussed the case with the clinical psychologist and it was agreed that the patient would be managed jointly to facilitate progress. The clinical psychologist helped the patient to manage the effects of his depressed mood (e.g., reduced motivation) and also to address relevant issues in his marital relationship. His physical function improved such that he was able to attend an intensive Pain Management Programme.

In this example, the physiotherapist recognised a level of pain-related depression which posed both a barrier to physical progress, and which required specific attention in its own right. The clinical psychology intervention allowed the patient to make better use of the physiotherapy input.

Case 4: clinical psychologist draws upon physiotherapy to enhance the patient's management

The clinical psychologist was working with a 62-year old man to help him increase his social functioning. During these sessions the patient complained that a particular movement appeared to trigger severe spasm, restricting his daily activities. He asked whether there was anything he could do to reduce the occurrence of the spasm. The clinical psychologist wondered whether graded exercises involving the 'trigger movement' may help.

315

This was discussed with the physiotherapist who jointly assessed the patient with the clinical psychologist. The physiotherapist noted guarded movement resulting in loss of function and altered posture. The patient was shown a graded lumbar extension exercise, and was helped to establish an initial baseline so that he could introduce this into his daily exercise routine. Continuing psychology sessions with periodic physiotherapy review enabled the patient to achieve his goals of leaving his flat on a daily basis and returning to regular swimming. The improved tolerance of the problematic movement was key to facilitating progress toward the goals of the clinical psychology sessions.

These case examples illustrate ways in which the quality of treatment can be enhanced by drawing upon the specific skills of a colleague when working at the limits of one's own expertise. Recognising the need to enlist the input of another clinician optimises patient care by ensuring relevant issues are addressed.

Implications for practice

Choosing the appropriate form of team working

Whilst the case examples illustrate the interface between physiotherapy and clinical psychology in the process of interdisciplinary teamwork, the particular form of joint working is a separate issue. The different options for joint working may be graded by level of intensity, and include:

1. Full joint working involving both professions treating the patient together.
2. Occasional joint working with one profession taking the overall lead.
3. Assessment and consultation by one profession on the other's case.
4. Discussion / consultation by one profession upon the other's case with no patient contact.

There is a balance to strike between effectiveness and efficiency. Choosing an insufficiently intensive form of joint work risks less than optimal outcome, whilst an overly intensive form risks unnecessary duplication and thereby inefficiency.

Avoiding pitfalls in teamwork

The case examples bring a perspective on the potential benefits of team-working. However, there are pitfalls as well as benefits to team-working. Problematic blurring of professional boundaries can occur in clinical fields, such as pain management, where an overlap of skills exists.

The professional practice guidelines of clinical psychologists (Division of Clinical Psychology, 1995), and the rules of professional conduct of the Chartered Society of Physiotherapy (The Chartered Society of Physiotherapy, 2002) make it clear that members of both professions have a responsibility to recognise and observe the limits of their professional competence. If limits of competence are exceeded, then the quality of care will be undermined.

In relation to patient care in pain management, examples may include a clinical psychologist too readily attributing a patient's complaint of pins & needles to psychological and behavioural causes (e.g., anxiety and hyperventilation), thereby running the risk of possible serious pathology being missed. Similarly, a physiotherapist may make a judgement about the 'normality' of a patient's response to a traumatic event and inadvertently leave a problematic post-traumatic stress disorder untreated. Even if the blurring of professional boundaries does not lead to such negative patient outcomes, it may still contribute to inter-professional tensions and thereby damage to working relationships.

In order to avoid these pitfalls it is important that clinicians pay attention to developing and maintaining high quality team-working. Several methods may be helpful in achieving these aims:

Training. If joint working occurs, each discipline may wish to outline their professional knowledge base, and the hallmarks of clinical presentations that they are skilled in assessing and treating. This will facilitate the physiotherapist's recognition of clinical material that may appropriately fall into the clinical psychologist's unique area of expertise and vice versa.

Agreement on generic pain management skills. We have suggested here that there is an overlap between the pain management expertise of physiotherapists and clinical psychologists. In our setting, for example, it is generally agreed that both professions are skilled in working with patients on interventions such as activity pacing and goal-setting. Each team will need to negotiate the extent of such shared expertise amongst themselves. Furthermore, it will be necessary to establish a consistent approach to this material across members of the team, and to re-visit this periodically to avoid "drift" in the way such areas are addressed clinically.

Agreement on boundaries of work outside each profession's expertise. Clearly it is neither feasible nor desirable that boundaries are so rigid that physiotherapists feel unable to discuss mental health concerns with their patients, or that clinical psychologists feel unable to discuss physical symptoms. The key here may be whether one is making a clinical decision that is outside ones expertise. In case example (1), it is perfectly appropriate for the physiotherapist to acknowledge the patient's trauma, to listen empathically and validate her distress. It would be inappropriate for the physiotherapist to assess whether the post-traumatic and grief issues require treatment. In case example (2) it is appropriate for the clinical psychologist to ask the patient to list the new physical symptoms she has noticed since she left the programme, but inappropriate to decide whether or not they require further assessment.

Communication. In a pain management setting, it is inevitable that clinicians will frequently encounter issues which fall either at the boundary of their own expertise, or within their colleague's area of expertise. It is important that the team fosters an environment in which every member feels readily able to approach colleagues to discuss such issues. Such open communication will ensure that important clinical issues are properly addressed.

A more complex model

We have focused specifically on the integration of physiotherapy and clinical psychology work, but recognise that the model is more complex than this. In reality the model may include a range of different disciplines including physiotherapists, clinical psychologists, medical doctors, nurses and occupational therapists. We would suggest that the principles discussed within this chapter apply to the relationship between all disciplines working within interdisciplinary pain management, and perhaps to other teams working closely together in other clinical areas.

Conclusion

The aim of this chapter has been to consider how physiotherapists and clinical psychologists may effectively work together within the area of pain management, ensuring that both physical and psychological aspects of the patients' pain problem are addressed. A model of the interface between physiotherapy and clinical psychology knowledge and skills has been outlined, and the importance of having a clear understanding of the contributions of each other's discipline has been emphasised. Reference to case examples has illustrated the process of effective teamwork.

We would point out that simply working together does not automatically lead to effective teamwork. When the intervention provided by different disciplines within a team is not truly integrated, then clinical effectiveness and efficiency may be compromised. Dissatisfaction and professional disharmony may also result. However, once high quality teamwork is established, which effectively combines the expertise of each discipline, a powerful therapeutic approach results optimising clinical outcome and creating a rewarding and stimulating environment in which to work. We hope that this chapter provides ideas that may help clinicians to establish and maintain high quality teamwork.

References

British Pain Society Pain Management Programme Directory. www.britishpainsociety.org / February 2005

Division of Clinical Psychology 1995 Professional Practice Guidelines. The British Psychological Society

Flor H, Fydrich T, Turk DC 1992 Efficacy of multidisciplinary pain treatment centres: A meta-analytical review Pain 49:221-230

Kendal NAS, Linton SJ, Main CJ 1997 Guide to assessing psychosocial yellow flags in acute low back pain: risk factors for long term disability and work loss. Accident rehabilitation and compensation insurance corporation of New Zealand and the National Health Committee. Wellington, New Zealand

Klaber Moffet J, Frost H 2000 Back to fitness programme: the manual for physiotherapists to set up the classes. Physiotherapy 85:295-305

Linton SJ 2000 A review of psychological risk factors in back and neck pain. Spine 25(9):1148-1156

Main CJ, Spanswick CC 2000 Pain Management: An Interdisciplinary Approach. Churchill Livingstone, Edinburgh

Melvin JL 1980 Interdisciplinary and multidisciplinary activities and the ACRM. Archives of Physical Medicine and Rehabilitation 61:379-380

Morley S, Eccleston C, Williams A C de C 1999 Systematic review and meta-analysis of randomized controlled trials of cognitive-behaviour therapy and behaviour therapy for chronic pain in adults, excluding headache. Pain 80:1-13

Pain Society 1997 Report of a working party of the Pain Society of Great Britain and Ireland: Desirable Criteria for Pain Management Programmes. Pain Society, London

Roland M, Waddell G, Klaber Moffet J, Burton AK, Main CJ, Cantrell T 1996 The Back Book: Stationery Office

Rossy LA, Buckelew SP, Dorr N, Hagglund KJ, Thayer JF, McIntosh MJ, Hewett JE, Johnson JC 1999 A meta-analysis of fibromyalgia treatment interventions. Annals of Behavioral Medicine 21(2):180-191

The Chartered Society of Physiotherapy 2002 Rules of professional conduct. Blackwell Science

Underwood M, O'Meara S, Harvey E 2004 United Kingdom back pain exercise and manipulation (UK BEAM) randomised trial: effectiveness of physical treatments for back pain in primary care. British Medical Journal Dec 11: 329-1377

Waddell G, Burton AK, McClune T 2001 The Whiplash Book. Stationery Office

Watson PJ 2000 Psychosocial predictors of outcome from low back pain In: L Gifford (Ed) Topical Issues in Pain 2, Physiotherapy Pain Association Yearbook. CNS Press, Falmouth 85-109

5

Pathophysology

18

Making Sense of "S1 mania"; Are things really that simple?

LORIMER MOSELEY

Introduction

The brain, it seems, is the new frontier for pain researchers. Substantial progress in technology has opened up the brain to investigation and the results have been met by some with excitement, by others with measured interest and by others still, with disdain.

Neuroimaging studies certainly produce captivating data. Pretty multicoloured 'blobs' ooze through folds of brain tissue. Such novel and technologically impressive data can easily be compelling. Functional magnetic resonance imaging (fMRI), electroencephalography (EEG), magnetoencephalography (MEG), photon emission topography (PET) and transcranial magnetic stimulation (TMS) have acronymed our lexicon and provided a mountain of information about brain state and activity across a range of activities, contexts, conditions and groups. For example, fMRI studies have shown that men have greater blood oxygen level dependent (BOLD) signal in the amygdala and hypothalamus while watching pornographic videos than women, which supposedly 'explains' why men are more aroused than women by that material (Hamann et al 2004); patients with schizophrenia show less BOLD signal in left anterior cingulate cortex than matched controls, which 'explains' why schizophrenia is associated with reduced inhibitory capacity (Rubia et al 2001); men show BOLD signal in the left medial prefrontal cortex and hippocampus, whereas women show BOLD signal in the left amygdala, when they are shown unpleasant words concerning body image, which 'explains' why women are more susceptible to eating disorders (Shirao et al 2005). So it is not all bells and whistles. But at the end of the day, does all this brain research amount to anything more than neophrenology?

This paper will discuss (i) the evidence that the primary sensory cortex, S1, is organised differently in chronic pain, (ii) whether or not changes in S1 organisation could and do cause pain, and (iii) the implications of cortical reorganisation for treatment of people in pain.

S1 ORGANISATION IN PEOPLE WITH CHRONIC PAIN

The brain is obviously of critical importance for pain. There are many studies that investigate different aspects of brain activity and organisation in association with pain e.g. (Apkarian 1999, Bromm 1995, Condes-Lara et al 2000, Creac'h et al 2000, Derbyshire & Jones 1998, Derbyshire et al 1994, Flor 2000, Flor et al 1998, Hsieh et al 1999, Huse et al 2001, Ingvar 1999, Karl et al 2001, Knecht et al 1998, May et al 2000, Petrovic et al 2000, Peyron et al 2000), see Flor (2000) for review), and many investigate cortical and sub-cortical regions aside from S1. Those studies that compare people with chronic pain to control subjects offer varying and in some cases contrasting results, but with regard to S1, there seems to be some consensus.

How is S1 organisation investigated?

First things first – what is cortical *reorganisation*? In some respects, it depends who you talk to. Here, cortical reorganisation refers to a reasonably labile change in the way cortical neurones respond to input such that the pattern of neuronal activity, or the 'representation', evoked by a particular stimulus changes over time. Care should be taken here too, however, because cortical cells can produce excitatory and inhibitory post-synaptic potentials without being large enough to produce an action potential. Conceding that limitation, the 'organisation' of S1 is investigated:- by stimulating the body part in question and recording electrical signal (EEG) or electromagnetic field (MEG) via electrodes placed on the outside of the skull; by 'imaging' areas in which there is a change in the relationship between oxygenated haemoglobin and de-oxygenated haemoglobin, the so-called BOLD signal (fMRI); or, by imaging blood flow, via detection of radioactive isotopes carried in the blood, throughout the brain (PET). Each technique has benefits and limitations and interpretation of data is often based on a number of assumptions. For example, imaging blood flow assumes that the change in blood flow reflects neuronal activity and often assumes that the neuronal activity is necessarily excitatory, which is difficult to verify. Nonetheless, these methods permit researchers to 'map' the body in S1 – the so-called 'virtual body' or sensory homunculus. Therefore it is possible to detect changes in S1 activity in response to standardised stimuli applied to the physical body – distortions of the sensory homunculus.

How is S1 organisation different in chronic pain?

Phantom limb pain.

Despite the differences between techniques and notwithstanding their limitations and underlying assumptions, the majority of available studies suggest that people with chronic pain have a change in the S1 representation of the affected body part. Most data relate to phantom limb pain in amputees. The impetus for investigating S1 activity in amputees appears to be an early anecdotal report that phantom sensations could be evoked in upper limb amputees by stimulating the face (Ramachandran et al 1992), known since Penfield and Rasmussen's landmark work (1950) to lie adjacent in the sensory homunculus to the upper limb. Ramachandran's group postulated that sensory referral of this type might reflect S1 reorganisation such that invasion of the virtual hand or arm by the virtual face meant that stimulation of the face would activate neurons responsible for evoking sensation in the arm. Their postulation was supported by the modality-specific nature of the referred sensations, but early imaging studies were not supportive – while they showed changes in cortical representation of the amputated and adjacent area, these changes occurred in patients both with and without sensory referral (Elbert et al 1994, Knecht et al 1996, Knecht et al 1998a, Yang et al 1994). Subsequently, Flor et al (1995) showed that phantom limb pain, rather than sensory referral, might be the perceptual correlate of S1 reorganisation – only amputees with phantom limb pain demonstrated a shift in S1 representation and the intensity of phantom limb pain related to the extent of the shift in representation. Those findings have been replicated by other studies (Birbaumer et al 1997, Flor et al 1998, Grusser et al 2001) and, taken together, provide strong evidence that S1 reorganisation and phantom limb pain are related. However, does one cause the other?

Relevant to this issue are intriguing data obtained in a study, again by Flor's group, in which amputees with phantom limb pain underwent anaesthetic block of the brachial plexus (Birbaumer et al 1997). In that study, 3/6 patients reported *elimination* of phantom limb pain and 3/6 patients reported *no change* in phantom limb pain. Notably, those in whom pain was eliminated showed a big shift in S1 organisation and those in whom pain was unchanged showed a negligible shift in S1 organisation. Although a small sample, the likelihood of this relationship being due to chance is less than 10%. At first glance, that finding appears to suggest that pain may actually cause S1 changes, rather than the other way around. That would be consistent with MEG data from a study in which healthy volunteers were given acute (< 20 minutes) and severe (mean maximum on a 0 – 10 scale = 8.5) experimental hand pain via an injection of capsaicin (Soros et al 2001). Subjects showed a decrease (1 – 6 mm) in the distance between the S1 hand and lip representations – thus the capsaicin injection, and presumably the pain, appeared to induce the change. Not that there are not other possible explanations. Perhaps the severity of the pain instigated some sort of unconscious or conscious coping strategy to reduce the evoked pain – possibly via information processing systems, which would seem consistent with the finding that the allocation of attention is important for changes in S1 (Braun et al 2002). That is, is the change produced by attentional changes relating to the injection? If so, the shift or increase in representation is a function of pain and attentional style. Perhaps less severe pain would not engage these processes and not impart the effect. Notably the magnitude of the shift (1 – 6 mm) was less than that reported in Birbaumer et al's (1997) phantom limb pain patients for whom changes were normalised by anaesthesia (~ 18 mm).

A further consideration is that it is actually not possible to stimulate an absent body part, which means that a shift in S1 representation of an amputated body part is assumed because S1 representation of the somatotopically adjacent body part is shifted. This assumption may not be valid. It is possible that S1 maps don't shrink but become responsive to input from both areas, such as is the case in focal dystonia[1], notably a non-painful (albeit highly disabling) condition. In that group, invasion of adjacent S1 representation is not associated with decrease in that area, but rather a 'smudging' in which S1 representations begin to overlap (Byl et al 2000, Byl et al 1996). At present, it is not possible to determine whether evidence of S1 reorganisation in amputees with phantom limb pain constitutes a decrease in representation or smudging of formerly discrete representations, or neither, or both.

Data from populations in which sensory input from the body part is removed suggest that the changes observed in phantom limb pain may be caused by this de-afferentation rather than by pain. That would be consistent with the mantra 'use it or lose it'. For example, Tinazzi et al (1997) reported expanded S1 response to median nerve stimulation after anaesthetic block of the ulnar nerve – remove the ulnar nerve input and neurons previously responsive only to ulnar nerve input now become responsive to median nerve stimulation.

In summary, there is strong evidence that phantom limb pain is associated with a change in organisation of S1. It is most likely that the change reflects 'smudging' between S1 receptor fields, but it is also possible that it simply reflects shrinkage of the S1 representation of the absent part. At this stage, we don't really know.

---

[1] Focal dystonia can occur in association with repetitive fine motor tasks and manifests as increasing difficult performing those movements.

Chronic back pain

There are initial data that suggest changes similar to those described for phantom limb pain also occur with chronic pain in which the body part is still intact. For example, Flor et al (1997) recorded evoked magnetic fields in the brain in response to electrical stimulation just under the skin. They concentrated on the post-stimulus period thought to best reflect S1 activity, i.e. from 0 – 100 ms post-stimulus (Elbert & Flor 1999, Elbert et al 1995), and applied the stimuli to the back, within the area of pain, or to the index finger, which was pain-free. They compared patients with chronic back pain to patients with sub-acute back pain and to asymptomatic healthy controls and reported two major findings. First, the centre of the S1 response evoked by back stimulation was ~ 2.5 cm more medial in the chronic back pain patients than it was in the asymptomatic controls. Second, the magnitude of the S1 response evoked by back stimulation was ~ 1.5 times greater in the chronic back pain patients than it was in the controls and the magnitude of the response related to the duration of symptoms. Two considerations are relevant to the magnitude data. First, although the authors stated that there was no difference in pain threshold between groups, mean --± SD of the pain threshold was 1.19 ± 0.28 mA for chronic pain patients and 0.54 ± 0.21 mA for the control group, which means that pain threshold for patients was three standard deviations greater than that for control subjects. The authors' conclude that there is greater S1 reactivity and larger S1 representation of the back in chronic pain patients than there is in sub-acute patients or control subjects appears sustainable. That said, I suggest caveats to those conclusions. For example, it is not possible to isolate the cause of the changes just to S1, nor indeed to the brain. Perhaps changes in S1 activity simply reflect peripheral, spinal, midbrain or thalamic changes. Could the changes reflect compensation for elevated pain and perceptual thresholds? Could leakage of inflammatory mediators from an injury site in the back impart the effect?

One further issue makes interpretation of S1 reorganisation in chronic back pain difficult to interpret and that is that back pain is seldom felt superficially. The skin is seldom damaged, nor inflamed, yet S1 provides a somatotopic representation of the body *surface*, not deeper tissues. Representation of deeper tissues may involve other cortical regions, for example insular cortex (Craig 2002), and although it seems likely that reorganisation could occur in such regions, it remains to be verified.

In summary, S1 representation of the skin over the back seems to be expanded in people with chronic back pain, although further studies should be undertaken to verify this. It is notable that expansion of S1 representation also occurs with use, according to the use it or lose it principle, and those changes can occur quickly and be continually modified (Pascual Leone et al 1993, Sterr et al 1998).

Although larger with use, S1 fields seem to remain discrete, whereas S1 fields may become smudged in chronic low back pain. Finally, it seems likely that brain areas that represent deeper tissues may also undergo reorganisation and that this would be more consistent with the type of pain experienced in back pain. Those possibilities remain to be established.

Complex regional pain syndrome

Complex regional pain syndrome (CRPS) is a debilitating and atypical chronic pain, which makes it frustrating for clinicians and interesting for researchers. There is evidence of S1 reorganisation in CRPS, but the pattern of change appears opposite to that observed in chronic low back pain. For example, an initial MEG study in six patients with CRPS1 showed a greater S1 response to tactile stimulation for the affected hand than for the unaffected hand and reduced distance between the centre of the S1 responses for stimulation of the thumb and the fifth finger (Juottonen et al 2002). Thus, although they show a shift in S1 representation, it seems to become smaller, which is opposite to that observed in low back pain. Those data have been replicated using EEG by Pleger et al (2004) and using MEG by Maihofner et al (2003), the latter also reporting reduced distance between what they proposed to represent the middle of the hand (midway between digits one and five) and the lip.

In addition to imaging studies, there are intriguing clinical phenomena associated with CRPS1 that imply reorganisation of S1 and that have also been reported in groups characterised by sensory loss. First, modality-specific sensory referral to the adjacent zone on the sensory homunculus has been reported. McCabe et al (2003) have done some excellent and innovative work in this area and quantified sensory response to stimulation of the affected hand: evoking simultaneous sensation at the face, and stimulation of the affected foot: evoking simultaneous sensation at the knee. The pattern of referral was very similar to that reported in amputees (Ramachandran et al 1992a). Second, our group has observed that people with CRPS1 of one limb perceive the affected limb to be bigger than it really is (Moseley 2005), which has also been observed after anaesthesia and after cutaneous stimulation (Gandevia & Phegan 1999) and anecdotally after amputation and stroke.

Taken together, the imaging and clinical data provide strong evidence that S1 reorganisation also occurs in CRPS1, but the pattern of reorganisation seems different to that observed for chronic back pain. There are clinical findings that are common to CRPS1 and conditions in which sensory input is lost. Further work is required to determine the importance and meaning of these similarities.

THE RELATIONSHIP BETWEEN PAIN AND S1 ORGANISATION IN CHRONIC PAIN

Evidence that S1 reorganisation could cause pain

This is an important question primarily because S1 mania seems to be riding on the back of the presumption that S1 reorganisation does in fact cause pain. Three arguments have been made to support this presumption; (i) a theoretical argument that S1 reorganisation causes incongruence between motor commands and sensory feedback that then causes pain, (ii) a logical argument based on clinical and experimental data that show relationships between pain and reorganisation and resolution of pain and normalisation of organisation, and (iii) a postulation based on experimental data that suggest distinct cortical networks involving S1 mediate pathological pain.

Sensory-motor incongruence theories

Harris (1999) proposed that in the same way that motion sickness might result from discordant sensory input (from vestibular apparatus and proprioceptors), pain may result from changes in the cortical representation of somatic input, which falsely signal incongruence between motor intention and movement. That the central nervous system (CNS) detects such incongruence has long been established. The reafference principle (Von Holst 1950), whereby an exact copy of the command for movement (the "efferent copy") is subtracted from sensory input about the actual movement ("reafference") to yield an error signal ("exafference"), and the corollary discharge model (Sperry 1950) are early examples. Since then, an impressive amount of research has been undertaken (see Gandevia 1996 for review). However, much of this has been concerned with the role that detection of sensory-motor incongruence has in the control of movement and in proprioception, rather than in generation of pain.

That such incongruence could cause pain appears feasible. That would be consistent with modern notions of pain in which pain is conceptualised as an output of the brain that motivates the individual to get out of a situation that the brain concludes to be dangerous (Moseley 2003). There is also some experimental support. In a novel study, McCabe et al (2005) simulated sensory-motor incongruence by placing a mirror between the limbs of healthy subjects while they moved their limbs. The mirror was positioned so that one limb was out of sight and the subject then 'concentrated' on watching the mirror image of their other limb. When subjects moved the in-view limb and watched the mirror image of it while they performed the opposite movement with the hidden limb behind the mirror, 59% reported symptoms in an open-ended response. Notably, 15% of subjects reported low level pain during this task.

329

Further support can be drawn from clinical trials that aim to reconcile this incongruence by getting patients to perform identical movements of both limbs while watching the mirror image of the unaffected limb where the affected limb should be. Thus, they receive visual feedback that 'everything is OK', even when the affected limb is absent (i.e. in patients with amputations and phantom limb pain), dystonic or 'looking dysfunctional' as is often the case in CRPS1. Several trials have used this strategy. For example, Ramachandran's group presented anecdotal data that some patients with phantom limb pain reported a reduction in pain after performing mirror movements (Ramachandran & Rogers-Ramachandran 2000). McCabe's group (2003a) undertook a randomised clinical trial in which patients with CRPS1 performed mirror movements and they reported a reduction in pain in patients with acute or subacute CRPS1. Finally, our group has incorporated mirror movements into management of patients with chronic CRPS1 and we have found substantial reductions in pain and disability at the end of that program (Moseley 2004a, Moseley 2005a), although we do not attribute the effects of that program solely to mirror movements.

A close relationship between S1 changes and pain

Most studies report that the greater the change in S1 representation of the affected part, the greater the pain, although there are exceptions. Some studies report a relationship between the magnitude of the S1 responses and the intensity of pain (table 1). That general message is corroborated by data that document a change in S1 representation over the course of treatment. For example, Maihofner's group compared one-year follow-up MEG data to pre-treatment data and reported that S1 reorganisation reversal was coincident with clinical improvement ($r \sim 0.9$, $p < 0.05$) (Maihofner et al 2004). Similar data were reported from a shorter study with chronic low back pain patients in which reduction in low back pain correlated with reversal of S1 changes ($r \sim 0.75$, $p < 0.05$). Finally, in phantom limb pain patients given a regional block reversal of S1 reorganisation only occurred in those who also reported elimination of pain (Birbaumer et al 1997).

Although the studies outlined in this section present a solid argument that S1 reorganisation and pain are related, the data offer fragile support for a causative link. What data there are might as easily suggest a causative link in the opposite direction. Thus, it seems that the jury on this issue is still out.

Could distinct cortical networks involving S1 cause pain?

Animal studies suggest that there are distinct clusters of neurons within S1, that are confined to deeper layers, that respond only to high intensity stimuli and may be specifically involved in pain (Kenshalo & Douglass 1995). This finding has not been reported in humans, but raises the possibility that expanded S1 receptive fields associated with use may involve different neuronal clusters to those associated with chronic pain. Other animal studies show that amputation can be associated with neuronal sprouting in S1 (Florence et al 1997), similar to neuronal sprouting that occurs in the dorsal horn after peripheral nerve injury (Nakatsuka et al 1999, Woolf et al 1992). As has been observed by Flor (2002) if one was to assume that the somatic representation held within the high-threshold neurons in the deeper layers of S1 was reasonably 'hard wired', which seems possible, then the processes observed in animals could evoke pain in humans. Flor suggests that this would also explain why patients with more intense chronic pain prior to amputation would suffer greater phantom pain after amputation, a relationship that has been reported (Grusser et al 2001, Huse et al 2001).

Obviously, theories such as these are difficult to test in humans and as a result remain to be verified, but they provide theoretical justification for why changes in S1 representation could cause pain. Although the devil's advocate has few friends, the emergence of S1 mania suggests that it is appropriate to present the contrary evidence – data that suggest S1 reorganisation doesn't cause pain.

Evidence that S1 reorganisation doesn't cause pain

The strongest evidence that S1 reorganisation doesn't necessarily cause pain comes from the large number of studies that show substantial and dynamic S1 changes in people who are pain free e.g. (Elbert et al 1998, Elbert & Flor 1999, Elbert et al 1995, Pearce et al 2000, Reddy et al 2002). Review of that literature is well beyond the scope of this paper, but suffice to reemphasise the "use it or lose it" principle that appears to underpin S1 changes and neither increased nor decreased S1 representation is *necessarily* associated with pain.

There are other observations relevant to many of the studies discussed earlier and which warrant a mention here. First, sensory-motor incongruence isn't always associated with pain, for example in focal dystonia there can be marked changes in cortical proprioceptive representations (Elbert et al 1998), yet no pain; our group and others have experimented with wearing prism glasses, applying tendon vibrations that evoke illusions of substantial and sometimes impossible body movements, none of which cause pain (Craske 1977, Gandevia 1985, Moseley 2004).

Second, the Birbaumer et al (1997) study in which the stump was anaesthetized and elimination of pain also reversed S1 changes, and the Soros et al study in which experimental hand pain caused S1 changes (Soros et al 2001) offer compelling evidence that S1 changes may occur in response to pain, rather than as a cause of pain. Third, emerging data that implicate glial mechanisms in the thalamus (Banati 2002), widespread changes in sensory processing probably mediated by thalamic or midbrain structures (Rommel et al. 1999), alterations in processing of somatically-targeted information in CRPS (Moseley 2004b) and in experimentally induced pain (Hudson et al 2005, Moseley et al 2005), raise the possibility that both pain and S1 reorganisation may be epiphenoma of some other process. Regardless, the wealth of literature in this area suggests that the physiological processes that underpin chronic pain are complex and, although S1 reorganisation may play a part, the proposal that chronic pain is caused by S1 reorganisation seems overly simplistic. Simplicity doesn't mean we should disregard it - there may be benefit in exploring new treatments for pain that may tap into some of the systems that underpin cortical changes.

IMPLICATIONS FOR TREATMENT OF PEOPLE WITH CHRONIC PAIN

Despite the gradual emergence of S1 mania, very few attempts have been made to target S1 organisation as a pain treatment strategy. One exception is a clinical trial undertaken, not surprisingly, by Herta Flor's group (Flor et al 2001). In that study, amputees with phantom limb pain took part in a training program in which they had to discriminate the location or intensity of mild cutaneous stimuli applied to the stump. Treatment consisted of a 90 minute session each day for two weeks and patients in the treatment group reported a 60% reduction in phantom pain and also demonstrated reversal of S1 reorganisation.

We are currently undertaking a three-armed randomised controlled trial of sensory discrimination training similar to that outlined by Flor et al (2001), in people with chronic low back pain. Initial data appear promising – improvements in spatial discrimination seem to be matched by reductions in spontaneous and movement-related pain – but definitive conclusions are premature. Another treatment that has gained some support is that of mirror movements for phantom limb pain (Ramachandran & Rogers-Ramachandran 2000) and more recently for CRPS1 (McCabe et al 2003a). The use of mirror movements is based on the sensory-motor incongruence theory formally presented by Harris (1999). It is proposed that by placing the phantom or affected limb behind the mirror, sensory-motor incongruence is removed because visual input involves the mirror image of the unaffected limb. McCabe et al (2003) undertook a controlled trial of mirror movements where CRPS1 patients performed mirror movements between four and nine times per day. There was a gradual but substantial reduction in spontaneous pain (mean change ~ 70 mm on a 100 mm VAS) and in temperature difference between sides (mean change ~ 1.8° C) in those patients with acute or intermediate disease, although those with chronic CRPS1 had no response.

That study provided the first robust evidence that mirror movements may impart pain relief in CRPS1 and corroborates anecdotal data from patients with phantom limb pain (MacLachlan et al 2004, Ramachandran & Rogers-Ramachandran 2000). However, another possible explanation for the effects relates more to activation of cortical mechanisms rather than reconciliation of sensory and motor processes. Our group applied an established principle of psychological and physical training – graded exposure – to people with chronic CRPS1. In two clinical trials, we first established that a motor imagery program, starting with hand laterality recognition, followed by imagined movements and then mirror movements, reduced pain and disability in people with chronic CRPS1 following wrist fracture (Moseley 2004a). We then established that the order of components was important for the effect, which is consistent with graded exposure but not consistent with a simple attentional engagement effect or reconciliation of sensory-motor incongruence (Moseley 2005a).

Although there are only a few documented attempts to directly 'train the brain', this line of investigation and therapeutic approach appears promising and raises the possibility that the proposed mechanism of some successful therapeutic strategies may lie in an effect on cortical changes. For example, electromyographic biofeedback training is established as an effective method to reduce low back pain (McQuay et al 1997), but the effect probably doesn't depend on how muscle activity is changed so much as the fact that patients concentrate on changing it (Blanchard et al 1982, Blanchard et al 1986, Holroyd et al 1984, Holroyd et al 1999). Perhaps the mechanism of effect lies in cortical reorganisation. Could similar mechanisms underpin the effect of specific motor control exercises for spinal pain (Richardson et al 1999) or knee pain (Cowan et al 2003)?

Summary

With the rapid progress in imaging technologies and in our understanding of pain, S1 mania may very well come to be known as the 'thin edge of the wedge'. Not that such a situation would be necessarily bad – there is strong evidence that S1 organisation is different in people with chronic pain and that when S1 organisation returns to normal pain usually resolves. That said, researchers and clinicians alike must exercise caution when interpreting such findings. The evidence that S1 reorganisation causes pain is fragile and there are plenty of examples where S1 reorganisation does not cause pain. It is possible that 'smudging' of S1 fields rather than expansion is important in pain, but again smudging has been observed in people who are pain-free. Rapid development in imaging technology may soon permit researchers to verify such proposals. However, and in any case, the literature seems clear on one thing – that the cortical mechanisms involved in pain are extremely complex, highly variable and dynamic. I suggest that we must balance our creativity and opportunism with measured appraisal of the literature so that we don't end up clearing the forest despite the trees.

Study	Subjects	Finding
(Flor et al 1995)	Phantom limb pain	Extent of S1 shift relates to pain intensity
(Birbaumer et al 1997)	Phantom limb pain	S1 normalisation and pain elimination with regional anaesthesia
(Flor et al 1997)	Back pain	Magnitude of S1 response relates to pain duration but not intensity
(Flor et al 1998)	Phantom limb pain	Extent of S1 shift relates to pain intensity
(Knecht et al 1998)	Phantom limb pain	Extent of S1 shift relates to sensory referral to phantom
(Grusser et al 2001)	Phantom limb pain	Extent of S1 shift relates to pain intensity
(Karl et al 2001)	Phantom limb pain	Extent of S1 shift relates to pain intensity
(Soros et al 2001)	Experimentally induced pain in healthy subjects	S1 shift evoked by pain.
(Juottonen et al 2002)	Complex regional pain syndrome	Extent of S1 shift NOT related to intensity or duration
(Maihofner et al 2003)	Complex regional pain syndrome	Extent of S1 shift related to pain intensity and hyperalgesia
(Giesecke et al 2004)	Back pain	Magnitude of S1 response related to pain intensity
(Maihofner et al 2004)	Complex regional pain syndrome	Extent of S1 normalisation related to pain reduction
(Pleger et al 2004)	Complex regional pain syndrome	Extent of S1 shift related to pain intensity

Table 1. Studies of S1 representation and pain.

Acknowledgements:

Nicole Acerra and Dr Tina Souvlis contributed to concepts presented in this work.
Lorimer Moseley is on leave from the School of Physiotherapy, University of Sydney, Australia.

Reference list

Apkarian AV 1999 Functional Magnetic Resonance Imaging of Pain Consciousness: Cortical Networks of Pain Critically Depend on What is Implied by "Pain". Curr Rev Pain 3:308-315

Banati RB 2002 Brain plasticity and microglia: is transsynaptic glial activation in the thalamus after limb denervation linked to cortical plasticity and central sensitisation? J Physiology-Paris 96:289-299

Birbaumer N, Lutzenberger W, Montoya P et al 1997 Effects of regional anesthesia on phantom limb pain are mirrored in changes in cortical reorganization. J Neurosci 17:5503-5508

Blanchard EB, Andrasik F, Arena JG, Teders SJ 1982 Variation in meaning of pain descriptors for different headache types as revealed by psychophysical scaling. Headache 22:137-139

Blanchard EB, Andrasik F, Appelbaum et al 1986 Three studies of the psychologic changes in chronic headache patients associated with biofeedback and relaxation therapies. Psychosom Med 48:73-83

Braun C, Haug M, Wiech K et al 2002 Functional organization of primary somatosensory cortex depends on the focus of attention. Neuroimage 17:1451-1458

Bromm B 1995 Consciousness, pain, and cortical activity. In: Bromm B, Desmedt JE (Eds). Pain and the brain: from nociception to cognition. Vol. 22. Raven Press, New York 35-60

Byl NN, Merzenich MM, Jenkins WM 1996 A primate genesis model of focal dystonia and repetitive strain injury: I. Learning-induced dedifferentiation of the representation of the hand in the primary somatosensory cortex in adult monkeys. Neurology 47:508-520

Byl NN, McKenzie A, Nagarajan SS 2000 Differences in somatosensory hand organization in a healthy flutist and a flutist with focal hand dystonia: a case report. J Hand Ther 13:302-309

Condes-Lara M, Barrios FA, Romo JR et al 2000 Brain somatic representation of phantom and intact limb: a fMRI study case report. Eur J Pain, 4:239-245

Cowan SM, Bennell KL, Hodges PW et al 2003 Simultaneous feedforward recruitment of the vasti in untrained postural tasks can be restored by physical therapy. J Orthop Res 21:553-558

Craig A 2002 How do you feel? Interoception: the sense of the physiological condition of the body. Nature Rev Neurosci 3:655-666

Craske B 1977 Perception of Impossible Limb Positions Induced by Tendon Vibration. Science 196:71-73

Creac'h C, Henry P, Caille JM, Allard M 2000 Functional MR imaging analysis of pain-related brain activation after acute mechanical stimulation. Am J Neuroradiol 21:1402-1406

Derbyshire SW, Jones AK 1998 Cerebral responses to a continual tonic pain stimulus measured using positron emission tomography. Pain 76:127-135

Derbyshire SW, Jones AK, Devani P et al 1994 Cerebral responses to pain in patients with atypical facial pain measured by positron emission tomography. J Neurol Neurosurg Psychiatry 57:1166-1172

Elbert T, Flor H 1999 Magnetoencephalographic investigations of cortical reorganization in humans. Electroencephalogr Clin Neurophysiol Suppl 49:284-291

Elbert T, Flor H, Birbaumer N, et al 1994 Extensive Reorganization of the Somatosensory Cortex in Adult Humans after Nervous-System Injury. Neuroreport 5:2593-2597

Elbert T, Pantev C, Wienbruch C, et al 1995 Increased cortical representations of the fingers of the left hand in string players. Science, 270:305-307

Elbert T, Candia V, Altenmuller E, et al 1998 Alteration of digital representations in somatosensory cortex in focal hand dystonia. Neuroreport 9:3571-3575

Flor H 2000 The functional organization of the brain in chronic pain. Prog Brain Res 129:313-22

Flor H 2002 The modification of cortical reorganization and chronic pain by sensory feedback. App Psychophysiol Biofeedb 27:215-227

Flor H, Elbert T, Knecht S et al 1995 Phantom-limb pain as a perceptual correlate of cortical reorganization following arm amputation. Nature 375:482-484

Flor H, Braun C, Elbert, T, Birbaumer N 1997 Extensive reorganization of primary somatosensory cortex in chronic back pain patients. Neurosci Lett 224:5-8

Flor H, Elbert T, Muhlnickel W et al 1998 Cortical reorganization and phantom phenomena in congenital and traumatic upper-extremity amputees. Exp Brain Res 119:205-212

Flor H, Denke C, Schaefer M, Grusser S 2001 Effect of sensory discrimination training on cortical reorganisation and phantom limb pain. Lancet 357:1763-1764

Florence SL, Jain N, Kaas JH 1997 Plasticity of somatosensory cortex in primates. Sem Neurosci 9:3-12

Gandevia S 1985 Illusory Movements Produced by Electrical-Stimulation of Low-Threshold Muscle Afferents from the Hand. Brain 108:965-981

Gandevia S 1996 Kinesthesia: roles for afferent signals and motor commands. In: Rothwell L, Shepherd J (Eds.): Handbook of physiology, section 12, Exercise: Regulation and integration of multiple systems. Oxford University Press, New York 128-172

Gandevia S, Phegan C 1999 Perceptual distortions of the human body image produced by local anaesthesia, pain and cutaneous stimulation. J Phys (Lond) 514:609-616

Giesecke T, Gracely RH, Grant MAB et al 2004 Evidence of augmented central pain processing in idiopathic chronic low back pain. Arth Rheumatism 50:613-623

Grusser SM, Winter C, Muhlnickel W et al 2001 The relationship of perceptual phenomena and cortical reorganization in upper extremity amputees, Neuroscience, 102:263-272

Hamann S, Herman RA, Nolan CL, Wallen K 2004 Men and women differ in amygdala response to visual sexual stimuli. Nature Neuroscience 7:411-416

Harris AJ 1999 Cortical origin of pathological pain. Lancet 354:1464-1466

Holroyd KA, Penzien DB, Hursey et al 1984 Change mechanisms in EMG biofeedback training: cognitive changes underlying improvements in tension headache. J Consult Clin Psychol 52:1039-1053

Holroyd KA, Malinoski P, Davis MK, Lipchik GL 1999 The three dimensions of headache impact: pain, disability and affective distress. Pain 83:571-578

Hsieh JC, Meyerson BA, Ingvar M 1999 PET study on central processing of pain in trigeminal neuropathy. Eur J Pain 3:51-65

Hudson M, McCormick K, Zalucki N, Moseley GL 2005 Expectation of pain replicates the effect of pain in a hand laterality recognition task: Bias in information processing toward the painful side? Euro J Pain In press

Huse E, Larbig W, Flor H, Birbaumer N 2001 The effect of opioids on phantom limb pain and cortical reorganization. Pain 90:47-55

Ingvar M 1999 Pain and functional imaging. Philos Trans R Soc Lond B Biol Sci 354:1347-1358

Juottonen K, Gockel M, Silen T et al 2002 Altered central sensorimotor processing in patients with complex regional pain syndrome. Pain 98:315-323

Karl A, Birbaumer N, Lutzenberger W et al 2001 Reorganization of motor and somatosensory cortex in upper extremity amputees with phantom limb pain. J Neurosci 21:3609-3618

Kenshalo DR, Douglass DK 1995 The Role of the Cerebral-Cortex in the Experience of Pain. In: Bromm B, Desmedt JE (Eds) Pain and the Brain. Advances in pain research and therapy Vol. 22. Raven Press, new York 21-34.

Knecht S, Henningsen H, Elbert T et al 1996 Reorganizational and perceptional changes after amputation. Brain 119:1213-1219

Knecht S, Henningsen H, Hohling C et al 1998 Plasticity of plasticity? Changes in the pattern of perceptual correlates of reorganization after amputation. Brain 121:717-724

Knecht S, Soros P, Gurtler S et al 1998a Phantom sensations following acute pain. Pain 77:209-213

MacLachlan M, McDonald D, Waloch J 2004 Mirror treatment of lower limb phantom pain: A case study. Disabil Rehab 26:901-904

Maihofner C, Handwerker HO, Neundorfer B, Birklein F 2003 Patterns of cortical reorganization in complex regional pain syndrome. Neurology 61:1707-1715

Maihofner C, Handwerker HO, Neundorfer B, Birklein F 2004 Cortical reorganization during recovery from complex regional pain syndrome. Neurology 63:693-701

May A, Bahra A, Buchel C, et al 2000 PET and MRA findings in cluster headache and MRA in experimental pain. Neurology 55:1328-1335

McCabe CS, Haigh RC, Halligan PW, Blake DR 2003 Referred sensations in patients with complex regional pain syndrome type 1. Rheumatology 42:1067-1073

McCabe CS, Haigh RC, Ring EFJ et al 2003a A controlled pilot study of the utility of mirror visual feedback in the treatment of complex regional pain syndrome (type 1). Rheumatology 42:97-101

McCabe CS, Haigh RC, Halligan PW, Blake DR 2005 Simulating sensory-motor incongruence in healthy volunteers: implications for a cortical model of pain, Rheumatology 44:509-516

McQuay HJ, Moore RA, Eccleston C, Morley S, Williams AC 1997 Systematic review of outpatient services for chronic pain control. Health Technol Assess 1 i-iv:1-135

Moseley GL 2003 A pain neuromatrix approach to patients with chronic pain. Man Ther 8:130-140

Moseley GL 2004 Cortical issues with rehabilitation and learning. 8th International Congress of the Australian Physiotherapy Association. Adelaide, Australia

Moseley GL 2004a Graded motor imagery is effective for long-standing complex regional pain syndrome. Pain 108:192-198

Moseley GL 2004b Why do people with CRPS1 take longer to recognise their affected hand? Neurology 62:2182-2186

Moseley GL 2005 Distorted body image in complex regional pain syndrome type 1. Neurology In press

Moseley GL 2005a Is successful rehabilitation of complex regional pain syndrome due to sustained attention to the affected limb? A randomised clinical trial. Pain 114:54-61

Moseley GL, Sim DF, Henry ML, Souvlis T 2005 Experimental hand pain delays recognition of the contralateral hand - evidence that acute and chronic pain have opposite effects on information processing? Cog Brain Res. In Press

Nakatsuk, T, Park JS, Kumamoto E et al 1999 Plastic changes in sensory inputs to rat substantia gelatinosa neurons following peripheral inflammation. Pain 82:39-47

Pascual Leone A, Cammarota A, Wassermann EM, et al 1993 Modulation of motor cortical outputs to the reading hand of braille readers. Ann Neurol 34:33-37

Pearce AJ, Thickbroom GW, Byrnes ML, Mastaglia FL 2000 Functional reorganisation of the corticomotor projection to the hand in skilled racquet players. Exp Brain Res 130:238-243

Penfield W, Rasmussen T 1950 The cerebral cortex of man; a clinical study of localization of function. Macmillan, New York

Petrovic P, Petersson KM, Ghatan PH et al 2000 Pain-related cerebral activation is altered by a distracting cognitive task. Pain 85:19-30

Peyron R, Laurent B, Garcia-Larrea L 2000 Functional imaging of brain responses to pain. A review and meta- analysis. Neurophysiol Clin 30:263-288

Pleger B, Tegenthoff M, Schwenkreis P et al 2004 Mean sustained pain levels are linked to hemispherical side-to-side differences of primary somatosensory cortex in the complex regional pain syndrome I. Exp Brain Res 155:115-119

Ramachandran VS, Rogers-Ramachandran D 2000 Phantom limbs and neural plasticity. Arch Neurol 57:317-320

Ramachandran VS, Rogers-Ramachandran D, Stewart M 1992 Perceptual correlates of massive cortical reorganization. Science 258:1159-1160

Ramachandran VS, Stewart M, Rogers-Ramachandran DC 1992a Perceptual correlates of massive cortical reorganization. Neuroreport 3:583-586

Reddy H, Bendahan D, Lee MA et al 2002 An expanded cortical representation for hand movement after peripheral motor denervation. J Neurol Neurosurg Psychiatry 72:203-210

Richardson C, Jull G, Hodges P,Hides J 1999 Therapeutic exercise for spinal segmental stabilization in low back pain. Churchill Livingstone, London

Rommel O, Gehling M, Dertwinkel R et al 1999 Hemisensory impairment in patients with complex regional pain syndrome. Pain 80:95-101

Rubia K, Russell T, Bullmore ET et al 2001 An fMRI study of reduced left prefrontal activation in schizophrenia during normal inhibitory function. Schizophrenia Res 52:47-55

Shira N, Okamoto Y, Mantani T, Yamawaki S 2005 Gender differences in brain activity generated by unpleasant word stimuli concerning body image: an fMRI study. Brit J Psychiat 186:48-53

Soros P, Knecht S, Bantel C, et al 2001 Functional reorganization of the human primary somatosensory cortex after acute pain demonstrated by magnetoencephalography. Neurosci Lett 298:195-198

Sperry R 1950 Neural basis of the spontaneous optokinetic responses produced by visual neural inversion. J Comp Physiol Psychol 43:482-489

Sterr A, Muller MM, Elbert T et al 1998 Perceptual correlates of changes in cortical representation of fingers in blind multifinger Braille readers. J Neurosci 18:4417-4423

Tinazzi M, Zanette G, Polo A, et al 1997 Transient deafferentation in humans induces rapid modulation of primary sensory cortex not associated with subcortical changes: a somatosensory evoked potential study. Neurosci Lett 223:21-24

Von Holst H 1950 Relations between the central nervous system and the peripheral organs. Br J Anim Behav 2:89-94

Woolf CJ, Shortland P, Coggeshall RE 1992 Peripheral nerve injury triggers central sprouting of myelinated afferents. Nature 355:75-78

Yang TT, Gallen C, Schwartz B et al 1994 Sensory Maps in the Human Brain. Nature 368:592-593

19

Muscle Activity and Back Pain

GEORGE A KOUMANTAKIS

Introduction

A significant amount of research has focused on different functional aspects of muscles surrounding the lumbar spine and pelvis under normal pain-free conditions and under acute, chronic pain and post-pain conditions in the lumbopelvic area. Different theories attempt to explain the nature of alterations in muscle activity by examining muscle function under various postural tasks, different time-lengths and additionally under diverse physical and psychological stress situations. The ambiguity in the source of pain in the area (Cavanaugh 1995) presents inherent difficulties as one structure or many in combination may affect the type and duration of altered muscle activation in many different ways.

In order to assess muscle activity, some research has concentrated on monitoring the motor output of certain muscle groups of the thoracolumbar area by measuring their strength output capability. This is an indirect method of muscle assessment and has some disadvantages compared to more detailed muscle activity analysis via the use of electromyography (EMG).

The basic EMG principles have been described in detail in two important textbooks (Basmajian & DeLuca 1985, Kumar & Mital 1996). In brief, the EMG signal can be defined as "the electrical manifestation of the neuromuscular activation associated with a contracting muscle". This signal is rather complex, affected by the anatomical and physiological properties of muscles, the control scheme of the peripheral nervous system and the characteristics of the equipment used to collect the signal (Basmajian & DeLuca, 1985).

A recording of an EMG signal has three types of application. It can be used to:

1. Determine the activation timing of a muscle, in order to appreciate when the excitation to the muscle begins and ends.
2. Estimate the force produced by the muscle (percent of maximum activation).
3. Provide an index of the rate at which a muscle fatigues, through the analysis of the frequency and the time domain of the signal (De Luca 1997). The raw EMG signal from a static contraction can be subjected to two separate types of analysis, one in the frequency domain and the other in the amplitude domain, yielding important information about the endurance characteristics of the underlying muscle (Basmajian & DeLuca 1985).

EMG assessment provides the distinct advantage of being able to concurrently monitor many different muscles. It therefore allows the relative contribution of each muscle involved in a given motor task to be easily assessed (Basmajian & DeLuca 1985). Another advantage, compared to the maximal assessment of strength method, is that EMG monitoring can be performed under submaximal conditions (Kumar & Mital 1996).

Notwithstanding the many advantages that EMG analysis offers in the study of muscle activity, it also possesses several limitations, which at times make interpretation of results problematic. EMG data are relatively repeatable over time in the hands of one experienced examiner (i.e. good intra-raterreliability) but usually less repeatable between different examiners (i.e. poorer inter-rater reliability). Thus, high accuracy is not always easy to achieve (Elfving et al 1999, Koumantakis et al 2001). Also, the EMG activity during certain tasks needs to be "normalised"(standardised) against a set task, due to a number of technical issues concerning EMG data collection. This means that EMG data needs to be repeatedly "benchmarked" at every new application of EMG recording electrodes over the same body area, in order to control for day-to-day variability within the same participant but also between participants (Basmajian & DeLuca 1985). Usually the normalisation procedure followed is against a maximal task, however this may not be valid most of the time. Normalisation against set submaximal tasks may also be achieved (Dankaerts et al. 2004) and may be more valid in low back pain participants that do not, as a rule, activate their muscles fully, to achieve a true maximum effort. Also, EMG data alone cannot always describe the atrophy level of trunk muscles of patients with LBP and some studies have been concerned with the degree of correlation between EMG and muscle biopsy data (Mannion et al 1998).

This review does not attempt to list every EMG analysis technique performed in the trunk muscles, its purpose is to analyse and critically appraise some of the most common techniques that have been widely used and provide some areas for future study.

There are at least four main areas of EMG research that have identified alterations in activity between controls and patients:
1. Amount of muscle activity (Amplitude analysis and Pattern recognition analysis)
2. Load-sharing patterns between muscles (Substitution strategies)
3. Onset of muscle activity
4. Fatigue resistance of muscular system
These will be discussed and interpreted later in the chapter.

An interesting point to consider when interpreting data from EMG studies is the timing when data were obtained. Several aspects of musculoskeletal dysfunction have been identified through cross-sectional (also called *case-control*) studies in low back pain (LBP) patients of varying chronicity. Cross-sectional studies, although relatively informative, provide a "snapshot" view of the LBP problem, at a particular stage of its process. In this sense, these studies are not able to demonstrate whether the pathological phenomena described are short-term and perhaps secondary to the pain experience or more-long term and possibly even a cause of the pain and disability cycle (Bombardier et al 1994). At the moment nearly all experimental evidence suggesting that certain altered neuromuscular activity is evident in LBP patients, fall under this category of study. The development and maintenance of LBP and the role of muscle activity in both may be complex to untangle and prospective studies are necessary to verify such cause and effect relationships. Also, EMG findings should be presented more under a prism of clinical significance, not solely rely on statistical significance, as significent (p) values denoting the latter can often be misleading (Feinstein 1998). Therefore, classification accuracy (sensitivity and specificity) results should be additionally presented in any new study demonstrating more clearly the discriminant ability of those techniques, with clear cut-off values, discriminating between low-back pain participants and pain-free control subjects.

Questions that still remain to be answered involve the different possible alterations in muscle activity of patients with LBP, the timing of these alterations, the most efficient rehabilitation methods to reverse altered muscle activation and finally whether back pain is improving or presents less recurrences only when all possible muscle dysfunctions resolve.

Structure and function of low back neuromuscular system without pain

In order to study muscle activity in patients with LBP, a brief introduction on neuromuscular pain-free function and its interdependence with some structural characteristics of the lumbar spine is required. Theoretically, all muscles surrounding the trunk can contribute to spinal stability. From an *anatomical and biomechanical* point of view, some studies have shown an increased significance of the deep back and abdominal muscles in the provision of active stabilisation to the lumbar spine. Bergmark (1989) utilised a mathematical *optimisation* model to distribute and study muscle forces. He concluded that the deep inter-segmental muscles that have direct attachments to the lumbar vertebrae are more ideally placed to provide inter-segmental stability and belong to the *local* system. Muscles included in this group are transversus abdominis (TrA), multifidus (MULT), internal oblique (IO) and according to some quadratus lumborum (QL) and iliopsoas (ILP) also. These muscles seem ideally situated to protect the lumbar functional spinal units from uncontrolled shearing forces, especially in the neutral zone (Panjabi 1992). Larger muscles are considered to generate movements in the lumbar spine and were classified as the *global* system (Bergmark 1989). Muscles under this category are rectus abdominis (RA), external oblique (EO), longissimus thoracis (LT) and iliocostalis lumborum (IL).

So, under normal pain-free conditions, deeper intersegmental muscles are considered to be primarily involved in stability provision to the inherently unstable non-contractile structures and more superficial trunk muscles are more involved in serving movement requirements of the spine (Basmajian & DeLuca 1985, Panjabi 1992a) as well as serving a secondary stabilising role (Cholewicki & Van Vliet IV 2002, McGill et al 2003).

Activation of the trunk muscles from the nervous system in order to respond to disturbances in equilibrium and stability is not sufficiently understood to permit detailed modelling, however several strategies for activation of the muscular system have been presented as valid: The *optimisation* strategy hypothesis maintains that the nervous system selects the pattern of muscular activity that provides the optimum load distribution parameters between the spinal structures. The *each muscle king* model supports the idea that the activity in a muscle is dependent on its mechanical state, ie. sudden small alterations in the length of the muscle result in an increase in force. Another concept is that the onset of the muscle activity follows a *ready-made programme*. The "real" control mechanism was suggested to be most probably a combination of these three strategies (Bergmark 1989).

The inherent weakness of optimisation models is that they provide the same set of muscle forces for every subject executing the same task, however we are all aware from clinical practice that each patient moves in their own way, dictated by personal and task specific factors. Therefore, optimisation analysis is lacking the biological sensitivity to various possible muscle recruitment and co-contraction patterns (Cholewicki et al 1995). Cholewicki & McGill (1996) in a study combining an EMG-assisted approach with optimisation aimed to quantify the stability of the lumbar spine in vivo. Their calculations showed that the spine would be unstable and therefore prone to injury if the activity of *multifidi* and lumbar erector spinae was zero, even when the controlling forces in large muscles were substantial. Instability could be prevented by increasing the activity (stiffness) of small muscles *bilaterally* to a minimum of 1-3% of a maximum voluntary contraction (MVC) or by increasing passive joint stiffness (Cholewicki & McGill 1996). It is interesting to note that in this study it was reported that there was an ample stability safety margin during tasks that demanded a high muscular effort. However, lighter tasks presented a potential hazard of spinal instability, especially if some reduction in passive joint stiffness was present. It seems that for the efficient handling of stability the nervous system should allocate the appropriate amount of muscle activity to the deep intersegmental muscles for light tasks in particular, but also for heavy tasks, while progressively increasing the activity of the torque producing muscles. All tasks seem to require a similar, low-activation level of background activity from the intersegmental muscular system. Cholewicki & McGill (1996) hypothesised that people employing erroneous motor control skills during light activities sustain and repeat injuries to the same tissues.

Recent *in vivo* data provide some further support to Bergmark's muscle classification system. Daneels et al (2001) have analysed the EMG patterns of activity of muscles belonging to the stabilising and mobilising spinal muscle systems during low-load assymetrical lifts performed by healthy subjects (Danneels et al 2001). Their data showed that muscles from the two systems behaved differently, with mobilisers exibiting a more assymetrical pattern of activation demonstrating task-specific activation patterns, while the stabilisers (IO, MULT and psoas) were activated in symmetric co-contraction patterns even during the performance of assymetric movements. However, joint moments were not measured in this study and therefore the functional subdivision between the muscles investigated could only be postulated, thus not precluding global muscles also from a (global) stabilising role.

Perhaps the most important strategy employed by the neuromuscular system to control stability is *co-contraction*. (Crisco & Panjabi 1990). These states are directly related to the agonist-antagonists relative activity controlled by the nervous system. In situations where both agonists and antagonists are activated simultaneously (co-activation) the stiffness of the joint will be high and the net torque low. If the antagonists are relaxed (reciprocal inhibition) the opposite will apply (Basmajian & DeLuca 1985).

The neural control system seems to make use of the co-contraction stabilising strategy in order to provide appropriate support to the passive structures. At least three different co-activation patterns are considered.

1. The first one is between the abdominal and back muscles. This pattern of activation has been observed prior to sudden loading of the torso (Lavender et al 1993) and also in rapid upper limb (Hodges & Richardson 1996) and lower limb (Hodges & Richardson 1997) movements, inducing trunk perturbations. A high level of antagonistic co-activation of the trunk musculature has been reported for isometric contractions in neutral trunk postures. Thelen et al (1995) estimated that co-contractions were contributing 16-19 % to the sum of muscle forces at the L3-4 level, during attempted extension of the trunk (Thelen et al 1995). Granata & Marras (2000) have recently confirmed that co-contraction between flexors and extensors is associated with a 12-18% increase in spinal compression, accompanied by a 34-64% increase in spinal stability (Granata & Marras 2000). Therefore, this strategy appears to have an adequate cost/benefit ratio.

2. The second co-contraction strategy is between the back muscles of either side (right-left). An experimental study of muscle activity in standing showed that about 75% of subjects used only their back muscles to counteract the force of gravity. The rest used mainly abdominal muscles, which might have been a manifestation of an overall different posture (Asmussen & Klaussen 1962). Back muscles are characterised as anti-gravity, postural (phasic) muscles, always bilaterally activated during movement in the sagittal plane to control and guide movement. Some differences in activity of the transversospinal muscles at the same levels has been noted during quiet sitting, standing and with movements in the sagittal plane. Jonsson (1970) explained these differences of electrical activity as being manifestations of postural assymetry (Jonsson 1970).

3. The third co-contraction strategy concerns the relative activation patterns between the stabilising and mobilising muscles employed in a particular task. Vink et al (1988) studied the relationship between force development and rectified & averaged surface EMG (RA-SEMG) of the multifidus, longissimus and iliocostalis muscles, under isometric conditions in standing. Muscles were activated bilaterally and the force to EMG relationship was close to linear for multifidus and curvilinear for the other two muscles. The results suggested that the activity of the multifidi increased proportionally during

increasing force exertions, signifying a possible postural role of those muscles, especially in counteracting forces in the sagittal plane. The other two more laterally placed muscles increased their activity mainly above 50% of the maximum force exertion, denoting a movement-related activation of those muscles (Vink et al 1988).

Even more significant co-contraction patterns are present during isometric lateral bending and axial twisting exertions of the trunk. Thelen et al (1995) calculated co-contraction moments during both activities to be 2-3 times greater than co-activation patterns in the sagittal plane. Consequently, the loading of lumbar joints associated with such torques is much higher than for equivalent trunk isometric extension moments. McGill (1991) proposed that the high levels of muscle co-activity observed during the generation of isometric axial torques may suggest that stabilisation of the lumbar joints is critical, because it is achieved at the expense of torque production (McGill 1991).

Co-contraction, therefore, is a complex muscle activation strategy, present during several different spinal movements. The contributory role of the deep trunk muscles in spinal stability, primarily in the sagittal but also in other planes of movement, is deemed important on the basis of these experimental findings. However, more recently, it has been demonstrated with use of EMG-assisted biomechanical models that in healthy volunteers performing a variety of stabilisation exercises the relative contribution of many muscles was important for appropriate exercise execution and also that the relative contribution of each muscle was dependent on the individual moment requirements of each exercise (McGill et al 2003). Very similar findings have also been reported, whereby stability was equally compromised by sequentially removing the contribution of different muscles active in a number of certain motor tasks (Cholewicki & Van Vliet IV 2002, McGill et al 2003). These authors are encouraging a view of stability as a dynamic objective of appropriate and safe movement execution.

The role of continuous muscle support to the passive spinal structures has also been emphasised. The anti-gravity function of the back muscles dictates that endurance capacity may be an important parameter for those muscles (Kalimo et al 1989, Mannion 1999).

Skeletal muscles consist of two main fibre types, according to their contractile properties. Type I (slow-twitch, ST) fibres have a large potential for endurance and type II (fast-twitch, FT) have a capacity for forceful contractions (Jones & Round 1990). Indeed, a number of studies have shown that in healthy subjects the cross-sectional area (CSA) of individual ST fibres is larger than the FT fibres in the paravertebral muscles, with the mean type I/II number of fibres ratio between them generally in favour of type I (Mannion et al 1997, Sirca & Kostevc 1985, Thorstensson & Carlson

1987). The fact that type I fibres in the paraspinals have larger diameters than type II is in contrast with extremity and abdominal muscles - except the transversus abdominis (Hägmark 1979) - where the FT fibres generally have larger diameters (Jørgensen et al 1993). The increase in relative size of type I fibres in the paraspinals appears to be an adaptive mechanism to resist fatigue (Mannion 1999).

Maximal methods of assessment: Muscle strength & classical endurance performance

Strength *performance* measurement, either isokinetically or isometrically, is a widely used method of assessment. Strength is defined as "the ability of a muscle or a muscle group to generate a force or a moment of force about a joint or body axis" (Smidt 1994). This definition, however, *does not* equate to strength performance, as strength output is dependent on several parameters (physiological and psychological).

Most of the studies in healthy subjects conclude that the trunk extensors can generate the largest torque, followed in order by the trunk flexors, trunk side-flexors and trunk rotators (Beimborn & Morrissey 1988). Several studies have shown that LBP patients present with lower strength values for the back and/or abdominal muscles (Grabiner & Jeziorowski 1992, Kishino et al 1985, Mayer et al 1985, Pope et al 1985). As previously indicated, low trunk strength does not seem to predispose to LBP development. Such trunk muscle weakness has initially been attributed to generalised muscle fibre atrophy of the paraspinals, documented in chronic LBP populations.

Other studies tested both strength and fatigue development in the paraspinal muscles. Suzuki & Endo (1983) found extensor and flexor strength and flexor endurance to be decreased in LBP subjects compared to controls. Similar studies though have shown that maximum strength was almost unaltered in chronic low back pain (CLBP), but endurance capacity was reduced for the extensors, (Holmström et al 1992, Nicolaisen & Jørgensen 1985, Roy et al 1989) or both the extensor and flexor muscle groups (Ito et al 1996).

Generally, assessment of muscle strength has produced inconsistent results in the literature. Low trunk strength results have been explained either in terms of generalised whole-body deconditioning arising from LBP or behavioural factors (fear of injury) (Lee et al 1995). Strength assessment has more recently been clearly recognised to be influenced by psychological parameters such as excessive illness behaviour (3-5 Waddell signs) (Hirsch et al 1991), fear of movement/ (re-) injury (Vlaeyen et al 1995), self-efficacy beliefs (Estlander et al 1994, Lackner & Carosella 1999) and pain anticipation (Al-Obaidi et al 2000). Beimborn & Morrissey (1988) point out that pain may interfere with the ability of a subject to produce a maximum voluntary contraction (MVC) and Mannion et al (1996) calculated that pain may also interfere in endurance assessments involving prolonged contractions to complete exhaustion. Thus, they suggest that classical strength and endurance tests may actually be a measure of pain tolerance rather than muscle function. All these factors may explain the widely overlapping sets of data between healthy (non-LBP) and LBP participants, as identified by large reviews of the trunk strength assessment literature (Coulter & Langridge 1997, Newton & Waddell 1993, Smidt 1994)

Classical measures of strength and endurance can only be considered "gross" measures of functional capability. Due to the large number of muscles surrounding the trunk and their unique architecture, it is simplistic to use generalised measures such as these to infer about complex neuromuscular phenomena involved in strength generation and fatigue resistance. Van Dieën et al (1993) has demonstrated in a small study involving 7 healthy participants that in those subjects with the longest endurance times there was a large shift of activity between the paraspinal muscles (Van Dieën et al 1993). These "load-sharing" phenomena may complicate paraspinal muscle fatigue or strength measurement and can be analysed in more detail with EMG.

It can be concluded that muscle *strength* and classical *endurance* assessments are inaccurate measures of the true maximal performance of the trunk muscles as well as indirect measures of the muscle activation required. This is for two reasons:
1. Muscle strength performance is not only dependent on actual muscle state but also on pain and psychology (willingness to perform).
2. It is uncertain which set of muscle synergies, at what timing and especially for how long - are contributing to muscle strength performance.

Maximal muscle *strength* performance measurement is only giving information re maximally achievable activation states of the neuromuscular system, while most every-day activities for most LBP sufferers are submaximal.
Two possible useful reasons for measuring maximal muscle strength or performance are:
1. For research purposes. For example, in prospective studies analysing the role of muscle strength and classical endurance as a predisposing factor in LBP development. Maximal muscle performance would therefore be assessed in initially healthy participants that are likely to perform close to their maximum strength levels.

349

2. As a possible screening tool for initial employment or for return to work after a low back injury in individuals having to deal with heavy and repetitive load handling.

However, it would be unwise to routinely test it in the majority of our patients. Here, it is important to note that prospective studies have shown no predictive effect of strength in the development of LBP (Adams et al 1999, Leino et al 1987) but that decreased strength is rather a consequence of LBP and specifically part of the deconditioning effect arising from it (Mannion 1999).

Some predictive value of classical paraspinal muscle endurance has been reported in two prospective studies, although the particular test used seemed to be more predictive for a subgroup of poor performers only. This test, called the Biering-Sørensen (BS) test, has been described as a useful measure for predicting first time occurrence of LBP in men (Biering-Sørensen 1984; Luoto et al. 1995). The test measures the time a person can sustain the prone alignment of the upper body with a static contraction of the back muscles, while firmly strapped from the pelvis downwards to an examination table (Biering-Sørensen 1984). Good isometric back muscle endurance was found to prevent first time occurrence of back pain in men only (Biering-Sørensen 1984). Luoto et al (1995) confirmed and extended Biering Sørensen's findings by demonstrating that fatigue in both men and women is a risk factor only for those subjects in the lowest performance tertile (Luoto et al 1995). However, Gibbons et al (1997) were not able to demonstrate any predictive effect of endurance time with this test in a smaller scale study (Gibbons et al 1997).

The four main areas of EMG research mentioned earlier will now be discussed. Recall that these were:
1. Amount of muscle activity (Amplitude analysis and Pattern recognition analysis)
2. Load-sharing patterns between muscles (Substitution strategies)
3. Onset of muscle activity
4. Fatigue resistance of muscular system

Alterations in the normal amount of muscle activity (Amplitude analysis & Pattern recognition analysis)

This is detected with EMG by performing 'amplitude' analysis of the EMG signal, denoting the ratio of activation of a certain muscle during a movement or a static posture over the activation of the same muscle during a maximal task. With this method characterisation of muscles as 'hyper-active', 'hypo-active' or even 'inhibited' have been attempted. However, different studies, mostly of case-control design, have reported results ranging across the full spectrum of possible muscle altered activity, as reviewed elsewhere (Dolce & Raczynski 1985, Fryer et al 2004, Fryer et al 2004a, Van Dieen et al 2003).

From a physiological point of view, contrasting effects of *spinal pathology* (pain, injury and degeneration) on muscle activity have been reported. For example, in large enough doses, some chemical mediators of inflammation can be neurotoxic (Cavanaugh et al 1997), and hence have a possible inhibitory effect on proprioceptive signals which then leads to decreased muscle activation.

Indahl et al (1997) described a complex reflex neuronal network in a porcine lumbar spine model between the disc, the facet joints and surrounding dorsal musculature. In their experiment, saline injections affecting proprioceptive discharge from the facet joint capsule were shown to decrease paraspinal muscle activation elicited by electrical stimulation of the disc (Indahl et al 1997). In contrast, electrical stimulation of the the joint capsule produced reflex multifidus activity on the same side and segmental level, whereas unilateral annulus stimulation produced activity on both sides and at different levels. Other researchers have also shown increased EMG activity (muscle spasms) in the multifidus muscle provoked by mechanical deformations or electrical stimulation of spinal ligaments in animal as well as human models (Solomonow et al 1998, Stubbs et al 1998, Williams et al 2000). Indahl et al (1997) concluded that joint capsule sprain could activate the paraspinal musculature and that LBP could be due to a combination of pain from injured structures and long-standing contraction of the multifidus muscles. However, this latter idea that pain in the spine is myogenically enhanced through muscle spasms limiting the blood circulation in an already painful area, the *spasm-pain-spasm* model, has gradually fallen out of favour. Certain research findings that weaken this model are the failure of the majority of studies to demonstrate elevated EMG activity at rest in pain patients compared to pain free participants and where increased EMG activity was present it was insufficient to cause increase in the levels of intramuscular pressure able to reduce muscle circulatory perfusion and thus lead to pain (Watson 2002).

351

More research findings seem to support the *"pain-adaptation model"*, although not unequivocally (Van Dieen et al 2003a). This model is suggesting that, as an adaptation to pain, EMG activity in agonist muscles during movement (ie. the extensors if trunk extension is performed concentrically) is reduced, but increased in antagonist muscles. In so doing the force production over a painful joint may reduce and also the range and velocity of movent causing pain will decrease (Lund et al 1991). High-threshold sensory afferents were proposed to regulate this model of altered activation via a phasic modulatory effect of the excitatory and inhibitory interneurons they supply. This was considered to be a reflex adaptation to pain (Lund et al 1991). It has subsequently been shown that chemical products of inflammation in the facet joints (Cavanaugh et al 1997), or intramuscular injection of bradykinin into the paraspinals (Pedersen et al 1997), will increase the excitatory state of the fusimotor system innervating the muscle spindles. Also, certain psychological states like fear can lead to increase fusimotor drive, a phenomenon that has been described as "fusimotor set" (Prochazka & Hulliger 1988).

The *flexion-relaxation phenomenon* is a term that describes the complete cessation of activity of the paraspinal muscles in full forward flexion, when the trunk is fully 'suspended' from the passive tension of the posterior ligamentous system combined with the passive tension of the paraspinal muscles. A number of studies have convincingly shown that the normal flexion-relaxation phenomenon dissapears in full forward flexion when back pain is present. In other words, the paraspinal muscles remain contracted when they would normally relax. This effect still occurs and is not diminished even when the full active range of flexion is achieved in LBP subjects or in subjects under experimentally-induced pain conditions (Kaigle et al 1998, Watson et al 1997, Zedka et al 1999)! Most authors propose that the increased paraspinal muscle activation is a protective response (reflex or voluntary) to some underlying injury of a spinal structure.

Among the various propositions of the mechanisms regulating this phenomenon two additional ones have been put forward in the literature: In a study that applied an experimental pain model to uninjured pain-free human subjects (injection of saline into the erector spinae), it was shown that pain caused similar adaptations to those described in the 'pain-adaptation model' (no paraspinal muscle relaxation in full flexion, decreased activity during re-extension and decreased velocity and range of trunk motion). This paraspinal response, however, was *not voluntary* because the response from the paraspinals could not be overcome when participants were asked to move faster or farther in the range of flexion. It was also *not a simple reflexively-mediated phenomenon*, as the changes in EMG activity were not associated with an increased gain of the paraspinals stretch reflex. Interestingly, these muscular adaptations to the pain were *considered to be alterations in the whole organisation of the neuronal circuitry,* with pain signals arising from any lumbar structure transmitted to the paraspinal motorneurones through a common channel, making the muscle work in a 'pain mode' to protect the spine from extreme movement (Zedka et al 1999).

This is in line with the view of Panjabi (1992) that "dysfunction" may arise for several painful conditions (injury, physiological degeneration or disease) in *any of three subsystems* (passive stability, active stability and neural control). It has been proposed that the nervous system attempts to correct the dysfunction by either:

a) An immediate response from other subsystems to successfully compensate. This response results in normal function.

b A long term adaptation response of one or more subsystems, resulting in normal function but with an altered stabilising system. This option may accelerate the degeneration of the system and also manifest as an increase in *muscle fatigue* due to over-activity of certain components of the muscular system, trying to compensate .

If these alterations cannot adequately compensate for the dysfunction, an injury to one or more components of any subsystem is hypothesised to follow, leading to overall system dysfunction and possibly LBP (Panjabi 1992.

Without precluding the above hypothesis, Watson et al (1997) offered an expanded viewing for the explanation of the flexion-relaxation phenomenon, demonstrating that *the hyperactivity observed in some muscles may be psychologically mediated* as it strongly correlated to fear-avoidance and self-efficacy beliefs in a chronic LBP population that they tested. This corroborates the biopsychosocial viewing of LBP and provides similar findings with previous research showing that pshychological fears and anxiety states increase the activation (Flor et al 1992) or reduce the ability for relaxation (Vlaeyen et al 1999) of muscles in the low back area of chronic LBP subjects. These influences of psychological state to EMG activity are believed to be a more long-term adaptation of the human organism, enhancing the initial influence of the re-organisation of the nervous system to motor output, which starts in the acute stage of symptoms.

Other studies have dealt with the analysis of a whole 'pattern' of activation (pattern recognition analysis) under more dynamic conditions. This was in order to reveal whether muscle usage patterns were altered in dynamic activities. Such studies have used standardised functional movements, concentrating on the temporal characteristics of EMG (looking to see whether certain muscles were 'hyper'- or 'hypo-active' during certain periods of the movement cycle). Analysis of EMG activity during normal walking revealed that 'out of phase' activity-increased when muscles acted as antagonists and reduced when acting as agonist (Arendt-Nielsen et al

1995). "Decoupling" (out of phase) patterns were also identified for the paraspinal muscles during dynamic high load isokinetic contractions of these muscles (Grabiner et al 1992). However, for EMG activity during flexion, extension & lateral bending tasks poor sensitivity was reported in a small sample size (Lariviere et al 2000).

Finally, recent research studies have started to consider changes in the motor output during the performance of several different tasks. Recent reviews conclude that the changes observed are probably task-dependent, related to the individual problem the body has to solve during a particular movement, and therefore highly variable between but also within individuals (McGill et al 2003, Van Dieen et al 2003a). Under this view, the changes noted are functional, reducing the probability of mechanical stresses to painful tissues by limiting range of movement and providing stabilisation of the spine (Van Dieen et al 2003a). To come to this conclusion with relative certainty, many different motor tasks have to be compared within and between subjects and many muscles have to be considered in order to assess their relative contribution within each of the tasks analysed. This has been attempted in some of the studies presented under the three EMG analysis methods that follow.

Load-sharing patterns between muscles (Substitution strategies)

As described in the previous section, both hyperactivity and hypoactivity have been reported in muscles surrounding the lumbar spine under clinical and experimental pain conditions. However, each movement or maintained posture in the low back activates several muscles, each having a different contribution to the execution of a given motor task. Therefore, it is possible for different muscles co-activated in a motor task to present differential alterations due to pain in the area, irrespective of their role as agonists or antagonists, and there is support for this hypothesis. There are theories as to the patterns these alterations in activation follow and these are presented here. Usually the relative activation of synergistic muscles are presented as ratios (percentage of activation of one muscle against the activation of another).

In healthy subjects, co-activation of both stabilising and mobilising muscles is the norm (Arokoski et al 1999, Ng & Richardson 1994), with some similar findings reported in patients also (Flicker et al 1993). There is some evidence that the empirically observed substitution strategies in the back muscular system occur in LBP patients. The "muscle substitution" theory suggests that when a muscle or group of muscles is weakened there is a tendency for subtle shifts in the patterns of motor activity, enabling the synergistic muscles to generate the forces required for functional tasks (Edgerton et al

1996, Panjabi 1992a). Such deviations from the normal activation pattern due to possible "inhibition" in certain muscles could, according to Panjabi (1992), cause fatigue in the active compensation muscles. Evidence of these changes, both between trunk muscle synergies in the back muscles (Edgerton et al 1996) and even within segmental sections of a single muscle (Lindgren et al 1993) have been detected with EMG.

Edgerton et al (1996) have examined altered motor control patterns for the back extensors in several relatively low-demand physiological postures (Edgerton et al 1996) (figure 1). These investigations reveal that such patterns may be influenced by several factors, such as nociceptive input to the spinal cord, a deficit in force generating capacity of selected muscles due to tissue injury or conscious/subconscious re-education of the motor system as a means of adapting to or accommodating pain. Also, they forewarn that investigations of muscle ratios can be potentially complex as one or both EMG amplitudes could contribute to an aberrant ratio.

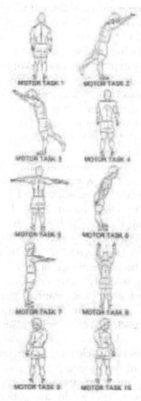

Figure 1. EMG activity patterns from 7 muscle pairs under 9 low-demand physiological postures(Reprinted with permission from Edgerton et al (1996) *Int J Rehabil Health*, 2, page 4).

Edgerton et al (1996) maintained that in order to detect such shifts, which most probably reflect changes in neural inputs to the motorneuron pools responsible for specific motor task generations, a number of carefully set criteria should be adhered to: many muscle pairs should be recorded (they recommend 7 pairs), in a number of motor tasks (9 tasks); for a muscle group to be categorised as hypo- or hyper-active in a motor task, the ratio between it and at least two muscle groups must be aberrant; a muscle group identified as having altered muscle recruitment patterns must exibit either hypo-/hyper-activity in *at least* 3 motor tasks. Of course, reproducibility of the methods employed should be high (Edgerton et al 1996). Analysis of the data from this classification scheme provided a specificity of 90% (correct identification of healthy subjects) and a sensitivity of 70% (correct identification of patients with LBP), with an overall classification accuracy of 88%.

Similar alterations in the activation ratio between the IO and RA have also been identified, using one motor task (bilateral leg-lift from supine lying) (O'Sullivan et al 1997). The validity of these findings is reduced though, as these aberrant ratios could only be demonstrated when the non-normalised EMG data were used but not with normalised data to a submaximal task. The difficulties of normalising data when a substitution strategy is present between two muscles may explain the findings of this study. Here, if motor output from both is equally affected an imbalance may well be revealed during the particular manoeuvre that is used for normalisation, hence the "imbalance" is concealed due to the fact that the relative activation of those two muscles remains similar in all examined tasks. Note that none of the criteria set by Edgerton (1996), that may have minimised these technical problems, were applied and the classification accuracy of the method was not reported. Intrestingly, in a subsequent study the same research group presented data suggesting that with specific stabilisation training these "abnormal" motor recruitment ratios normalised (O'Sullivan et al 1998).

A more recent study(Van Dieen et al 2003), has presented somewhat opposite results regarding the direction of 'imbalance' between the deep and superficial abdominal muscles found by O'Sullivan et al (1997). Trunk muscle recruitment in 16 patients with LBP and 16 matched control subjects were compared during the performance of slow trunk motions about the neutral posture and progressively increasing isometric contractions while seated upright. Ratios of electromyographic amplitudes and estimated moment contributions of antagonist over agonist muscles and of segmentally inserting muscles over muscles inserting on the thorax and pelvis were calculated. In addition, model simulations were performed to assess the effect of changes in muscle recruitment on spinal stability. Results denoted that the ratios of antagonist over agonist, and of lumbar over thoracic erector spinae electromyographic amplitude and estimated moment contributions were greater in the patients than in the control subjects. In other words, this latter study indicated that the relative activation of the deep muscles was higher compared to the more superficial

356

in patients than in control participants. These changes were explained as most likely functional, to effectively increase spinal stability (Van Dieen et al 2003). Note that the isometric nature of contraction in the O'Sullivan et al. study and the partly isotonic data in the Van Dieen et al (2003) experiment, as well as the different muscles tested precludes a direct comparison of those two studies.

Onset of muscle activity analysis

Another aspect of muscle activation research assesses neuromuscular control state, i.e. it evaluates rapid, pre-programmed responses of the nervous system to external or internal perturbations applied to the body that increase active stability of the joints through the appropriate muscle recruitment. The nervous system deals with the imposed stability requirements through two main mechanisms: *anticipatory postural adjustments* (APAs) which occur before or up to 50-70 milliseconds (msecs) after the onset of activity in a prime mover muscle (feed-forward control) and *reflex responses* which occur after 70 msecs (feedback control) (Bouisset & Zattara 1990). Other authors, however, accept less strict limits for APAs and suggest that these are present up to 100 msecs after activity detection in a prime mover/movement initiation, with feedback strategies (postural reactions) coming into play after this time-point (Alaranta et al 1994). Panjabi (1992) mainly referred to the feedback (reflex) mechanisms for stability provision. Most probably, both mechanisms work in parallel (Bergmark 1989) and have been the object of several EMG studies.

One of the first studies to show an alteration of the normal APAs activation patterns in patients with LBP was performed about a decade ago. The onset of activity in several abdominal (TrA, IO, EO, RA) and one back muscle (MULT) during *rapid* upper limb (UL) movements was monitored in 15 patients with LBP and 15 matched control subjects, using fine-wire and surface EMG techniques (Hodges & Richardson 1996). Primary findings indicated that TrA was invariably the first active muscle irrespective of UL movement direction in pain-free subjects (*24-39 msecs* before the onset of the UL prime mover activity), whereas its activity was significantly delayed in the patient group with all movements. Differences in delay between the two groups were *between 61-165 msecs*. Onset of trunk muscle activity up to 50 msecs after the onset of the prime mover activity was regarded as anticipatory (feed-forward) and any onset beyond that cut-off point were interpreted as true delays in anticipatory responses (Hodges & Richardson 1996).

In pain-free participants, the other abdominals and MULT were all activated between 9-84 msecs after the onset of deltoid muscle activity, with the exception of IO (-11 msecs) for one of the movements. Earlier contraction of MULT was seen with UL flexion (9.3 msecs pain-free; 11.0

msecs LBP) than extension (74.1 pain-free; 69.7 LBP) and this is consistent with the maintenance of the alignment of the trunk against the reactive force producing spinal flexion to the spine. Surprisingly, MULT was found to be active earlier in the LBP group with UL abduction (56.8 pain-free; 16.9 LBP). For UL flexion only, generalised delays in all LBP subjects' abdominal muscles were present, being statistically significant for IO, EO but not for RA due to large standard deviation in the patient group (Hodges & Richardson 1996).

It would be reasonable to assume that with *increasing load* demands on the lumbar spine stabilising system, the motor strategies would become more pronounced. Indeed, a second study applying the same principle as the above experiment was tested for rapid lower limb (LL) movements in 15 healthy subjects (Hodges & Richardson 1997). In this experiment, *all* trunk muscles analysed (stabilisers *and* mobilisers) formed part of the feed-forward control mechanism, all contracting before or concurrently with the prime mover for the three movements analysed. The activation of TrA, IO and EO also were independent of movement direction of the LL. Again, the response of TrA was much faster than all other muscles and significantly faster than the ones documented in the UL experiment (reaction times between -113 and -70 msecs). MULT displayed a longer reaction time associated with hip extension compared with the other two directions of movement, which is consistent with the need for this muscle to control the trunk flexion moment (Hodges & Richardson 1997). A subsequent case-control study utilising 3 rapid LL movements has shown generalised delays in most muscles in chronic LBP subjects, with significant delays in TrA present in all three movements, whereas in the other muscles there were delays in one (IO, RA) or two (ES) of the movements (Hodges & Richardson 1998). Despite these initial interesting findings, it was difficult to accept how such small delays could be the primary source of LBP in the patients tested. This concern is reflected in a commentary by Hasan (1997) who suggested that because of the large inertias of the skeletal segments involved in the LL studies, an onset timing difference of a few tens of msecs would not have a major kinematic significance (Hasan 1997).

In another investigation involving patients, Hodges and Richardson (1999) have found these generalised delays (in TrA, IO and ES) in APAs to be related to multidirectional movement of the UL *under both rapid and functional speeds* and also *decreased frequency of response* from the abdominals in the patient group. These delays in the onset of activity were less pronounced between-groups for functional than with rapid speeds of limb movement. Hodges et al (2003) has further employed the onset of activity in a number of trunk muscles during conditions of increased task complexity. Results of this study showed that delayed reaction time of TrA in patients with LBP in relation to healthy participants was the most consistent effect of increased task complexity, indirectly denoting a change in the organisation of the postural response of TrA (Hodges 2001).

The role of the deep segmental fascicles of multifidus (MULT) in APAs was clarified in subsequent research that differentiated between the superficial and the deep fibres of this muscle, with the deep fibres contributing to the feedforward control of movement (Moseley et al 2002). Therefore, the deep fibres of MULT with TrA were invariably activated before or almost concurrently with the prime-mover muscle.

A more recent study was concerned with the effect of acute experimentally induced pain on the feedforward onset and amount of recruitment of trunk muscles (Hodges et al 2003). A variable change in the onset and amplitude of most trunk muscles was reported, with activation of TrA consistently reduced in amplitude or delayed. The other muscles monitored presented variable responses. Interestingly, in this study the onset of deep multifidus was earlier after the painful injection. Also, although delayed, the onset of activity of TrA was within normal APA limits (before the onset of activity of prime mover directly after injection of hypertonic saline and only 2.6 milsecs delayed on average 20 minutes after the painful injection). Those statistically significant EMG alterations in healthy participants, which were still within 'normal' feedforward control limits were possibly due to differences between experimentally induced muscle pain and acute/chronic pain conditions arising from deep spinal structures.

Finally, the authors attributed the between-subject variability in motor responses to pain to either the non-homogeneity of clinical LBP, but perhaps more correctly, since the injection site was the same for all subjects, to factors associated with the variability in the experience and report of LBP and/or the variability in possible responses from the motor system under different conditions and motor tasks . According to the authors, even the splinting phenomenon provided by the more superficial muscles might have led to a decreased need for TrA to spinal control contribution, offering a 'mechanical' explanation to their results.

Recent experimental findings additionally indicate that alterations in recruitment of TrA seem to be present in pelvic pain patients also, presumably due to the contribution of TrA in the stability enhancement of the sacroiliac joints (Hungerford et al 2003, O'Sullivan et al 2002).

Another study (Moseley et al 2004a) examined the differential effect of experimentally induced pain and attention-demanding and stressful tasks on the reaction times of several trunk muscles. It showed that stress as well as pain can delay the reaction times of several of the deep trunk muscles. Interestingly, far more muscles were affected by stress (TrA, deep and superficial MULT, IO and EO) than by pain only (delay only in TrA) (Moseley et al 2004a). A further study on the same participants (Moseley et al 2004) examined the effect of *anticipation* of painful stimuli on alterations in APAs and showed that anticipation of pain led to *delayed* activation of the *deep* trunk muscles and *increased* the activity of at least one *superficial* trunk muscle. Therefore, psychological factors have again been shown to alter motor control strategies of the nervous system.

359

In studies examining the effect of pain on the feedback control mechanisms of the low-back neuromuscular system, some similarities were observed to the studies concerned with alterations in APAs. Two studies have been performed, in which participants with LBP or with pain under remission and pain-free participants were pulling isometrically against a cable in trunk flexion, extension, and lateral bending directions. Load was applied to subjects' trunks by suddenly releasing the cable during each maximal pull performed. The first study involved 17 subjects with chronic LBP and 17 controls (Radebold et al 2000). The second involved 17 athletes in the recovery stage of an acute LBP injury compared with 17 pain-free athletes (Cholewicki et al 2002). Individuals with chronic LBP and those recovering from acute LBP exhibited similar neuromotor control alterations: a delay in the shut-off of their agonists and switch-on of their antagonists in response to the cable release in each of the 3 directions. Furthermore, in comparison with healthy controls, patients with chronic LBP demonstrated that a significantly smaller number of trunk muscles responded to sudden loading.

However, it has to be pointed out that other research findings suggest that in CLBP patients functional speed of movement execution is generally decreased, either due to patient deconditioning or due to the 'distracting' effects of pain (Luoto et al 1996, Luoto et al 1998, Marras & Wongsam 1986). Therefore, it may be unrealistic to suggest that dysfunctional components in the stabilising muscles' onset of activity are maintaining the LBP, especially when these muscles have been primarily identified as being activated during rapid movement tests. It just does not take into account the 'normal' physiological speed range of CLBP sufferers.

This type of research may be more applicable to the study of risk factors for re-injury in special populations, like those involved in athletics (Cholewicki et al 2002). Athletes are often involved in sudden purturbations that may be of sufficient loading to set off new LBP episodes. Another limitation of these studies is that the innervation zones of TrA, IO and EO have not been identified and thus the distance between these points and the electrode detection surfaces is unknown and possibly different between the two groups of participants. However, the delays described, apparent even in studies that have used healthy participants and experimental pain was induced, seem consistent enough to overcome this detail.

Since alterations in the motor control of the deep stabilising muscles have been shown to occur in unselected groups of patients with low back pain even after the remission of their symptoms, it may be proposed that all low back pain patients will benefit from stabilisation exercise re-training. However, this hypothesis has not been confirmed by our group's research which we conducted on patients with recurrent non-specific low back pain. We found very similar overall between-group results in a randomised controlled trial (RCT) that investigated the adjunct effect of trunk stabilization exercises when added to general trunk muscle exercises for a number of outcome measures (pain, disability, back function and psychological state) (Koumantakis et al 2005, Koumantakis et al 2005a). Two other studies that have shown a superiority of trunk muscle stabilisation re-training have been conducted in specific populations of LBP patients but they have not compared stabilisation training against another standardised form of trunk muscle training (Hides et al 1996, O'Sullivan et al 1997). Therefore, stabilisation muscle exercise re-training may be more relevant for populations with overt instability manifestations.

It is important to state that at this time, no study has so far demonstrated that LBP amelioration is directly dependent on normalisation of activity onset in stabilising muscles. Some preliminary work in two individual patients did not fully support reversal of these patterns to 'normal' levels after intensive training with specific stabilising exercises (Jull et al 1998). Another study looking at the improvement of feedback activation of paraspinal muscles after a 2-week rehabilitation programme has demonstrated an improvement in the onset of activation in less than half (45%) of the participants (Panagiotacopulos et al 1998). Furthermore, studies looking only at the onset of activity of the stabilising muscles do not address the issue of whether this early activation in healthy subjects is of sufficient magnitude to provide the desired stability (Hasan 1997). The theoretical purpose of early activation of the stabilising muscles is to contain abnormal ranges of joint movement, yet no human in-vivo study has clearly shown such a relationship under functional demands. Finally, although the methods used for determination of EMG onset in this line of experiments seems to follow a certain tested methodology (Hodges & Bui 1996), there seem to be different analysis methods affecting the results and also the magnitude of EMG activity seems to be more informative about stability provision rather than just the onset of activity (Morey-Klapsing et al 2004).

EMG Fatigue Analysis

A number of experimental studies point to the fact that healthy subjects have greater endurance capacity of the trunk flexor and extensor muscles compared to chronic LBP patients with static and dynamic tests for each of the muscle groups. Endurance deficits in patients with back pain may be present either due to disuse of trunk muscles (Mannion et al 2000) or as a secondary phenomenon to increased excitation in low back musculature (lack of adequate relaxation intervals) leading to early fatigue development. It has been additionally demonstrated that trunk muscle fatigue has a negative effect in the motor control strategies employed to execute movements (Parnianpour et al 1988, Sparto et al 1997), also impairing the proprioceptive acuity of the trunk muscles (Taimela et al 1999).

Fatigue however, as outlined so far, is as complex a phenomenon to assess as subjects' performance, similar to strength and every other maximal performance test, – as it is influenced by a number of confounding variables. Even the predictive value of the Biering-Sørensen (BS) test in prospective studies of healthy asymptomatic individuals can be viewed as relative, under this framework. Alternative, reliable and valid fatigue assessment techniques are needed to overcome these problems. Through mathematical transformations of the raw signal (Fourier analysis) the magnitude of the signal at each firing frequency of the muscle fibres (from type I-low frequency to type II-high frequency) can be graphically depicted as shown in figure 2. This figure represents the power spectrum of the muscle at a particular contraction level and at a particular point in time. The Mean Power Frequency (MPF) or the Median Frequency (MF), the latter being the frequency value that divides the *power spectrum* in two equal halves, appear to provide an appropriate representation of biochemical events within the muscle that is believed to be a consistent descriptor of time-dependent changes, with a shift towards lower frequencies noted during relatively short contractions, ranging from 30 seconds to 2-3 minutes (Basmajian & DeLuca 1985, Mannion & Dolan 1994).

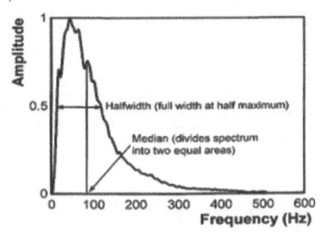

Figure 2. Schematic representation of the frequency spectrum of differentially detected EMG signal. From Nargol et al (1999) "Factors in the reproducibility of electromyographic power spectrum analysis of lumbar paraspinal muscle fatigue." *Spine*, 24(9), page 885, with permission.

DeLuca (1985) has proposed that *the rate of decrease in MF*, as expressed by the least squares linear regression (slope) from the beginning to the end of a contraction *signifies the endurance capacity of a muscle* (figure 3), with a steeper slopes indicating greater muscle fatiguability (De Luca 1985). Good correlations (r=-0.60 to -0.88) between the MF slopes and endurance time from tests kept to complete exaustion seem to support this hypothesis for the paraspinal muscles of healthy well-motivated subjects (Kankaanpää et al 1997, Mannion & Dolan 1994, Van Dieën et al 1993a). Also, some moderate correlations were reported between MF slopes and scores from scales of perceived exertion administered during the test in healthy well-motivated subjects: r= -0.54 to -0.90, p<0.01 (Kankaanpää et al 1997) and in another study r= -0.41 to -0.50, p<0.01 (Dedering et al 1999). This latter association is not a consistent finding in all studies, with no association also reported (Elfving et al 2000). Furthermore, a recent study tested the association between muscle fibre composition and objective EMG power spectral analysis endurance findings (Mannion et al 1998), with the results suggesting a significant moderately strong correlation (r=0.60, p<0.001) between the relative area occupied by type I fibres with MF slopes. Associations between the number of type I and type II fibres with EMG measures were weaker, though. The obvious advantage of this technique is that one can infer the muscle fiber composition of a muscle from its MF slopes, unfortunately though, the correlation between muscle histomorphometric characteristics and MF slopes was not very strong.

Many studies focusing on the analysis of the time-dependent characteristics of the EMG frequency spectrum, have established an association between steeper MF slopes of low back muscles and LBP (Biedermann et al 1991, Roy et al 1989, Roy et al 1990, Tsuboi et al 1994). Those studies have shown that MF parameters can generally provide a valid measure of fatigue by discriminating between LBP and healthy subjects, with the former having higher fatigue rates. However, causal relationships between fatigue and LBP remain unknown. On the contrary, opposite results have also been obtained, with MF slopes of patients with LBP being less steep than those of healthy participants (Elfving et al 2003, Oddsson & De Luca 2003, Peach & McGill 1998) but with equally good classification accuracy!

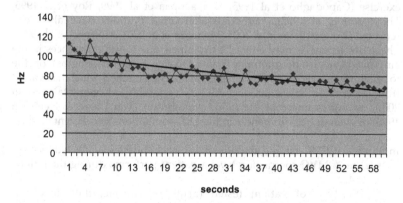

seconds

Figure 3. Schematic representation of the median frequency (MF) decrease with time (over a 1-minute contraction).

363

The advantage of the EMG-assisted endurance assessment over the mechanical capacity ("holding-time to complete exhaustion") endurance testing is apparent. The duration of the contraction sustained with the classic endurance tests is linked to subjects' willingness to maintain the requested posture (Mannion et al 1996), whereas EMG fatigue measures are independent of subjects *volitional* effort, as the firing frequency of motor units cannot be perceived nor regulated (Basmajian & DeLuca 1985). However, it is also logical to assume that *non-volitional* alterations in the organisation of the motor commands from the CNS, as in muscle inhibition phenomena or alterations in load-sharing between synergistic muscles, can offer alternative interpretations of EMG-related endurance indices (possibly inhibited muscles are phenomenically more fatigue resistant) (Peach & McGill 1998, Roy & Oddsson 1998). Another explanation for the apparently 'opposite' results for less fatigue in patients with LBP is that the MF-slope is affected by load carried (individuals with less strength performance show less fatigue). Setting the level of contraction for an EMG fatigue test at a certain percentage of an MVC may mean that patients in pain will present with slopes of 'equal steepness' or 'shallower' if the level of the test is not appropriate. Also, slope steepness is affected by age, sex (women have more fatigue-resistant muscles) and body mass index (BMI) (Kankaanpaa et al 1998).

Finally, a transformation of type I to type II fibres of the paraspinals with increasing symptom duration in chronic LBP patients (Mannion et al 2000) may not demonstrate apparent fatigue development when compared to acute LBP patients until the fiber transformation occurs. These points may present problems with the validity of the EMG fatigue method, when applied in acute patients with LBP.

Some previous studies have demonstrated that the EMG fatigue assessment method is able to monitor significant improvements in endurance following exercise (Capodaglio et al 1995, Kankaanpaa et al 1999, Roy et al 1995, Thompson et al 1992), although alternative findings have also been reported (Koumantakis et al 2005, Mannion et al 2001, Moffroid et al 1993). These discrepancies may either be explained due to the differences in the employed exercise programmes (type of exercises or time-lengths), or due to reliability issues of the power spectral analysis method which has varied from acceptable levels (around 33-34% variability) (Koumantakis et al 2001), to rather unacceptable (>50% variability) (Van Dieen & Heijblom 1996) or even due to differences in the LBP populations in different studies.

In Summary, EMG fatigue analysis of low-back muscles is affected by:
- The % MVC contraction level a patient performs during the fatigue test.
- The type of patient tested (acute or chronic, their levels of disability/immobility, their age, sex and body type).
- The reliability of the technique, which is far more difficult to achieve compared to the previous 3 methods of EMG analysis described.

It is likely that the occasional 'atypical' and 'conflicting' results obtained when comparing normals and back pain sufferers is due to the different forces endured by the two groups in the test. Patients are may not be tested at an equally high sustained force level, so are contracting 'less' hard than their healthy counterparts – hence, the shallower fatique slopes shown in some of them. It is important that results are presented alongside all the data gathered (e.g. forces sustained during testing/pain history and patient details) so that fair comparisons can be made.

Conclusions and future directions

All muscles surrounding the lumbar spine contribute to its normal and painless function, depending on their anatomical profile and their pre-programmed activation from the CNS, mainly through a co-contraction strategy in all planes of movement. It seems that the muscles close to the spine need to maintain a low activation level, whereas the activation of the more superficial muscles is more task-orientated, and dependent on movement direction and task load.

When pain occurs muscle activity is affected in a manner that does not conform to a specific model. It seems, from more recent EMG studies, that the muscle activity changes observed are not only dependent upon the effect of the pain stimulus at spinal cord level, but also upon the interaction of this stimulus with the higher motor centres of the central nervous system, as well as its perception from the emotional system (fear, stress etc.) (see figure 4 below). Apart from the immediate changes in muscle activity observed, diminished endurance capacity (limitations in ability for sustained contractions) is most likely established in a more long-term timescale and is a consequense of disuse.

Muscle activity hypertonicity may be a contributing factor to the pain experience, - obviously not during relaxation time, but likely more during moderate or heavy manual work where some muscle groups demonstrate increased activity or sustained muscle activation, i.e. muscle spasms. If the spinal system is required to function in increased speed mode, the delays from the neuromuscular response that have been noted may well contibute to inadequate spinal joint protection. Studies so far are yet to show that some of the changes in muscle fibre function are a definite risk factor for repeated injury.

EMG has a variety of applications in patients with LBP. One is to assess for deviations in muscle function assumed to be caused by pain. Indeed, EMG studies have identified several and sometimes contrasting differences between patients with LBP and healthy subjects in a number of indices.

The diversity of the findings may well be due to the different methods of EMG assessment available and their individual methodological problems, like: direct comparison of EMG activity in the same muscle groups of healthy participants and patients without utilising the muscle-ratio method from different muscle groups (see figure 1), or low reliability (repeatability) of some EMG methods, with others also having questionable validity (eg. the contrasting results from EMG fatigue studies).

In general, methodological problems tend to be overcome with more recent and detailed EMG methods. The SENIAM (Surface Electromyography for the Non-Invasive Assessment of Muscles) is a European collaborative effort in the Biomedical Health and Research Programme (BIOMED II) of the European Union. Details of the project can be found on a relevant web-page (www.seniam.org). This project has resulted in European recommendations for EMG recording and signal processing methods, a set of simulation models for education and testing, a set of test signals, eight books, 1 CD, publications and a European network for surface EMG.

Findings depend not only on the quality of EMG data combined with good knowledge of the normal function of the low-back muscular system, but also on the research design of the reviewed studies. Physiotherapists need a basic understanding of both in order to assess the importance of those findings.

The variety of results, obtained mainly from case-control studies (with the inherent inability to prove cause & effect relationships), occurred for three possible reasons. Firstly, because absolute matching between patients and controls is difficult to achieve, and secondly, due to the fact that different spinal pain aetiologies may have a differential effect on muscle activity. Thirdly, some consideration needs to be given to the between-subject variation in the response of the neuromuscular system to pain.

As a general point for all studies, it may not be sufficient to only report statistical significance between healthy participants and patients with LBP for the following two reasons. First, clearer 'cut-off' levels for dysfunction (discriminant validity) should be additionally presented, beyond which a patient will have an established muscle dysfunction that requires treatment. Secondly, because statistical significance is not always equivalent to clinical significance. Thus, any new research should present whether the differences found experimentally can be detected by clinicians.

To many, past EMG research appears somewhat 'fragmented'. This is probably due to the efforts and reporting of the researchers who were attempting to make their findings fit a predictable model of muscle activity disorganisation due to pain. A more current view, is that the changes observed with LBP are probably *task-dependent*. Thus, the level of muscle activity may vary depending on the relative contribution of a particular muscle to a particular task, and therefore be highly variable between, but also within, individuals when different tasks are involved. The current idea is to consider EMG activity changes in LBP as *functional*, reducing the probability of mechanical stresses to painful tissues by limiting range of movement and providing stabilisation of the spine.

366

The author proposes that all past research findings need re-evaluation, making use of the higher-quality studies conducted under the prevailing views discussed. Joint re-testing in much larger populations to assess the relative importance of all EMG indices may be required, as interractions may or may not exist between different EMG indices.

For instance, hyperactivity and hypoactivity phenomena of trunk muscles, if maintained sufficiently, may have detrimental effects on spinal pain. Hyperactivity in certain muscles, possibly caused by hypoactivity in some of their synergists or their antagonistic muscles, if not given the adequate relaxation intervals, may lead to increased muscular fatigue of the hyperactive muscles (Panjabi 1992) and then in turn to delayed activation onsets. Effusion of the facet joints, probably through the mechanical effect of capsule distension, causes altered proprioceptive feedback and subsequently decreased muscle activation to the lumbar spine. This may combine with asynchronous activation of the back muscles which then renders spinal segments more vulnerable to further injury during everyday functional tasks.

This research effort possibly has to be co-ordinated as a multi-centre type of study, to then be able to sub-classify participants according to their LBP chronicity, physical job requirements, fitness levels, psychosocial factors and any other parameter that might be affecting their EMG indices.

It may be that different mechanical abnormalities in patients may require different muscle re-training programmes. On the other hand, 'broad' categories of patients may benefit from the same neuromuscular rehabilitation programme. Other types of measurement, like proprioception assessment (Koumantakis et al 2002) or more general body postural control and balance (Luoto et al 1998) may be relevant to validate some of the EMG methods against and in this way broaden our understanding of the LBP problem. The possibility again is equivocal, as these impairments may either occur due to pain or be potential risk factors for the development of LBP through provision of insufficient or inaccurate information of the positioning of body parts. More integrated approaches have recently been favoured, promoting the notion that pain may have direct influence on the motor centres, fear-avoidance or be due to changes in the sensory (including the proprioceptive) system (Hodges & Moseley 2003).

The timing of muscle dysfunction, whether it precedes or it follows pain in the area, is not always clear. Research with experimentally-induced muscle pain has shed some light onto the impairments that appear immediately after a short-term painful stimulus(Arendt-Nielsen et al 1995, Hodges et al 2003, Zedka et al 1999). Future research may also correlate the short & long-term history (mechanical & psychosocial stressors) prior to and around the time of the initiation of pain and establish the relative importance of the physical and psychological causes of pain initiation and maintenance during the course of LBP in different populations and settings. Evidence so far from prospective studies conducted in healthy participants show that some of the physical parameters associated with EMG were either not predictive (Adams et al 1999) or minimally predictive (Stevenson et al 2001) of LBP development.Also, in patients with non-specific LBP, report of pain and disability improvement was not concomitant with EMG normalisation (Koumantakis et al 2005, Koumantakis et al 2005a, Mannion et al 2001).

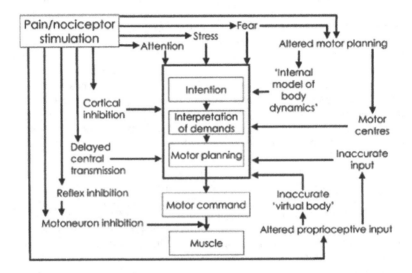

Figure 4. Flow diagram of a multitude mechanisms that may affect motor control. Inhibitory pain pathways (shown on left side) were regarded as less likely contributors to dysfunction. The more direct influence of nociception and pain on the motor centres, on the development of fear and on altering normal sensory feedback are seen as more likely candidates of motor control problems related to pain. (From Hodges & Moseley (2003) 'Pain and motor control of the lumbopelvic region: effect and possible mechanisms.' J Electromyogr Kinesiol, 13, page 364, with permission).

It is likely that a great deal more than neuromuscular re-setting is required for successful tackling of back pain. An important issue is the integration of psychosocial components to our physiotherapy interventions which may well lead to normalisation of asynchronous muscle activity.

Treatment techniques that are thought to be able to normalise the detected dysfunctions need to be thoroughly tested, so as to answer questions like 'Are all our muscle rehabilitation approaches helping our patients'? Or 'Which type of patients are more suited for certain muscle re-education techniques'? Another debatable issue that remains is whether the normalisation of impaired activation of the neuromuscular system in LBP is actually desirable. Researchers are suggesting that alterations in recruitment noted may actually be offering increased stability to the lumbar spine (Van Dieen et al 2003a).

368

To conclude, the primary role of physiotherapy should be to promote patient re-activation through controlled therapeutic exercises in order to avoid the deleterious consequences of disuse. A primary objective is to foster positive effects on pain and disability which may occasionally require skilled muscle activity normalisation.

References

AdamsM, Mannion A, Dolan P 1999 Personal risk factors for first-time low back pain. Spine 24(23):2497-2505

Al-Obaidi SM, Nelson RM et al 2000 The role of anticipation and fear of pain in the persistence of avoidance behavior in patients with chronic low back pain. Spine 25(9):1126-1131

Alaranta H, Moffroid M et al 1994 Postural control of adults with musculoskeletal impairment. Critical Reviews in Physical and Rehabilitation Medicine 6(4):337-370

Arendt-Nielsen L, Graven-Nielsen et al 1995 The influence of low back pain on muscle activity and coordination during gait: A clinical and experimental study. Pain 64:231-240

Arokoski JPA, Kankaanpää M et al 1999 Back and hip extensor muscle function during therapeutic exercises. Archives of Physical Medicine and Rehabilitation 80(7):842-850

Asmussen E, Klaussen K 1962 Form and function of the erect human spine. Clinical Orthopaedics & Related Research 25:55-63

Basmajian JV, DeLuca CJ 1985 Muscles alive. Their functions revealed by electromyography. 5th Edn Williams and Wilkins,Baltimore

Beimborn D, Morrissey M 1988 A review of the literature related to trunk muscle performance. Spine 13(6):655-660

Bergmark A 1989 Stability of the lumbar spine. A study in mechanical engineering. Acta Orthopaedica Scandinavica 60 Supp 230:5-54

Biedermann H, Shanks G et al 1991 Power spectrum analyses of electromyographic activity. Discriminators in the differential assessment of patients with chronic low-back pain.Spine 16(10):1179-1184

Biering-Sørensen F 1984 Physical measurements as risk indicators for low back trouble over a one year period. Spine 9(2):106-119

Bombardier C, Kerr M et al 1994 A guide to interpreting epidemiologic studies on the etiology of back pain. Spine 19(18S):2047S-2056S

Bouisset S, Zattara M 1990 Segmental movement as a perturbation to balance? Facts and concepts. In: Winters J, Woo S-J (Eds), Multiple Muscle Systems. Biomechanics and Movement Organisation. Springer-Verlag, New York 498-506

Capodaglio P, Nilsson J, Jurisic DH 1995 Changes in paravertebral EMG spectum parallel to strength increases after rehabilitation in chronic low back pain patients. Clinical Rehabilitation 9:354-362

Cavanaugh J 1995 Neural mechanisms of lumbar pain. Spine 20(16):1804-1809

Cavanaugh J, Ozaktay A et al 1997 Mechanisms of low back pain. A neurophysiologic and neuroanatomic study. Clinical Orthopaedics and Related Research 335:166-180

Cholewicki J, McGill SM, Norman RW 1995 Comparison of muscle forces and joint load from an optimization and EMG assisted lumbar spine model: Towards development of a hybrid approach. Journal of Biomechanics 28:321-331

Cholewicki J, McGill SM 1996 Mechanical stability of the in vivo lumbar spine: implications for injury and chronic low back pain. Clinical Biomechanics 11(1):1-15

Cholewicki J, Greene et al 2002 Neuromuscular Function in Athletes Following Recovery From a Recent Acute Low Back Injury. Journal of Orthopaedic and Sports Physical Therapy 32:568-575

Cholewicki J, Van Vliet IV JJ 2002 Relative contribution of trunk muscles to the stability of the lumbar spine during isometric exertions. Clinical Biomechanics 17(2):99-105

Coulter A, Langridge J 1997 Iso-machines in the physiotherapy management of low back pain. British Journal of Therapy and Rehabilitation 4(10) :536-540-557-558

Crisco J, Panjabi M 1990 Postural biomechanical stability and gross muscular architecture in the spine. In: Winters JM, Woo S-LY (Eds), Multiple Muscle Systems. Biomechanics and Movement Organisation. Springer-Verlag, New York

Dankaerts W, O'Sullivan P et al 2004 Reliability of EMG measurements for trunk muscles during maximal and sub-maximal voluntary isometric contractions in healthy controls and CLBP patients. Journal of Electromyography and Kinesiology 14(3):333-342

Danneels LA, Vanderstraeten GG et al 2001 A functional subdivision of hip, abdominal, and back muscles during asymmetric lifting. Spine 26(6):E114-E121

Dedering _, Németh G, Harms-Ringdahl K 1999 Correlation between electromyographic spectral changes and subjective assessment of lumbar muscle fatigue in subjects without pain from the lower back. Clinical Biomechanics 14:103-111

De Luca C 1985 Myoelectrical manifestations of localised muscular fatigue in humans. Critical Reviews in Biomedical Engineering 11(4):251-279

De Luca C 1997 The use of surface electomyography in biomechanics. Journal of Applied Biomechanics 13:135-163

Dolce J, Raczynski J 1985 Neuromuscular activity and electromyography in painful backs:psychological and biomechanical models in assessment and treatment. Psychological Bulletin 97(3):502-520

Edgerton V, Wolf S et al 1996 Evaluating patterns of EMG amplitudes for trunk and neck muscles of patients and controls. International Journal of Rehabilitation and Health 2(1):1-18

Elfving B, Nemeth G et al 1999 Reliability of EMG spectral parameters in repeated measurements of back muscle fatigue.Journal of Electromyography and Kinesiology 9:235-243

Elfving B, Németh G, Arvidsson I 2000 Back muscle fatigue in healthy men and women studied by elecromyography spectral parameters and subjective ratings. Scandinavian Journal of Rehabilitation Medicine 32(3):117-123

Elfving B, Dedering A, Nemeth G 2003 Lumbar muscle fatigue and recovery in patients with long-term low-back trouble-Electromyography and health-related factors. Clinical Biomechanics 18(7):619-630

Estlander A-M, Vanharanta H et al 1994 Anthropometric variables, self-efficacy beliefs, and pain and disability ratings on the isokinetic performance of low back pain patients. Spine 19(8):941-947

Feinstein A 1998 P-values and confidence intervals: two sides of the same unsatisfactory coin. Journal of Clinical Epidemiology 51(4):355-360

Flicker PL, Fleckenstein JL et al 1993 Lumbar muscle usage in chronic low back pain. Magnetic resonance image evaluation.Spine 18(5):582-586

Flor H, Birbaumer N et al 1992 Symptom-specific psychophysiological responses in chronic pain patients. Psychophysiology 29:452-460

Fryer G, Morris T, Gibbons P 2004 Paraspinal muscles and intervertebral dysfunction: Part one. Journal of Manipulative and Physiological Therapeutics, 27(4):267-274

Fryer G, Morris T, Gibbons P 2004a Paraspinal muscles and intervertebral dysfunction: Part two. Journal of Manipulative and Physiological Therapeutics, 27(5):348-357

Gibbons L, Videman T, Battié M 1997 Isokinetic and psychophysical lifting strength, static back muscle endurance, and magnetic resonance imaging of the paraspinal muscles as predictors of low back pain in men. Scandinavian Journal of Rehabilitation Medicine 29:187-191

Grabiner M, Jeziorowski J 1992 Isokinetic trunk extension discriminates uninjured subjects from subjects with previous low back pain. Clinical Biomechanics 7:195-200

Grabiner M, Koh T, Al Ghazawi A 1992 Decoupling of bilateral paraspinal excitation in subjects with low back pain. Spine 17:1219-1223

Granata K, Marras W 2000 Cost-benefit of muscle cocontraction in protecting against spinal instability. Spine 25(11:1398-1404

Hägmark T 1979 Fibre types in human abdominal muscles. Acta Physiologica Scandinavica 107:319-325

Hasan Z 1997 Invited commentary. Physical Therapy 77(2):142-143

Hides JA, Richardson CA, Jull GA 1996 Multifidus muscle recovery is not automatic after resolution of acute, first-episode low back pain. Spine 21(23):2763-2769

Hirsch G, Beach G et al 1991 Relationship between performance on lumbar dynamometry and Waddell score in a population with low-back pain. Spine 16(9):1039-1043

Hodges P 2001 Changes in motor planning of feedforward postural responses of the trunk muscles in low back pain. Experimental Brain Research 141:261-266

Hodges P, Bui B 1996 A comparison of computer based methods for the determination of onset of muscle contraction using electromyography. Electroencephalography and Clinical Neurophysiology 101:511-519

Hodges PW, Richardson CA 1996 Inefficient muscular stabilisation of the lumbar spine associated with low back pain. A motor control evaluation of transversus abdominis. Spine 21(22):2640-2650

Hodges PW, Richardson CA 1997 Contraction of the abdominal muscles associated with movement of the lower limb. Physical Therapy 77(2):132-144

Hodges PW, Richardson CA 1998 Delayed postural contraction of transversus abdominis in low back pain associated with movement of the lower limb. Journal of Spinal Disorders 11(1):46-56

Hodges PW, Richardson CA 1999 Altered trunk muscle recruitment in people with low back pain with upper limb movement at different speeds. Archives of Physical Medicine and Rehabilitation 80(9):1005-1012

Hodges P, Moseley G 2003 Pain and motor control of the lumbopevic region: effect and possible mechanisms. Journal of Electromyography and Kinesiology 13:361-370

Hodges P, Moseley G et al 2003 Experimental muscle pain changes feedforward postural responses of the trunk muscles. Experimental Brain Research 151:262-271

Holmstrøm E, Moritz U, Andersson M 1992 Trunk muscle strength and back muscle endurance in construction workers with and without low back disorders. Scandinavian Journal of Rehabilitation Medicine 24:3-10

Hungerford B, Gilleard W, Hodges P 2003 Evidence of altered lumbopelvic muscle recruitment in the presence of sacroiliac joint pain. Spine 28(14):1593-1600

Indahl A, Kaigle A et al 1997 Interaction between the porcine lumbar intervertebral disc, zygapophysial joints, and paraspinal muscles.Spine 22(24):2834-2840

Ito T, Shirado O et al 1996 Lumbar trunk muscle endurance testing: An inexpensive alternative to a machine for evaluation. Archives of Physical Medicine and Rehabilitation 77(1):75-79

Jones DA, Round JM 1990 Skeletal muscle in health and disease. Manchester University Press, Manchester

Jonsson B 1970 The functions of individual muscles in the lumbar part of the erector spinae muscles. Electromyography 10:5-21

Jørgensen K, Mag C et al 1993 Muscle fibre distribution, capillary density, and enzymatic activities in the lumbar paravertebral muscles of young men. Significance for isometric endurance. Spine18(11)P:1439-1450

Jull G, Scott Q et al 1998 New concepts for the control of pain in the lumbopelvic region. In: Vleeming A et al (Eds), European Conference Organisers, Third Interdisciplinary World Congress on Low Back and Pelvic Pain, Vienna, Austria 128-131

Kaigle A, Wessberg P, Hansson T 1998 Muscular and kinematic behavior of the lumbar spine during flexion-extension. Journal of Spinal Disorders 11(2):163-174

Kalimo H, Rantanen J et al 1989 Lumbar muscles: Structure and function. Annals of Medicine 21:353-359

Kankaanpää M, Taimela S et al 1997 Lumbar paraspinal muscle fatigability in repetitive isoinertial loading: EMG spectral indices, Borg scale and endurance time. European Journal of Applied Physiology 76:236-242

Kankaanpää M, Laaksonen D et al 1998 Age, sex and body mass index as determinants of back and hip extensor fatigue in the isometric Sorensen back endurance test. Archives of Physical Medicine and Rehabilitation 79(9):1069-1075

Kankaanpää M, Taimela S et al 1999 The efficacy of active rehabilitation in chronic low back pain. Effect of pain intensity, self-experienced disability, and lumbar fatigability.Spine 24(10):1034-1042

Kishino N, Mayer T, Gatchel R 1985 Quantification of lumbar function: Part 4. Isometric and isokinetic lifting simulation in normal subjects and low back dysfunction patients. Spine 10:921-927

Koumantakis GA, Arnall F et al 2001 Paraspinal muscle EMG fatigue testing with 2 methods in healthy volunteers. Reliability in the context of clinical applications. Clinical Biomechanics 16(3):263-266

Koumantakis G, Winstanley J, Oldham J 2002 Thoracolumbar proprioception in individuals with and without low back pain: Intratester reliability, clinical applicability, and validity. Journal of Orthopaedic and Sports Physical Therapy 32:327-335

Koumantakis GA, Watson PJ, Oldham JA 2005 Supplementation of general endurance exercise with stabilisation training versus general exercise only. Physiological and functional outcomes of a randomised controlled trial of patients with recurrent low back pain. Clinical Biomechanics 20(5):474-482

Koumantakis GA, Watson PJ, Oldham JA 2005a Trunk muscle stabilization training plus general exercise versus general exercise only: Randomized controlled trial of patients with recurrent low back pain. Physical Therapy 85(3):209-225

Kumar S Mital A 1996 Electromyography in Ergonomics. Taylor & Francis, London

Lackner JM Carosella AM 1999 The relative influence of perceived pain control, anxiety, and functional self-efficacy on spinal function among patients with chronic low back pain. Spine 24(21):2254-2261

Lariviere C, Gagnon D, Loisel, P 2000 An application of pattern recognition for the comparison of trunk muscles EMG waveforms between subjects with and without chronic low back pain during flexion-extension and lateral bending tasks. Journal of Electromyography and Kinesiology 10(4):261-273

Lavender S, Marras W, Miller R 1993 The development of response strategies in preparation for sudden loading to the torso. Spine 18(14):2097-2105

Lee J-H, Ooi Y, Nakamura K 1995 Measurement of muscle strength of the trunk and the lower extremities in subjects with history of low back pain. Spine 20(18):1994-1996

Leino P, Aro S, Hasan J 1987 Trunk muscle function and low back disorders: A ten-year follow-up study. Journal of Chronic Diseases 40(4):289-296

Lindgren K-A, Sihvonen T et al 1993 Exercise therapy effects on functional radiographic findings and segmental electromyographic activity in lumbar spine instability. Archives of Physical Medicine and Rehabilitation 74:933-939

Lund J, Donga R et al 1991 The pain-adaptation model: A discussion of the relationship between chronic musculoskeletal pain and motor activity. Canadian Journal of Physiology and Pharmacology 69:683-694

Luoto S, Heliövaara M et al 1995 Static back endurance and the risk of low-back pain. Clinical Biomechanics 10(6):323-324

Luoto S, Taimela S et al 1996 Psychomotor speed and postural control in chronic low back pain patients. A controlled follow-up study. Spine 21(22):2621-2627

Luoto S, Aalto H et al 1998 One-footed and externally disturbed two-footed postural control in patients with chronic low back pain and healthy control subjects. A controlled study with follow-up. Spine 23(19):2081-2090

Mannion AF 1999 Fibre type characteristics and function of the human paraspinal muscles: Normal values and changes in association with low back pain. Journal of Electromyography and Kinesiology 9:363-377

Mannion AF, Dolan P 1994 Electromyographic median frequency changes during isometric contraction of the back extensors to fatigue. Spine 19(1):1223-1229

Mannion AF, Dolan P, Adams MA 1996 Psychological questionnaires: Do "abnormal" scores precede or follow first-time low back pain? Spine 21(22): 2603-2611

Mannion AF, Dumas GA et al 1997 Muscle fibre size and type distribution in thoracic and lumbar regions of erector spinae in healthy subjects without low back pain: Normal values and sex differences. Journal of Anatomy 190:505-513

Mannion AF, Dumas GA et al 1998 The influence of muscle fiber size and type distribution on electromyographic measures of back muscle fatigability. Spine 23(5):576-584

Mannion AF, Koser L et al 2000 Influence of age and duration of symptoms on fibre type distribution and size of back muscles in chronic low back pain patients. European Spine Journal 9:273-281

Mannion AF, Taimela S et al 2001 Active therapy for chronic low back pain. Part 1. Effects on back muscle activation, fatigability, and strength. Spine 26(8):897-908

Marras W, Wongsam P 1986 Flexibility and velocity of the normal and impaired lumbar spine. Archives of Physical Medicine and Rehabilitation 67:213-217

Mayer T, Smith S et al 1985 Quantification of lumbar function. Part 2: Sagittal plane trunk strength in chronic low-back pain patients. Spine 10(8):765-772

McGill SM 1991 Electromyographic activity of the abdominal and low back musculature during the generation of isometric and dynamic axial trunk torque: Implications for lumbar mechanics. Journal of Orthopaedic Research 9(1):91-103

McGill S, Grenier S et al 2003 Coordination of muscle activity to assure stability of the lumbar spine. Journal of Electromyography and Kinesiology 13:353-359

Moffroid MT, Haugh LD et al 1993 Endurance training of trunk extensor muscles. Physical Therapy 73(1):3-10

Morey-Klapsing G, Arampatzis A, Br_ggemann G 2004 Choosing EMG parameters: comparison of different onset determination algorithms and EMG integrals in a joint stability study Clinical Biomechanics 19:196-201

Moseley G, Hodges P, Gandevia S 2002 Deep and superficial fibers of the lumbar multifidus muscle are differentially active during voluntary trunk movements. Spine 27:E29-E36

Moseley G, Nicholas M, Hodges P 2004 Does anticipation of back pain predispose to back trouble? Brain 127:2339-2347

Moseley G, Nicholas M, Hodges P 2004a Pain differs from non-painful attention-demanding or stressful tasks in its effect on postural control patterns of trunk muscles. Experimental Brain Research 156:64-71

Nargol AVF, Jones et al 1999 Factors in the reproducibility of electromyographic power spectrum analysis of lumbar paraspinal muscle fatigue. Spine 24(9): 883-888

Newton M, Waddell G 1993 Trunk strength testing with iso-machines. Part 1: Review of a decade of scientific evidence. Spine 18(7):801-811

Ng J, Richardson C 1994 EMG study of erector spinae and multifidus in two isometric back extension exercises. Australian Journal of Physiotherapy 40(2):115-121

Nicolaisen T, Jørgensen K 1985 Trunk strength, back muscle endurance and low back pain trouble. Scandinavian Journal of Rehabilitation Medicine 17:121-127

Oddsson L, De Luca C 2003 Activation imbalances in lumbar spine muscles in the presence of chronic low back pain Journal of Applied Physiology 94(4):1410-1420

O'Sullivan PB, Twomey LT, Allison GT 1997 Evaluation of specific stabilising exercise in the treatment of chronic low back pain with radiologic diagnosis of spondylolysis or spondylolisthesis. Spine 22(24):2959-2967

O'Sullivan PB, Twomey L, Allison GT 1998 Altered abdominal muscle recruitment in patients with chronic back pain following a specific exercise intervention. Journal of Orthopaedic and Sports Physical Therapy 27(2):114-124

O'Sullivan P, Beales D et al 2002 Altered motor control strategies in subjects with sacroiliac joint pain during the active straight-leg-raise test. Spine 27(1):E1-E8

Panagiotacopulos N, Lee J et al 1998 Evaluation of EMG signals from rehabilitated patients with lower back pain using wavelets. Journal of Electromyography and Kinesiology 8:269-278

Panjabi M 1992 The stabilising system of the spine. Part II. Neutral zone and instability hypothesis. Journal of Spinal Disorders 5(4):390-397

Panjabi M 1992a The stabilising system of the spine. Part I. Function, dysfunction, adaptation and enhancement. Journal of Spinal Disorders 5(4):383-389

Parnianpour M, Nordin M et al 1988 The triaxial coupling of torque generation of trunk muscles during isometric exertions and the effect of fatiguing isoinertial movements on the motor output and movement patterns. Spine 13(9):982-992

Peach JP, McGill, SM 1998 Classification of low back pain with the use of spectral electromyogram parameters. Spine 23(10):1117-1123

Pedersen J, Sjölander P et al 1997 Increased intramuscular concentration of bradykinin increases the static fusimotor drive to muscle spindles in neck muscles of the cat. Pain 70:83-91

Pope M, Bevins T et al 1985 The relationship between anthropometric, postural, muscular, and mobility characteristics of males aged 18-55. Spine 10:644-648

Prochazka A, Hulliger M 1988 The continuing debate about CNS control of proprioception. Journal of Physiology 513:315

Radebold A, Cholewicki J et al 2000 Muscle response pattern to sudden trunk loading in healthy individuals and in patients with chronic low back pain.Spine 25(8):947-954

Roy SH, De Luca CJ, Casavant DA 1989 Lumbar muscle fatigue and chronic lower back pain. Spine 14(9):992-1001

Roy S, De Luca C et al 1990 Fatigue, recovery and low back pain in varsity rowers. Medicine and Science in Sports and Exercise 22(4):463-469

Roy SH, De Luca CJ et al 1995 Spectral electromyographic assessment of back muscles in patients with low back pain undergoing rehabilitation. Spine 20(1):38-48

Roy SH, Oddsson LIE 1998 Classification of paraspinal muscle impairments by surface electromyography. Physical Therapy 78(8):838-851

Sirca A, Kostevc V 1985 The fibre type composition of thoracic and lumbar paravertebral muscles in man. Journal of Anatomy 141:131-137

Smidt G 1994 Trunk muscle strength and endurance in the context of low-back dysfunction. In: Palastanga N, Boyling J (Eds), Grieve's Modern Manual Therapy, 2nd Edn. Churchill Livingstone, Edinburgh

Solomonow M, Zhou B-H et al 1998 The ligamento-muscular stabilizing system of the spine. Spine 23(23):2552-2562

Sparto P, Parnianpour M et al 1997 The effect of fatigue on multijoint kinematics, coordination, and postural stability during a repetitive lifting test. Journal of Orthopaedic and Sports Physical Therapy 25(1):3-12

Stevenson J, Weber C et al 2001 A longitudinal study of the development of low back pain in an industrial population. Spine 26(12):1370-1377

Stubbs M, Harris M et al 1998 Ligamento-muscular protective reflex in the lumbar spine of the feline. Journal of Electromyography & Kinesiology 8:197-204

Suzuki N, Endo S 1983 A quantitative study of trunk muscle strength and fatigability in the low back pain syndrome. Spine 8(1):69-74

Taimela S, Kankaanpoo M, Luoto S 1999 The effect of lumbar fatigue on the ability to sense a change in lumbar position. A controlled study. Spine 24(13):1322-1327

Thelen D, Schultz A, Ashton-Miller J 1995 Co-contraction of lumbar muscles during the development of time-varying triaxial moments. Journal of Orthopaedic Research 13(3):390-398

Thompson DA, Biedermann H-J et al 1992 Changes in paraspinal electromyographic spectral analysis with exercise: Two studies. Journal of Electromyography & Kinesiology 2(3):179-186

Thorstensson A & Carlson H 1987 Fibre types in human lumbar back muscles. Acta Physiologica Scandinavica, 131:195-202

Tsuboi T, Satou T et al 1994 Spectral analysis of electromyogram in lumbar muscles: fatigue induced endurance contraction. European Journal of Applied Physiology and Occupational Physiology 69:361-366

Van Dieën J, Oude Vrielink H, Toussaint H 1993 An investigation into the relevance of the pattern of temporal activation with respect to erector spinae muscle endurance. European Journal of Applied Physiology 66:70-75

Van Dieën J, Vrielink H et al 1993a Trunk extensor endurance and its relationship to electromyogram parameters.European Journal of Applied Physiology 66:388-396

Van Dieën JH, Heijblom P 1996 Reproducibility of isometric trunk extension torque, trunk extensor endurance, and related electromyographic parameters in the context of their clinical applicability. Journal of Orthopaedic Research 14:139-143

Van Dieën J H, Cholewicki J, Radebold A 2003 Trunk muscle recruitment patterns in patients with low back pain enhance the stability of the lumbar spine. Spine 28(8):834-841

Van Dieën J, Selen L, Cholewicki J 2003a Trunk muscle activation in low-back pain patients, an analysis of the literature. Journal of Electromyography and Kinesiology 13:333-351

Vink P, Van der Velde E, Verbout A 1988 A functional subdivision of the lumbar extensor musculature. Recruitment patterns and force-RA-EMG relationships under isometric conditions. Electromyography and Clinical Neurophysiology 28:517-525

Vlaeyen JWS, Kole-Snijders AMJ et al 1995 Fear of movement/ (re)injury in chronic low back pain and its relation to behavioral performance. Pain 62:363-372

Vlaeyen J, Seelen H et al 1999 Fear of movement/(re)injury and muscular reactivity in chronic low back pain patients: An experimental investigation. Pain 82: 297-304

Watson P 2002 Psychophysiological models of pain. In: Gifford LS (Ed), Topical Issues in Pain 4. CNS Press, Falmouth 191-198

Watson P, Booker C, Main C 1997 Evidence for the role of psychological factors in abnormal paraspinal activity in patients with chronic low back pain. Journal of Musculoskeletal Pain 5(4):41-56

Williams M, Solomonow M et al 2000 Multifidus spasms eleicited by prolonged lumbar flexion. Spine 25(22):2916-2924

Zedka M, Prochazka A et al 1999 Voluntary and reflex control of human back muscles during induced pain. Journal of Physiology 520(2):591-604

20

Clinical Pain, Experimental Evidence: Molecular Mechanisms within the Spinal Cord.

STEPHEN THOMPSON

"In the end, all we are really doing, is collecting butterflies".
Thus ran a typical subtle commentary by Patrick Wall describing the attempts of clinicians and scientists to understand pain by the ordering, naming and classification of observed phenomena. With the advent and application of the molecular revolution to the study of pain we appear to be taking this neuroscientific taxonomy to its logical extreme. Pat may have argued that this molecular dissection was further removing us from the true understanding of the nature of persistent pain. However, there is no doubt that the startling discoveries of the last decade, whilst certainly adding to the phenomenology, have shed enormous insight into the mechanisms that underlie the organic nature of persistent pain states in man.

Nociceptive pain.

Under normal circumstances, pain occurs in response to activation of a specific population of high threshold primary sensory neurons, or nociceptors, following transduction of an appropriate nociceptive stimulus into electrical activity. Propagation of the pain signal by activated nociceptors is accomplished by activation of key voltage gated Na+ channels (VGSC's) expressed by primary sensory neurons. Primary sensory neurons terminate within the dorsal horn of the spinal cord where transmission of information takes place at key synaptic connections with both local dorsal horn interneurons and ascending projection neurons. Under normal circumstances, activated nociceptors release the neurotransmitter glutamate from their central terminals.

Glutamate binds to and activates a number of postsynaptic receptor subtypes including the ionotropic NMDA and AMPA receptors and members of the metabotropic glutamate receptor family. Information reaches the brain from the spinal cord via several ascending pathways. Two pathways have been extensively investigated. One, the spinothalamic system, terminates within the ventroposterior and ventrobasal thalamus and is considered to relay information regarding the sensory or discriminative (where, how much) aspects of the stimulus (see Hunt & Mantyh 2001). The other terminates within pararbrachial areas and periaqueductal grey region and is considered to modulate the affective (pain quality) dimensions of the nociceptive stimulus. Nociceptive pain is the term used to categorized responses to activation of this transmission system. Nociceptive pain is considered to play a protective and adaptive role that permits the organism to respond to and avoid a damaging or potentially damaging stimulus. Within this pain transmission system, a diverse range of molecules have been identified that are responsible for transduction of the nociceptive signal, propagation of electrical activity and synaptic transmission of neuronal activity. Several recent reviews have highlighted recent developments in pain transduction and propagation (Costigan & Woolf 2000, Clapham et al 2003, Waxman et al 2000). This review will therefore only briefly mention the main players in these areas before focusing upon molecular aspects of activation and modification of synaptic transmission within the dorsal horn of the mammalian spinal cord that may lend new insight into the mechanisms of persistent pain.

Pain Transduction

The mammalian sensory nervous system detects a wide range of stimuli. We are able for example to detect temperature and small temperature changes. Temperatures below 15°C or above 43°C evoke thermal sensations accompanied by the sensation of pain. These stimuli are detected and transduced into electrical signals by members of a family of thermosensitive ion channels that act as an interface between the environment and nervous system. These channels are members of the TRP (transient receptor potential) family. Each channel member of the family exhibits distinct thermal activation thresholds and channel kinetics and receptor distribution (see Clapham et al 2003 and Wang & Woolf 2005 for recent reviews). For example TRPV1 (formerly VR1, capsaicin receptor) is activated by capsaicin, is sensitive to heat > 43°C, is relatively Ca^{2+} selective and current amplitude is increased by protons and modulated by PIP2. Following tissue damage and associated inflammation and acidification a further range of membrane receptors and ion channels that are located on the peripheral terminals of nociceptors are activated by specific components of the inflammatory response. Some components of the 'inflammatory soup' such as protons and ATP directly depolarise and activate nociceptor fibres through activation of ASIC or P2X3 receptors respectively and may give rise to the direct sensation of pain. Generally however, inflammatory mediators have the effect of sensitising the nociceptor terminal to further stimuli via the activation several families of serine-threonine and tyrosine protein kinases with subsequent posttranslational modification of ion channels and membrane receptors. This is the basis of peripheral sensitisation (see Woolf 2004 for review).

Pain propagation

Once action potentials are initiated by a noxious stimulus they are propagated from the peripheral terminal of a nociceptor to the central nervous system along the sensory neuron axon. Action potential propagation is mediated by the activation of VGSC's. Since the generation of action potentials in nociceptors is dependent upon such VGSC's, much emphasis has been placed upon the understanding of the expression and function of these channels for the understanding of pain transmission. At least eight different genes encode distinct VGSC's in the mammalian nervous system. Six different channels are expressed by sensory neurons of which two are unique to nociceptors $Na_v1.8$ (formely SNS, PN3) & $Na_v1.9$ (formerly SNS2, NaN). Following peripheral nerve injury or peripheral inflammation the patterns of expression of these two ion channels may be altered and ion channel properties may be influenced following activation of intracellular protein kinases leading to channel phosphorylation. For these reasons VGSC's have received much attention as possible targets for pharmacological manipulation in the search for new pain therapies.

Pain transmission in the dorsal horn.

Transmission of information from nociceptors into the central nervous system takes place at glutamatergic synapses with second order neurons in the dorsal horn of the spinal cord. There is a precise pattern of dorso-lateral and ventro-medial termination of sensory afferent fibres, including nociceptors, within the dorsal horn that mirrors the peripheral somatotopic distribution of sensory terminals. Fast excitatory synaptic transmission is mediated by the excitatory amino acid glutamate released from presynaptic terminals and activating postsynaptic AMPA and kainate ligand-gated ion channels (ionotropic receptors). Excitatory nociceptive signals entering the spinal cord may be modulated by local and descending inhibitory influences that may act either pre-synaptically, post-synaptically, or both. The central terminals of nociceptors express receptors for opioids, GABA, and cannabinoids (CB1), activation of which reduces transmitter release (pre-synaptic inhibition).

Dorsal horn neurons also express receptors for opioids and GABA, activation of which produces a postsynaptic hyperpolarisation (postsynaptic inhibition). Under certain circumstances the effectiveness of inhibitory mechanisms may be powerful, resulting in prevention of pain transmission within the dorsal horn. This physiological engram permits fast, faithful, transfer of input from nociceptors to the brain providing information relating to the duration, intensity, location and modality of peripheral noxious events and forms the basis of nociceptive pain.

Clinical pain.

In contrast to noiciceptive pain which is considered to play a protective role permitting avoidance and adaptation, clinical pain is chronic and may persist beyond the initial period of tissue injury. It may arise either following chronic inflammatory states (inflammatory pain) or following peripheral or central nerve injury (neuropathic pain). Both of these types of clinical pain are characterised by hypersensitivity to normal stimuli, both at the site of injury and away from the injury area (secondary hyperalgesia). By the appearance of spontaneous periods of pain dissociated from a stimulus. By the production of pain by stimuli that would not normally be associated with pain e.g. light touch or cooling (allodynia, cold allodynia) and by exaggerated pain in response to an adequate stimulus (hyperalgesia). The underlying principles and mechanisms in these chronic pain states are the same and are rooted in the phenomenon of activity-dependent neuronal plasticity. Clinical pain is indeed one of the direct (unpleasant) consequences of activity-dependent neuronal plasticity. This neuronal plasticity may occur at any point along the pain transfer system; within primary sensory nociceptor terminals, along nociceptor axons and within the synaptic transmission system in the spinal cord, the medulla or the cerebral cortex. The neuronal plasticity responsible for clinical pain has three distinct phases, modulation, modification and architectural alteration. Using synaptic transmission within the spinal dorsal horn as the example, I will highlight each of these three phases of synaptic plasticity in relation to amplification of the pain signal.

Modulation of the pain signal in the dorsal horn.

In general peripheral nociceptors behave as classical sensory transducers, the higher the stimulus intensity, the greater the action potential discharge. The more intense the peripheral noxious stimulus therefore, the greater the frequency and the longer the duration of action potentials induced within peripheral nociceptors. In addition, an increase in the excitability of the nociceptor terminal following sensitisation by inflammatory mediators results in a greater action potential discharge per stimulus. The overall result of this is that following persistent nociceptive stimuli a high frequency, long duration action potential barrage arrives at the central terminals of nociceptors within the spinal cord. In addition to the release of glutamate from central nociceptor terminals, high frequency discharge also results in the release of several neuropeptides, such as substance P (SP) and calcitonin-gene-related peptide (CGRP) as well as neurotrophins contained within C-fibre nociceptors such as brain-derived neurotrophic factor (BDNF). Neuropeptides and neurotrophins activate G-protein-linked postsynaptic peptide receptors and tropomyosin-related kinase receptors (trk) respectively. G-protein coupled receptor activation results in ion flux with slow kinetics. Activation of neuropetide receptors therefore evokes slow, sustained inward currents that result in prolonged slow depolarising postsynaptic potentials (Thompson & Woolf 1991, Thompson et al 1993). Together with the high rate of presynaptic activity, the ideal conditions are therefore met for a temporal summation of slow post-synaptic potentials that results in a cumulative post-synaptic depolarisation (Thompson et al 1990). This temporal summation of slow post-synaptic potentials underlies the phenomenon of Windup (Sivilotti et al 1993), first introduced by Lorne Mendell and Pat Wall in 1965. Windup is the first, acute form, of activity-dependent plasticity to manifest following sustained nociceptor input to the spinal cord (figure 1). It is characterised by a progressive increase in the input-output relationship of the central nervous system that is responsible for the slow build up pain responses experienced following repeated application of a noxious stimulus.

The persistent depolarisation of the postsynaptic membrane has a key affect upon the properties of post-synaptically located NMDA receptors. Under normal circumstances, at resting membrane potentials, NMDA receptors are characterised by voltage-dependent block by magnesium ions (Mg^{2+}) bound within the pore of the channel that prevents channel opening (Ozawa et al 1998). NMDA receptors are complex mulitmeric macromolecules consisting of three receptor subunits from related genes NR1, NR2 and NR3 (Hollmann & Heinemann1994). All NMDA channels that are functional must contain at least one NR1 subunit required for receptor activity. Regulation of the NMDA channel opening is now known to be remarkably complex (see Pláteník et al 2000 for review) involving requirement of the essential co-agonist glycine as well as glutamate, as well as modulation by Zn^{2+}, H^+ and redox active agents. A further key process regulating activity of membrane ion channels including NMDA and AMPA channels is by transfer of an inorganic phosphate group (phosphorylation). Phosphoryaltion of membrane proteins such as AMPA and NMDA receptors changes channel configuration, channel kinetics and hence potentiates channel activity.

How does glutamate receptor channel phosphorylation occur? NMDA channel opening is associated with Ca^{2+} influx. Calcium ions are extremely versatile and ubiquitous second messengers in the nervous system and are responsible for the activation of several intracellular signalling cascades that result in the activation of phosphorylation cascades within spinal dorsal horn neurons and the modulation of the nociceptive response. Many of these effects are mediated through the Ca^{2+} binding protein calmodulin (CaM). CaM mediates the Ca^{2+} activation of several enzyme signalling pathways that are crucial for the phosphorylation-mediated amplification of pain responses. One enzyme of particular

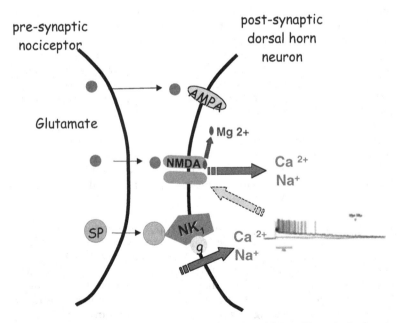

Figure 1 - Modulation of the pain signal in the dorsal horn. Phase 1, short term changes in the input/output relationships of the dorsal horn results from the temporal summation of slow synaptic potentials and the voltage-dependent properties of the NMDA receptor.

importance with respect to the NMDA receptor is the Ca^{2+}/calmodulin dependent kinase (CaMK) II (figure 2). Although CaMKII is present in low concentrations in the spinal dorsal horn, its role is well established in other models of persistent synaptic plasticity such as hippocampal long term potentiation (LTP) (see Malenka & Nicoll 1999, for review). Here it has been shown that when activated by Ca^{2+}/calmodulin and autophosphorylated, its activity outlasts the duration of the intracellular calcium signal, providing a continued trigger for downstream events. One such event is the direct phosphorylation of the GluR1 receptor subunit of the AMPA excitatory amino acid channel. This has the resultant effect of increasing ion current and postsynaptic depolarisation following glutamate activation of the AMPA receptor.

In addition to direct phosphorylation of AMPA receptors, CaMKII also increases the intracellular levels of another important second messenger, cyclic adenosine monophosphate (cAMP) through activation of the membrane associated molecule adenyl cyclase (AC). cAMP in turn activates a further downstream molecule, cyclic AMP-dependent protein kinase (PKA). PKA activates numerous downstream substrates including the NMDA receptor itself. PKA phosphorylation of the NMDA receptor occurs on a particular amino acid residue (serine -897) of the NR1 subunit, an established PKA-dependent modulatory site (Zou et al 2000, 2002). Similar to the AMPA receptors, phosphorylation of the NMDA NR1 subunit has potent effects upon its channel properties. The overall effect is a feed-forward increase in post-synaptic excitability (figure 2).

As mentioned above, CaMKII is expressed at low levels within the spinal dorsal horn. There is a strong possibility therefore that other serine/threonine protein kinases and/or tyrosine kinases may play an important role in postsynaptic excitability changes within the spinal cord. Protein kinase C (PKC) is a serine/threonine kinases that has been shown to directly modulate NMDA receptor activity. PKC exists in several isoforms. The PKCy (gamma) and PKC*d* (delta) isoforms are expressed by subpopulations of dorsal horn neurons (Polgar et al 1999, Brenner et al 2004) and have been implicated in pain processing (Malmberg et al 1997a, Brenner et al 2004, Dina et al 2000). PKC is activated in a Ca^{2+}-dependent manner and phosphorylates the NMDA NR1 subunit on a particular PKC-dependent amino acid residue (serine-896). This phosphorylation takes place within the endoplasmic reticulum (ER) and results in the suppression of an ER retention signal allowing NMDA receptor trafficking to the postsynaptic membrane. Synaptic plasticity under these circumstances therefore occurs via an NMDA-induced feed-forward trafficking of mature NMDA receptors to the synapse, ultimately enhancing the strength of the nociceptive signal.

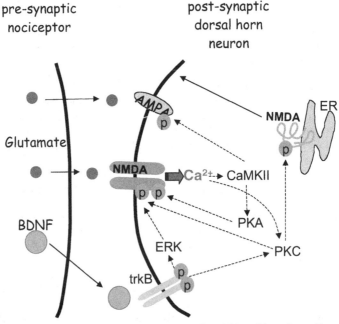

pre-synaptic
nociceptor

post-synaptic
dorsal horn
neuron

Figure 2 - Modulation of the pain signal in the dorsal horn. Phase 2, medium term changes in synaptic enhancement result from posttranslational modifications of existing proteins within dorsal horn neurons following the activation of intracellular kinase pathways. See text for details.

In addition to glutamate and neuropeptides, certain populations of primary sensory nociceptors constitutively express non-classical neuromodulators such as (BDNF) (Michael et al 1997). BDNF is contained in small diameter, trkA-expressing nociceptors and its expression is upregulated in an NGF-dependent manner following peripheral inflammation (Cho et al 1997). BDNF is released at central nociceptor terminals within the dorsal horn by particular high-frequency bursting activity (Lever et al 2001). Noxious stimulation results in activation of post-synaptic trkB receptors that are expressed by subpopulations of superficial dorsal horn neurons (Pezet et al 2002). trkB receptor activation may be mimicked by exogenous BDNF application (Pezet et al 2002) and exogenously delivered BDNF has been shown to be pro-nociceptive (Groth & Aanonsen 2002). Intrathecal injection of anti-BDNF antibodies or sequestering proteins on the other hand prevent the development of thermal hyperalgesia following peripheral inflammation or nerve injury (Kerr et al 1999, Fukuoka et al 2001). These data suggest that BDNF is a major mediator of central sensitisation (Mannion et al 1999, Thompson et al 1999). The BDNF receptor trkB is a receptor tyrosine kinase, whose activation results in the activation of signalling cascades with major consequences for ionotropic channel activity. Downstream signalling following BDNF binding and trkB receptor dimerisation is complex. I will highlight here two pathways that that been investigated within the spinal dorsal horn and shown to be involved in postsynaptic modulation of nociceptive responses.

The role of BDNF in the spinal cord is thought to be modulatory, enhancing NMDA receptor-mediated responses (Kerr et al 1999). Two particular trkB activated signalling pathways responsible for NMDA receptor modulation are the phospholipase-C (PLC) – PKC pathway and the ras/raf – ERK pathway (figure 2). Following BDNF binding, trkB receptors dimerise and autophosphorylate (each monomer has intrinsic protein tyrosine kinase activity). Phosphotyrosine residues in activated trkB serve as cytoplasmic docking sites for adapter proteins which contain src-homolgy motifs (SH2) and are involved in downstream signalling. PLC is one such SH2 containing adapter protein that is activated and which in turn activates PKC via the IP3/DAG pathway. There is good experimental evidence that BDNF-mediated synaptic plasticity of nociceptive reflex activity is mediated, at least in part, by this trkB-PKC pathway (Slack et al 2004). The second SH2 containing adapter protein known to be activated following trkB activation is GRB2. GRB2 activates the small G-proteins ras and raf via the exchange factor sos (son of sevenless). Signals then pass from activated ras to a cascade of protein kinases of the MAPK (mitogen activated protein kinase) family. In the mammalian CNS the best characterised MAPK's are the extracellular signal-regulated protein kinases (ERK's). Nociceptive input to the spinal cord is associated with the activation of ERK1/2 (Pezet et al 2002), an effect mimicked by the exogenous application of BDNF. Additionally, Injury-induced ERK1/2 activation may be inhibited by the BDNF inhibitor trkB-IgG (Pezet et al 2002). ERK1/2 has been shown to enhance NMDA receptor activation via NR1 phosphorylation (Slack et al 2004). BDNF therefore may lead to modulation of NMDA receptor function by NR1 phosphorylation via independent signalling pathways. It is highly likely therefore that, under conditions of peripheral inflammation when expression levels of BDNF are raised within nociceptors, BDNF modulation of NMDA receptor function is a relevant mechanism of synaptic plasticity.

The mechanisms outlined above represent medium-term changes in synaptic excitability that underpin medium-term changes in pain responses. These mechanisms are not exhaustive. Signalling from neurokinin receptors, metabotropic gluatamate receptors or ephrin tyrosine kinase receptors has not been considered in this discussion. Similarly, the important modulation of NMDA receptor activity by the non-receptor tyrosine kinase Src has been omitted. The underlying mechanisms involved in all pathways however are similar and require posttranslational modifications of existing proteins. These changes are often reversible and are dependent upon activities of different families of serine/threonine and tyrosine protein kinases with their associated phosphatases within posysynaptic elements. The overall effect is phosphorylation of membrane receptors or ion channels or translocation of translationary immature receptors to the postsynaptic membrane. The overall result is a medium term enhancement of nociceptive input.

Longer term modification of the pain signal in the dorsal horn.

How does pain sensitivity remain elevated following injury? In particular how does hypersensitivity often persist following apparent healing? The answer lies in the crucial understanding that noxious stimulation always induces new gene expression. Noxious stimulation not only induces new gene expression at every level of the neuraxis; sensory neurons, dorsal horn neurons, thalamic relay neurons and cerebral cortex, but also that the pattern of gene expression is dynamic and may change substantially with time. What are the mechanisms concerned with long term consolidation of nociceptive signalling? The key understanding here is that both NMDA and neurotrophin receptor activation and their associated signalling pathways induce transcriptional changes within dorsal horn neurons. We will consider two important signalling pathways that induce gene transcription, ERK and Ca^{2+}/Calmodulin dependent signalling pathways (figure 3). There is increasing evidence that in addition to promoting acute central sensitisation in dorsal horn neurons via posttranslational changes, ERK promotes alteration in gene transcription in the spinal cord (Ji et al 2002, Kawasaki et al 2004). In addition to phosphorylation of cytoplasmic and membrane bound proteins, ERK activity is coupled to activation of immediate early genes (IEG's). Many of these IEG's are transcription factors that control the subsequent expression of second, later transcribed genes called delayed response genes. Activated (phosphorylated) ERK forms an active homomeric complex and enters the nucleus where it controls the activity of many nuclear transcription factors. Transcription factors are DNA binding proteins that activate or suppress gene transcription. They may be divided into constitutive transcription factors (CTF's) and inducible transcription factors (ITF's). The prototypic member of the CTF family is $cAMP/Ca^{2+}$ response-element binding protein (CREB). CREB is activated by phosphorylation and regulates ITF transcription. ITF genes e.g. *c-fos, c-jun* are therefore IEG's whose expression is controlled by CTF's. The family of ITF proteins include Fos, Jun and Krox. These proteins dimerize to form the functional transcription factor known as activator protein 1 (AP1). The consensus DNA sequence recognised by AP1 and its trans-activation ability and consequently the target delayed response gene activated depends upon the homo- or heteromeric composition of AP1.

388

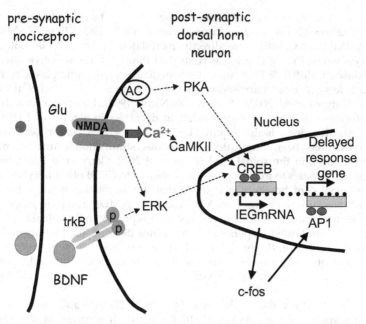

pre-synaptic
nociceptor

post-synaptic
dorsal horn
neuron

Figure 3 - Modification of the pain signal in the dorsal horn. Long term changes in pain processing occur within the dorsal horn following protein kinase mediated transcriptional modifications. See text for details of pathways.

ERK enters the nucleus to phosphorylate CREB on a serine residue (ser[133]). Several studies have shown that noxious stimulation is associated with CREB phosphorylation in the dorsal horn (Ji & Rupp 1997, Messersmith et al 1998). It is also long established that noxious inflammatory and neuropathic stimuli activate the IEG's *c-fos, c-jun* and *Zif268* (Abbadie et al 1994, Hunt et al 1987, Tolle et al 1994). It is now becoming clear that in the spinal cord the activation of CREB and several of these IEG's is ERK-dependent (Ji et al 1999, Kawasaki et al 2004, Slack 2003). Therefore capsaicin and C-fibre evoked CREB phosphorylation can be prevented by inhibition of ERK and importantly ERK inhibition also prevents capsaicin-induced secondary mechanical hyperalgesia (Kawasaki et al 2004). What is responsible for ERK activation in these neurons? There is evidence from other regions of the CNS that BDNF activates CREB in an ERK-dependent fashion (Finkbeiner et al 1997). Lately BDNF has been shown to induce IEG expression within dorsal horn neurons that is associated with CREB activation and therefore probably ERK mediated (Slack 2003). However multiple neurotransmitter/neuromodulator receptors are implicated with activation of ERK in the CNS. With particular relationship to chronic pain, NMDA receptor activation is strongly implicated in ERK activation (Ji et al 1999, Ji & Rupp 1997, Kawasaki et al 2004). Multiple pain pathways therefore converge upon ERK/CREB/IEG activation.

389

CREB phosphorylation may also be modulated via Ca^{2+}/calmodulin dependent kinases such as PKA, CAMKII and CaMKIV. CAMKII and CaMKIV are directly modulated by intracellular calcium levels whilst PKA activation is controlled through Ca2+ sensitive adenlyl cyclases. CaMKII & PKA are critical mediators of synaptic plasticity that leads to storage of information in the hippocampus (LTP) (Abel et al 1997, see Matynia et al 2002, Malenka & Nicoll 1999). Deletion of CaMKIV isoforms in the hippocampus result in decreases in a form of LTP that suggest this kinase is also required for long-term spatial memory formation. CaMKII has been implicated in noxious stimulation-induced central sensitisation in the spinal cord (Fang et al 2002, Garry et al 2003). Since CaMKII appears to make a minor contribution to CREB phosphorylation in the spinal cord however, it is likely that this facilitation is mediated via posttranslational changes of AMPA and/or NMDA receptor properties under these circumstances. In contrast PKA is present in the spinal cord and strongly implicated in persistent pain states (Sluka 2002, Malmberg et al 1997). Correspondingly PKA activation has been shown to make a significant contribution to noxious stimulation-induced CREB phosphorylation in the spinal cord (Miletic et al 2004; Kawasaki et al 2004).

What are the mechanisms by which IEG activation leads to the consolidation of the pain signal? IEG's control the expression of delayed response genes. Following nerve injury, inflammation and in disease states in which pain dominates, transcriptional changes occur within dorsal horn cells. These transcriptional changes involve alterations in the levels of dorsal horn neurotransmitters, e.g. tachykinins (Noguchi & Ruda 1992); dynorphin (Hylden et al 1992); enkephalin (Noguchi et al 1992), dorsal horn receptors, e.g. NK1 receptors (McCarson & Krause 1994); AMPA and NMDA receptors (Tomiyama et al 2005), ion channels e.g. Na channels (Hains et al 2004), as well as changes in more general mediators e.g. COX-2 (Samad et al 2001). It is obvious that transcriptional changes such as these within the pain processing pathway is likely to have a major impact upon synaptic integration of nociceptive signals. The overall result is a long term alteration of nociceptive input/output relationships of the spinal cord.

Architectural alteration in the dorsal horn

Can pain sensitivity remain permanently altered following peripheral injury? The answer is almost certainly yes and may have an anatomical basis within the spinal cord in architectural alterations (figure 4). As mentioned earlier, nociceptive synaptic input onto dorsal horn neurons is focused by an array of pre- and post-synaptic inhibitory mechanisms. Small intrinsic inhibitory neurons within the spinal cord release gylcine and GABA. The potent effect of these inhibitory neurotransmitters can be seen from the effect of GABA upon nociceptive responses (Hwang & Yaksh, 1997). Following peripheral nerve injury there is a significant reduction of GABA-mediated inhibitory currents in dorsal horn neurons (Moore et al 2002). GABA receptor loss within the spinal dorsal horn may underlie this phenomenon (Castro-Lopes et al 1993). However down regulation of GABA accompanied by preferential loss of small GABA-expressing dorsal horn neurons has been observed within the dorsal horn following both intense electrical stimulation of peripheral nerve and following nerve injury (Coggeshall et al 2001, Ibuki et al 1997). The mechanism of this cell loss is unknown at present but may involve apoptotic events (Moore et al 2002).

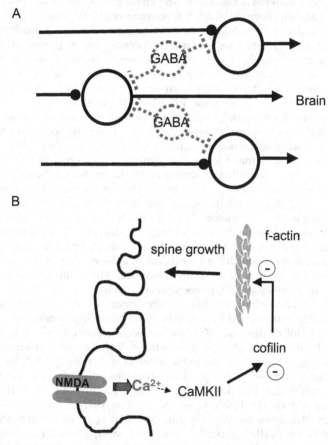

Figure 4 - Permanent modification of the pain signal in the dorsal horn may occur via loss of small inhibitory interneurons (A) or by architectural changes in postsynaptic spine morphology (B). Protein kinase pathways inhibit cofilin activity. Inhibition of cofilin activity may promote f-actin formation and alteration in cytoskeletal morphology.

The growth, elaboration and synaptic connectivity of developing sensory systems is now known to be crucially dependent upon pre- and post-synaptic activity patterns. This has been demonstrated within many regions of the somatosensory cortex as well as the dorsal horn of the spinal cord (Schlaggar et al 1993, Fox 1992, Beggs et al 2002). A mechanism has been proposed, common to all, whereby experience-dependent synaptic plasticity results from changes in synaptic transmission that shape synaptic circuits and store information. The molecular basis of this experience dependent plasticity involves activation of the NMDA receptor, and the establishment of synaptic LTP. Thus chronic pharmacological antagonism of the NMDA receptor or subunit knockout results in disruption of connectivity patterns in the developing visual cortex, somatosensory cortex and spinal cord (Beggs et al 2002, Yoshimura et al 2003, Fox 2002). It relies on the function of the NMDA as a co-incidence detector, signalling pre-synaptic activity with post-synaptic depolarisation. Synapses at which correlated activity is detected are preferentially strengthened whilst uncorrelated synapses are weakened and eliminated. What is the mechanism by which this synaptic strengthening may occur? One possible mechanism involves anatomical plasticity. At many locations within the CNS including the spinal cord, excitatory synapses are located at post-synaptic dendritic spines (Morris et al 2004). Dendritic spines are highly specialised subcellular compartments which can undergo dramatic changes in architecture with major functional significance for synaptic efficacy. For example stimuli such as high frequency stimulation that produce LTP cause a rapid formation of new spines at the location of synaptic drive (Engert & Bonhoeffer 1999). Dendritic spine architecture is determined by the underlying actin cytoskeleton. The cytoskeleton is not a static framework but may show extreme dynamic changes in structure. It is not surprising therefore that changes in actin dynamics alter dendritic spine morphology. Several lines of research have now revealed, at least some, of the molecules involved in the control of actin dynamics. The actin cytoskeleton is regulated by activation of transmembrane receptors via small GTP-binding proteins (GTP-ases) of the Rho family (figure 4). Actin assembly and disassembly is controlled by a variety of actin binding proteins ultimately under control of these Rho-GTPase molecules. (see Carlisle & Kennedy 2005). To date a number of extracellular ligands and transmembrane receptors have been identified in the nervous system that participate in co-ordinated control of actin dynamics. These include several extracellular matrix molecules that interact with the NgR/LINGO-1/p75 receptor complex and ephrin/Eph's. Over the last few years it has now become apparent that spine morphology and even new spine appearance may be regulated by NMDA receptor-dependent synaptic activity. Therefore NMDA receptor activation is associated with decreased treadmilling and stabilisation of actin filaments (Star et al 2002) and spine formation may be inhibited by NMDA antagonists (Jourdain et al 2003). The mechanism of such activity/NMDA determined architectural alterations in neurons is currently unclear but may involve a CaMKII mediated interaction with the actin-regulatory binding proteins (Jourdain et al 2003).

Can these mechanisms operate in the adult spinal cord following injury? The simple answer is that we currently do not know. Data from the hippocampus and visual cortex have shown however that the adult nervous system has a much greater potential for experience-dependent plasticity than was previously considered (Sawtell et al 2003). It will not be surprising therefore if in the next few years similar mechanisms are seen to underlie persistent pain hypersensitivity in the spinal cord.

Thus many new butterflies have been added to the pain collection. Exotic species previously thought to belong elsewhere have also crept into the cabinet. There is also no doubt that whole new drawers will have to be added to accommodate new arrivals in the very near future. The key challenge now is not just to order and annotate this collection but to use it to understand the holistic nature that is chronic pain. This will necessitate therapists, clinicians and basic scientists sharing an understanding of the complex mechanisms now known to operate at all levels of the nervous system following peripheral injury.

References

Abbadie C, Besson JM, Calvino B 1994 c-Fos expression in the spinal cord and pain-related symptoms induced by chronic arthritis in the rat are prevented by pretreatment with Freund adjuvant. J Neurosci 14(10):5865-5871

Abel T, Nguyen PV, Barad M et al 1997 Genetic demonstration of a role for PKA in the late phase of LTP and in hippocampus-based long-term memory. Cell 88(5):615-626

Beggs S, Torsney C, Drew LJ, Fitzgerald M 2002 The postnatal reorganization of primary afferent input and dorsal horn cell receptive fields in the rat spinal cord is an activity-dependent process. Eur J Neurosci 16(7):1249-1258

Brenner GJ, Ji RR, Shaffer S, Woolf CJ 2004 Peripheral noxious stimulation induces phosphorylation of the NMDA receptor NR1 subunit at the PKC-dependent site, serine-896, in spinal cord dorsal horn neurons. Eur J Neurosci 20(2):375-384

Carlisle HJ, Kennedy MB 2005 Spine architecture and synaptic plasticity. Trends Neurosci 28(4):182-187

Castro-Lopes JM, Tavares I, Coimbra A 1993 GABA decreases in the spinal cord dorsal horn after peripheral neurectomy. Brain Res 620(2):287-291

Cho HJ, Kim JK, Zhou XF, Rush RA 1997 Increased brain-derived neurotrophic factor immunoreactivity in rat dorsal root ganglia and spinal cord following peripheral inflammation. Brain Res 764(1-2):269-272

Clapham DE, Montell C, Schultz G, Julius D 2003 International Union of Pharmacology. XLIII. Compendium of voltage-gated ion channels: transient receptor potential channels. Pharmacol Rev 55(4):591-596

Coggeshall RE, Lekan HA, White FA, Woolf CJ 2001 A-fiber sensory input induces neuronal cell death in the dorsal horn of the adult rat spinal cord. J Comp Neurol 435(3):276-282

Costigan M & Woolf CJ 2000 Pain: molecular mechanisms. J Pain 1(3 Suppl):35-44

Dina OA, Barletta J, Chen X, Mutero A, Martin A, Messing RO, Levine JD 2000 Key role for the epsilon isoform of protein kinase C in painful alcoholic neuropathy in the rat. J Neurosci 20(22):8614-8619

Engert F, Bonhoeffer T 1999 Dendritic spine changes associated with hippocampal long-term synaptic plasticity. Nature 399(6731):66-70

Fang L, Wu J, Lin Q, Willis WD 2002 Calcium-calmodulin-dependent protein kinase II contributes to spinal cord central sensitization. J Neurosci 22(10):4196-4204

Finkbeiner S, Tavazoie SF, Maloratsky A et al 1997 CREB: a major mediator of neuronal neurotrophin responses. Neuron 19(5):1031-1047

Fox K 2002 Anatomical pathways and molecular mechanisms for plasticity in the barrel cortex. Neuroscience 111(4):799-814

Fukuoka T, Kondo E, Dai Y et al 2001 Brain-derived neurotrophic factor increases in the uninjured dorsal root ganglion neurons in selective spinal nerve ligation model. J Neurosci 21(13):4891-4900

Garry EM, Moss A, Delaney A et al 2003 Neuropathic sensitization of behavioral reflexes and spinal NMDA receptor/CaM kinase II interactions are disrupted in PSD-95 mutant mice. Curr Biol 13(4):321-328

Groth R, Aanonsen L 2002 Spinal brain-derived neurotrophic factor (BDNF) produces hyperalgesia in normal mice while antisense directed against either BDNF or trkB, prevent inflammation-induced hyperalgesia. Pain 100(1-2):171-181

Hains BC, Saab CY, Klein JP et al 2004 Altered sodium channel expression in second-order spinal sensory neurons contributes to pain after peripheral nerve injury. J Neurosci 24(20):4832-4839

Hollmann M, Heinemann S 1994 Cloned glutamate receptors. Annu Rev Neurosci 17:31-108

Hunt SP, Mantyh PW 2001 The molecular dynamics of pain control. Nat Rev Neurosci 2(2):83-91

Hunt SP, Pini A, Evan G 1987 Induction of c-fos-like protein in spinal cord neurons following sensory stimulation. Nature 328(6131):632-634

Hwang JH, Yaksh TL 1997 The effect of spinal GABA receptor agonists on tactile allodynia in a surgically-induced neuropathic pain model in the rat. Pain 70(1):15-22

Hylden JL, Noguchi K, Ruda MA. (1992) Neonatal capsaicin treatment attenuates spinal Fos activation and dynorphin gene expression following peripheral tissue inflammation and hyperalgesia. J Neurosci. May;12(5):1716-25.

Ibuki T, Hama AT, Wang XT et al 1997 Loss of GABA-immunoreactivity in the spinal dorsal horn of rats with peripheral nerve injury and promotion of recovery by adrenal medullary grafts. Neuroscience 76(3):845-858

Ji RR, Baba H, Brenner GJ, Woolf CJ 1999 Nociceptive-specific activation of ERK in spinal neurons contributes to pain hypersensitivity. Nat Neurosci 2(12):1114-1119

Ji RR, Befort K, Brenner GJ, Woolf CJ 2002 ERK MAP kinase activation in superficial spinal cord neurons induces prodynorphin and NK-1 upregulation and contributes to persistent inflammatory pain hypersensitivity. J Neurosci 22(2):478-485

Ji RR, Rupp F 1997 Phosphorylation of transcription factor CREB in rat spinal cord after formalin-induced hyperalgesia: relationship to c-fos induction. J Neurosci 17(5):1776-1785

Jourdain P, Fukunaga K, Muller D 2003 Calcium/calmodulin-dependent protein kinase II contributes to activity-dependent filopodia growth and spine formation. J Neurosci 23(33):10645-10649

Kawasaki Y, Kohno T, Zhuang ZY et al 2004 Ionotropic and metabotropic receptors, protein kinase A, protein kinase C, and Src contribute to C-fiber-induced ERK activation and cAMP response element-binding protein phosphorylation in dorsal horn neurons, leading to central sensitization. J Neurosci 24(38):8310-38321

Kerr BJ, Bradbury EJ, Bennett DL et al 1999 Brain-derived neurotrophic factor modulates nociceptive sensory inputs and NMDA-evoked responses in the rat spinal cord. J Neurosci 19(12):5138-5148

Lever IJ, Bradbury EJ, Cunningham JR et al 2001 Brain-derived neurotrophic factor is released in the dorsal horn by distinctive patterns of afferent fiber stimulation. J Neurosci 21(12):4469-4477

Malenka RC, Nicoll RA 1999 Long-term potentiation--a decade of progress? Science 285(5435):1870-1874

Matynia A, Kushner SA, Silva AJ 2002 Genetic approaches to molecular and cellular cognition: a focus on LTP and learning and memory. Annu Rev Genet 36:687-720

Malmberg AB, Brandon EP, Idzerda RL et al 1997 Diminished inflammation and nociceptive pain with preservation of neuropathic pain in mice with a targeted mutation of the type I regulatory subunit of cAMP-dependent protein kinase. J Neurosci 17(19):7462-7470

Malmberg AB, Chen C, Tonegawa S, Basbaum AI (1997a) Preserved acute pain and reduced neuropathic pain in mice lacking PKCgamma. Science 278(5336):279-283

Mannion RJ, Costigan M, Decosterd I et al 1999 Neurotrophins: peripherally and centrally acting modulators of tactile stimulus-induced inflammatory pain hypersensitivity. Proc Natl Acad Sci USA 96(16):9385-9390

McCarson KE, Krause JE 1994 NK-1 and NK-3 type tachykinin receptor mRNA expression in the rat spinal cord dorsal horn is increased during adjuvant or formalin-induced nociception. J Neurosci 14(2):712-720

Messersmith DJ, Kim DJ, Iadarola MJ 1998 Transcription factor regulation of prodynorphin gene expression following rat hindpaw inflammation. Brain Res Mol Brain Res 53(1-2):260-269

Michael GJ, Averill S, Nitkunan A et al 1997 Nerve growth factor treatment increases brain-derived neurotrophic factor selectively in TrkA-expressing dorsal root ganglion cells and in their central terminations within the spinal cord. J Neurosci 17(21):8476-8490

Miletic G, Hanson EN, Miletic V 2004 Brain-derived neurotrophic factor-elicited or sciatic ligation-associated phosphorylation of cyclic AMP response element binding protein in the rat spinal dorsal horn is reduced by block of tyrosine kinase receptors. Neurosci Lett 361(1-3):269-271

Moore KA, Kohno T, Karchewski LA et al 2002 Partial peripheral nerve injury promotes a selective loss of GABAergic inhibition in the superficial dorsal horn of the spinal cord. J Neurosci 22(15):6724-6731

Morris R, Cheunsuang O, Stewart A, Maxwell D 2004 Spinal dorsal horn neurone targets for nociceptive primary afferents: do single neurone morphological characteristics suggest how nociceptive information is processed at the spinal level. Brain Res Brain Res Rev 46(2):173-190

Noguchi K, Ruda MA 1992 Gene regulation in an ascending nociceptive pathway: inflammation-induced increase in preprotachykinin mRNA in rat lamina I spinal projection neurons. J Neurosci 12(7):2563-2572

Noguchi K, Dubner R, Ruda MA 1992 Preproenkephalin mRNA in spinal dorsal horn neurons is induced by peripheral inflammation and is co-localized with Fos and Fos-related proteins. Neuroscience 46(3):561-570

Ozawa S, Kamiya H, Tsuzuki K 1998 Glutamate receptors in the mammalian central nervous system. Prog Neurobiol 54(5):581-618

Pezet S, Malcangio M, Lever IJ et al 2002 Noxious stimulation induces Trk receptor and downstream ERK phosphorylation in spinal dorsal horn. Mol Cell Neurosci 21(4):684-695

Platenik J, Kuramoto N, Yoneda Y 2000 Molecular mechanisms associated with long-term consolidation of the NMDA signals. Life Sci 67(4):335-364

Polgar E, Fowler JH, McGill MM, Todd AJ 1999 The types of neuron which contain protein kinase C gamma in rat spinal cord. Brain Res 833(1):71-80

Samad TA, Moore KA, Sapirstein A et al 2001 Interleukin-1beta-mediated induction of Cox-2 in the CNS contributes to inflammatory pain hypersensitivity. Nature 410(6827):471-475

Sawtell NB, Frenkel MY, Philpot BD et al 2003 NMDA receptor-dependent ocular dominance plasticity in adult visual cortex. Neuron 38(6):977-985

Schlaggar BL, Fox K, O'Leary DD 1993 Postsynaptic control of plasticity in developing somatosensory cortex. Nature 364(6438):623-626

Sivilotti LG, Thompson SWN, Woolf CJ 1993 Rate of rise of the cumulative depolarization evoked by repetitive stimulation of small-caliber afferents is a predictor of action potential windup in rat spinal neurons in vitro. J Neurophysiol 69:1621-1631

Slack SE 2003 Mechanisms of BDNF-modulated synaptic plasticity in the spinal cord. PhD thesis, University of London

Slack SE, Pezet S, McMahon SB et al 2004 Brain-derived neurotrophic factor induces NMDA receptor subunit one phosphorylation via ERK and PKC in the rat spinal cord. Eur J Neurosci 20(7):1769-1778

Sluka K 2002 Stimulation of deep somatic tissue with capsaicin produces long-lasting mechanical allodynia and heat hypoalgesia that depends on early activation of the cAMP pathway. J Neurosci 22(13):5687-5693

Star EN, Kwiatkowski DJ, Murthy VN 2002 Rapid turnover of actin in dendritic spines and its regulation by activity. Nat Neurosci 5(3):239-246

Thompson SWN, Bennett DL, Kerr BJ et al 1999 Brain-derived neurotrophic factor is an endogenous modulator of nociceptive responses in the spinal cord. Proc Natl Acad Sci USA 96(14):7714-7718

Thompson SWN, King AE, Woolf CJ, 1990 Activity-dependent changed in rat ventral horn neurones in vitro summation of prolonged afferent evoked postsynaptic depolarizations produce a D-APV sensitive windup. Europ J Neurosci 2:638-649

Thompson SWN, Urban L, Dray A 1993 Contribution of NK1 and NK2 receptor activation to high threshold afferent fiber evoked ventral root responses in the rat spinal cord in vitro. Brain Res 625:100-108

Thompson SWN, Woolf CJ 1991 Primary afferent evoked prolonged potentials in the spinal cord and their central summation: Role of the NMDA receptor. Proceedings of the VIth World Congress on Pain. In: Bond MR, Charlton JE, Woolf CJ (Eds) Pain Research and Cinical Management Vol. 4 IASP Press, Seattle

Tolle TR, Herdegen T, Schadrack J et al 1994 Application of morphine prior to noxious stimulation differentially modulates expression of Fos, Jun and Krox-24 proteins in rat spinal cord neurons. Neuroscience 58(2):305-321

Tomiyama M, Furusawa K, Kamijo M et al 2005 Upregulation of mRNAs coding for AMPA and NMDA receptor subunits and metabotropic glutamate receptors in the dorsal horn of the spinal cord in a rat model of diabetes mellitus. Brain Res Mol Brain Res 136(1-2):275-281

Wang H, Woolf CJ 2005 Pain TRPs. Neuron 46(1):9-12

Waxman SG, Cummins TR, Dib-Hajj SD, Black JA 2000 Voltage-gated sodium channels and the molecular pathogenesis of pain: a review. J Rehabil Res Dev 37(5):517-528

Woolf CJ 2004 Pain: Moving from symptom control toward mechanism-specific pharmacologic management. Ann Intern Med 140(6):441-451

Yoshimura Y, Ohmura T, Komatsu Y 2003 Two forms of synaptic plasticity with distinct dependence on age, experience, and NMDA receptor subtype in rat visual cortex. J Neurosci 23(16):6557-6566

Zou X, Lin Q, Willis WD 2000 Enhanced phosphorylation of NMDA receptor 1 subunits in spinal cord dorsal horn and spinothalamic tract neurons after intradermal injection of capsaicin in rats. J Neurosci 20(18):6689-6997

Zou X, Lin Q, Willis WD 2002 Role of protein kinase A in phosphorylation of NMDA receptor 1 subunits in dorsal horn and spinothalamic tract neurons after intradermal injection of capsaicin in rats. Neuroscience 115(3):775-786

Index

descending pathways, pain relief, 18–19
developmental anomalies, asymmetry, 7
Diagnostic and Statistical Manual of mental Disorders - 4th edition (DSM IV)
    acute stress disorder, 263
    post-traumatic stress disorder, 258, 263
diagnostic labeling, 113–114
diagnostic reasoning, 290
"dialectical reasoning," 290–291
diffuse/distant noxious inhibitory control (DNIC), 19–20
directive questions, 71
disability
    chronic, 140
    lifestyle substitution, 185
    maintenance, 287
    models, 279
    patient cognition and, 274–275
    prevention, 217
    secondary gain from, 178–180
Disabled Living Allowance (DLA), 178
dissociation, peri-traumatic, 261
distal goals, proximal goals vs., 43
distress
    continuum in chronic pain, 285–287, 302
    maintenance, 287
    schema enmeshment, 284
doctor-patient relationship, communication issues, 56
dorsal horn
    central sensitisation, 14, 15
    modulation of pain signals, 383–388
        long-term, 388–390
        medium-term, 384–388
        short-term, 383–384
        structural alteration, 390–393
    pain transmission in, 381–382
    referred pain, 9
dynamic lifting capability, functional assessment, 226, 232

E
"each muscle king" model, 344
early retirement, 220
economic issues see costs
education/training
    clinical psychologists, 317
    cognitive-behavoural treatment, 245–246, 265–266, 333
    communication, 55, 82, 107, 116–117
        modeling, 116
        modelling, 116
        neurophysiology training, 97
        physiotherapists, 117–118
        practice, 116–117
        practicing key skills, 116–117
    employment services, 183, 188
    interdisciplinary approach to pain management, 317
    in neurophysiology, 97
    patients and return to work, 154
    see also learning

405

Review:Topical Issues in Pain 1: Whiplash Science and Management. Fear Avoidance Beliefs and Behaviour. Editor Louis Gifford

By Professor Patrick Wall, best known for the Gate control theory of pain and author of the best selling books 'The Challenge of Pain' (with Ronald Melzack),'Pain the Science of Suffering' and 'The Textbook of Pain' (with Ronald Melzack).

It is not an exaggeration to say that this book marks a milestone not only for an understanding of pain but also for the maturation of physiotherapy. For centuries physiotherapy has been placed in a minor subservient role among the medical arts. This low status encouraged a passive intuitive acceptance of therapy in a barren desert of intellectual questioning. The present rapid evolution of attitude no longer permits untested acceptance. The authors of this book and the organisers of the Physiotherapy Pain Association are clearly pioneers leading their profession out of the desert. They have been reading and experiencing and questioning everything to the conditions, which are treated rather than restricting themselves to the classical physiotherapy texts, which are often dull, repetitive and trivial. In addition to an open-minded education, they point to the almost unique opportunity characteristic of physiotherapy, which remains the close prolonged interaction with patients. Social pressure has removed this from almost every other branch of the medical arts.

The practical pragmatic obsession of old-school physiotherapy assigned questioning and investigation to a separate and distant other class who in practise in fact ignored the problems. Research was assigned to some non-existent class of intellectuals and thought to be beyond the scope of physiotherapists. A striking example is that to be found on page 94 where 20 therapies for whiplash are listed. Of these two are thought to be useless, two useful and the other 16 have not been adequately investigated. This vagueness is a threat to patients and to physiotherapists and to an understanding of pain. Research can not be the responsibility of others. It does not require huge high tech resources. The results are not to be feared. The discovery that a therapy depends on a placebo response should be welcomed with relief because it liberates the therapist into a positive area to explore the economics and the precise nature of the placebo component of the therapy.

Work over the past thirty years has rejected the model of a pain mechanism as caused by a fixed rigid modality-dedicated mechanism. The process, which produces pain, is plastic and changes sequentially with time. That essential mobility of mechanism exists in damaged tissue, in the peripheral nerves and spinal cord. This movement of pathology from periphery to centre proceeds with the triggering of reactive processes in the brain. It presents the therapist with a migrating distributed target. For that reason, I was particularly impressed by the chapter by Gifford on the "Mature Organism Model" which places pain in an integrated context without any permission to accept the old dualistic split that pain must be either in the body or in the mind.

I look forward to this series and to the activities of the Physiotherapy Pain Association because they promise to revolutionise the morale, dignity and way of thinking of physiotherapists and thereby to affect everyone concerned with pain.

Patrick Wall   26.11.98

Reproduced with permission from : Physiotherapy, February 1999/vol 85/no 2 page 101-102).

Review:Topical Issues in Pain 2: Biopsychosocial assessment and management; Relationships and pain Editor: Louis Gifford

By Gordon Waddell,Consultant Orthopaedic Surgeon and author of 'The Back Pain Revolution'.

The first year book from the Physiotherapy Pain Association was a hard act to follow, but this second year book is even better.

This a diverse collection of essays on selected aspects of pain which is inevitably somewhat disjointed and variable in style and quality, but that lets it explore a number of rarely visited, fascinating topics. Although the authors come from a range of professional backgrounds, they all have considerable "hands on" clinical experience of physiotherapy for patients with pain. Indeed, one of the major achievements and attractions of this book is the highly successful blend of the latest concepts and research on pain with practical illustrations of how that can be applied in practice. That practice ranges all the way from routine out-patient physiotherapy to a tertiary pain management clinic, and the one general criticism is that sometimes the setting of a particular essay is not made clear. For example, lessons from the highly selected patients in a pain management programme are not always applied to more routine practice. However, once the reader realises that different authors may sometimes be talking about different patients, it is possible to draw these lessons from oneself.

Altogether, this is a rich kaleidoscope of the latest thinking and research, which includes some real gems. Each reader will find their own favourites, but a very personal selection that tickled my fancy included the chapters on interpreting the results of treatment, the challenge of change in practice, the impact of patient preferences on treatment outcome, applying yellow flags in clinical practice, pain perceptions and attitudes, and most of the section on "relationships" including in particular pain stories, pain couples and the INPUT Patient Handout on Chronic Pain and Pregnancy. These include some original, highly pertinent and stimulating perspectives. The major achievement and value throughout the book are the many examples of how biopsychosocial principles can be applied in clinical practice.

This is a delightful little book for all physiotherapists and indeed all other health professionals who actually treat patients with pain, not only for those working in pain clinics. The Physiotherapy Pain Association and the editor, Louis Gifford, are once again to be congratulated on producing such a marvellous collection of essays.

Gordon Waddell DSc MD FRCS
(Reproduced with permission Physiotherapy Dec 2000 vol 86(12):665)

Topical Issues in Pain 1

Reader's comments:

'one of the best and most useful Physiotherapy books I've read'

'clinically relevant and up to date stuff'

'keep this sort of material coming!'

Topical Issues in Pain 2

Reader's comments:

'Excellent, another useful and extremely usable book'

'We have found the case history in chapter 4 invaluable in our in-service training of the biopsychosocial model and assessment'

'Should be a standard text in all Physiotherapy undergraduate and post graduate education programmes'

'Easy to read, easy to understand and I've read it from cover to cover (I don't normally get passed chapter 1!!)'.

Topical Issues in Pain 3

Reader's comments:

'congratulations on Topical Issues in Pain 3,
a tremendous piece of work.'

'a vital resource'

'I learnt some more very interesting things about the
sympathetic nervous system, a really comprehensive guide.'

'the usual high standard and easy to read'